Linda L. Oakes, MSN, RN-BC, CCNS, is currently a Pain Clinical Nurse Specialist at St. Jude Children's Research Hospital in Memphis, Tennessee. She obtained her undergraduate degree in nursing at the University of South Carolina and her master's in pediatric nursing at the University of Tennessee. During her 37 years as a nurse, her career has also included roles as a critical care nurse and as a nursing educator in the states of South Carolina, North Carolina, Florida, and Ohio. In 1987, she joined St. Jude Children's Research Hospital as the first intensive care unit (ICU) Clinical Nurse Specialist and gradually became aware of the need to improve the pain management for children with cancer. In 2003, she stepped out of her ICU role by developing the role of the institution's first advanced practice nurse in pain management. Her passion for pain management has been a key factor in developing a Pain Management Service at St. Jude for patients with complex pain conditions. However, her mission has always been to provide resources for all health care providers so they may use evidence-based assessment tools and interventions.

Linda is currently certified as an acute care clinical nurse specialist as well as a Pain Management Nurse. Her professional memberships include active involvement in the American Association of Critical Care Nurses with local and national level appointments, Sigma Theta Tau, International Association of Pain, American Pain Society, and American Society of Pain Management Nurses, for which she has served on national clinical expert consensus panels regarding the need to provide safe and effective pain management. At St. Jude, she has served as a coinvestigator of several research protocols involving pediatric pain assessment and management, outcomes of nursing procedures, and end-of-life decision making. Linda has had the opportunity to share these research efforts and her expertise in pain and critical care nursing through many publications and presentations nationally, as well as through St. Jude's international outreach efforts in South America and China.

Compact Clinical Guide to

INFANT AND CHILD PAIN MANAGEMENT

An Evidence-Based Approach for Nurses

Linda L. Oakes, MSN, RN-BC, CCNS

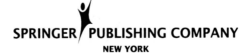

SPRINGER PUBLISHING COMPANY
NEW YORK

Springer Publishing Company, LLC
11 West 42nd Street
New York, NY 10036
www.springerpub.com

Acquisitions Editor: Margaret Zuccarini
Senior Editor: Rose Mary Piscitelli
Cover design: Steven Pisano
Composition: Absolute Service, Inc./Pablo Apostol, Project Manager

ISBN: 978-0-8261-0617-9
E-book ISBN: 978-0-8261-0618-6

13 14   5 4 3 2

The author and the publisher of this Work have made every effort to use sources believed to be reliable to provide information that is accurate and compatible with the standards generally accepted at the time of publication. Because medical science is continually advancing, our knowledge base continues to expand. Therefore, as new information becomes available, changes in procedures become necessary. We recommend that the reader always consult current research and specific institutional policies before performing any clinical procedure. The author and publisher shall not be liable for any special, consequential, or exemplary damages resulting, in whole or in part, from the readers' use of, or reliance on, the information contained in this book. The publisher has no responsibility for the persistence or accuracy of URLs for external or third-party Internet websites referred to in this publication and does not guarantee that any content on such websites is, or will remain, accurate or appropriate.

Library of Congress Cataloging-in-Publication Data
Oakes, Linda L.
  Compact clinical guide to infant and child pain management : an evidence-based approach / Linda L. Oakes.
    p. ; cm.—(Compact clinical guide series)
  Includes bibliographical references and index.
  ISBN 978-0-8261-0617-9—ISBN 978-0-8261-0618-6 (e-book)
  1. Pain in children–Treatment. 2. Analgesia. I. Title. II. Series: Compact clinical guide series.
  [DNLM: 1. Pain—therapy. 2. Adolescent. 3. Child. 4. Infant. WL 704]
  RJ365.O25 2011
  618.92'0472—dc22
                                        2010050803

Printed in the United States of America by Gasch Printing.

In memory of
Dr. Donna Wong
(1948–2008)

Developer of the Wong-Baker
FACES Pain Scale

Contents

Foreword

It is an honor to write the foreword for Linda Oakes's *Compact Clinical Guide to Infant and Child Pain Management.* It is particularly meaningful to me because my nursing career began out of a love for infants and children. I worked in a tertiary neonatal intensive care unit (NICU) for 13 years in the 1970s and 1980s and have never been able to forget the frustration I felt over the prevailing thinking that infants did not feel pain and, if they did, would not remember it, implying a lack of consequences later in life. Even when the presence of pain was acknowledged, it was assumed that infants could not tolerate analgesics and it would be dangerous to administer them. This thinking was used to justify the widespread failure on the part of health care providers to provide analgesics to infants, even to those who had painful congenital anomalies, underwent major surgery, or suffered terminal illness.

Pain is common in infants and children, particularly pain associated with procedures (American Academy of Pediatrics, 2001; American Academy of Pediatrics & Canadian Paediatric Society, 2006). A prospective study recorded all painful procedures in 151 neonates during the first 14 days of their stay in a tertiary NICU and found that each neonate experienced an average of 14 painful procedures per day (Simons, van Dijk, Anand, Roofthooft, van Lingen, & Tibboel, 2003). A multicenter epidemiologic study reported a similar very high number of painful procedures in the NICU, but only 20.8% were performed with analgesia before the procedures (Carbajal et al., 2008). Little is known about the impact of repeated painful procedures and early pain experiences on later quality of life, physiologic changes, and pain-related behavior and perception (Hermann, Hohmeister,

Demirakça, Zohsel, & Flor, 2006; Howard, 2003; Lidow, 2002; Taddio, Shah, Atenafu, & Katz, 2009). For example, there is heightened interest and ongoing research regarding the relationship between the development of chronic pain in children and their previous pain experiences (Hohmeister et al., 2010; Huguet & Miro, 2008).

Although it becomes immediately clear while reading the pages of this clinical guide that there have been major improvements in pediatric pain management since my early experiences as a NICU nurse, we continue to see examples of undertreated pain and its adverse effects in infants and children in all settings (Colleau & Lipman, 2004; Howard, 2003; Jacob et al., 2003). This is why Linda's clinical guide is both timely and a welcome addition to the growing body of resources available to clinicians who care for these vulnerable populations. It is exciting to review the content that she has organized into seven sections ranging from a chapter on pain assessment, which contains an excellent overview of tools for assessment in both verbal and preverbal patients, to several chapters devoted to specific therapies, such as epidural analgesia and peripheral nerve blocks, and pain associated with conditions such as sickle-cell disease and trauma. It is difficult to find a clinical guide that presents the evidence supporting the appropriate treatment of multiple aspects of pediatric pain in a way that can be applied so readily in the clinical setting, yet Linda has achieved this.

It was a defining moment for me in my career when I heard the great pediatric pain management pioneer, Dr. Donna Wong, state emphatically in a lecture, "Unless proven otherwise, babies and children can feel pain and deserve the same quality of pain treatment as adults!" Linda Oakes's clinical guide affirms this statement. It is particularly appropriate that she has dedicated it to Dr. Wong's memory.

Chris Pasero, MS, RN-BC, FAAN
Pain Management Educator and Clinical Consultant
El Dorado Hills, California

REFERENCES

American Academy of Pediatrics. (2001). The assessment and management of pain in infants, children, and adolescents. *Pediatrics, 108*(3), 793–797.

American Academy of Pediatrics & Canadian Paediatric Society. (2006). The prevention and management of pain in the neonate: An update. *Pediatrics, 118*(5), 2231–2241.

Carbajal, R., Rousset, A., Danan, C., Coquery, S., Nolent, P., Duerocq, S., & Bréart, G. (2008). Epidemiology and treatment of painful procedures in neonates in intensive care units. *Journal of the American Medical Association, 300*(1), 60–70.

Colleau, S. M., & Lipman, A. G. (2004). Progress and needs in pediatric palliative care pain management. *American Pain Society Bulletin, 14*(2), 1, 5.

Hermann, C., Hohmeister, J., Demirakça, S., Zohsel, K., & Flor, H. (2006). Long-term alternation of pain sensitivity in school-aged children with early pain experiences. *Pain, 124*(3), 278–285.

Hohmeister, J., Kroll, A., Wollgarten-Hadamek, I., Zohsel, K., Demirakça, S., Flor, H., & Hermann, C. (2010). Cerebral processing of pain in school-aged children with neonatal nociceptive input: An exploratory fMRI study. *Pain, 150*(2), 257–267.

Howard, R. F. (2003). Current status of pain management in children. *Journal of the American Medical Association, 290*(18), 2464–2469.

Huguet, A., & Miro, J. (2008). The severity of chronic pediatric pain: An epidemiological study. *Journal of Pain, 9*(3), 226–236.

Jacob, E., Miaskowski, C., Savedra, M., Beyer, J. E., Treadwell, M., & Styles, L. (2003). Management of vaso-occlusive pain in children with sickle cell disease. *Journal of Pediatric Hematology/Oncology, 25*(4), 307–311.

Lidow, M. S. (2002). Long-term effects of neonatal pain on nociceptive systems. *Pain, 99*(3), 377–383.

Simons, S. H., van Dijk, M., Anand, K. S., Roofthooft, D., van Lingen, R. A., & Tibboel, D. (2003). Do we still hurt newborn babies? A prospective study of procedural pain and analgesia in neonates. *Archives of Pediatric & Adolescent Medicine, 157*(11), 1058–1064.

Taddio, A., Shah, V., Atenafu, E., & Katz, J. (2009). Influence of repeated painful procedures and sucrose analgesia on the development of hyperalgesia in newborn infants. *Pain, 144*(1–2), 43–48.

Preface

The *Compact Clinical Guide to Infant and Child Pain Management* is intended to assist primary care providers caring for infants, children, and adolescents who experience pain. The reduction of pain must become a priority for all health care providers, with recognition that failure to do so amounts to substandard and unethical practice. Pain management for infants, children, and adolescents has made great strides in the past 3 decades. However, many pediatric and family practice health care providers need concisely written and evidence-based resources for guidance in using age-appropriate assessment tools as well as how to combine therapeutic pharmacologic modalities with appropriate nonpharmacologic techniques for common pediatric conditions associated with pain.

This book consists of seven sections: Section I: Overview of Pain in Infants and Children, describing the problems of pain and pain assessment tools; Section II: Common Medications for Managing Acute and Chronic Pain, including nonopioids, opioids, and coanalgesics; Section III: Regional Analgesia, including the increasing use of continuous epidural and peripheral nerve block infusions; Section IV: Nonpharmacologic Methods, describing the use of cognitive-behavioral techniques, cognitive techniques, and physical approaches to relieve pain; Section V: Integration of Methods of Treatment, explaining the multidisciplinary approach and the role of parents in reducing pain; Section VI: Special Treatment Considerations for Pain Including Impact on the Family, including the unique strategies needed to reduce pain associated with needle-related procedures, critical illness, and terminal illness; and Section VII: Managing Common Pain Conditions, describing the specific problem, assessment, and treatment of pain associated with surgery, trauma, sickle-cell disease, and cancer as well as chronic pain.

For the sake of providing a concise resource, the reader is to consider the following descriptions of common terms:

- The words *child* and *children* refer to infants, children, and adolescents unless otherwise specified.
- The singular pronoun *he* refers to a child who is either male or female.
- Babies are referred to as follows:
    - *Neonate:* an infant from birth to 1 month
    - *Infant:* an infant from 1 month to 1 year
- The content of this book does not refer to preterm infants unless otherwise noted.
- The word *parent* refers to all family and nonfamily caregivers who are not health care providers.
- The term *health care providers* refers to physicians, nurses, physical therapists, pharmacists, and other clinicians who have been educated to care for patients.
- The term *prescribing health care providers* refers to physicians and advanced practice nurses authorized to prescribe interventions including medications.
- The term *opioid* is the same as narcotic. In light of the negative connotations of the word "narcotic," the term opioid is used throughout this book when pertaining to medically prescribed narcotic analgesics.
- Specific medicines are included only if they are available in the United States.

In writing this book, I have made every effort to base my practice on the evidence available at the time, translating the literature about pediatric pain management with care to confirm the accuracy of the information presented and to describe generally accepted practice. Every effort has been taken to ensure that the medication selections offered in this book have been described in accordance with current recommendations and practices at the time of this publication. Application of this information for a specific patient remains the professional responsibility of the health care provider. Any recommendations regarding medication dosages are to be compared with recommendations of pharmaceutical sources. The health care provider is advised to check the package insert for each drug for any future changes in indications, precautions, contraindications, or dosages.

I am aware of many pain management issues that are not included or well covered in this book. I encourage others to pursue future research necessary to improve pain management in children by:

- Increasing the inclusion of viewpoints of older children and adolescents in studies;
- Examining the pharmacokinetics and pharmacodynamics of all analgesic drugs used in neonates and young children, not only with single doses but also with repeated doses;
- Evaluating the outcomes of various combinations of medications, as well as integrating nonpharmacologic techniques into treatment regimens;
- Evaluating the effects of analgesics on long-term growth and development;
- Incorporating the necessary emphasis on patient safety (e.g., the use of "smart pumps" with parameters appropriate for children) without compromising the efficacy of pain management;
- Understanding how to use opioids and antidepressants more safely for adolescents who may have underlying risk factors;
- Investigating the influence of pharmacogenetics and other biological variations in responses to analgesics; and
- Most importantly, determining factors that affect pain management practices, especially ways to improve the translation of well-conducted research to bedside practice.

Based on my experience as a nurse for 37 years, with the last 23 years as a clinical nurse specialist at St. Jude Children's Research Hospital, I have been privileged to care for many brave children and their courageous families who have stimulated my passion for relieving suffering, which I view as a central element of nursing's professional commitment to patient care. My patients continue to teach me that the assessment of their pain is not just a pain intensity rating, even with the most valid pain assessment tools; that their responses to opioid and other analgesic drugs can differ from those described in even the most carefully written textbook; and that children with serious and chronic illnesses experience much more than "only one little stick" as they struggle to cooperate with their caregivers. Because my patients have shared with me, with the utmost dignity and good humor, how we, as health care providers, have succeeded and failed in our efforts to provide comfort, I enthusiastically agreed to compile what I hope will serve future patients. So on behalf of all the children who need our caring touch, thank you Yvonne D'Arcy, Pain Management & Palliative Care Nurse Practitioner at Suburban Hospital–Johns Hopkins Medicine and series editor, as well as Margaret Zuccarini from Springer Publishing Company for asking me to join their efforts in providing such resources for health care providers. I am grateful for the encouragement of Chris Pasero who generously agreed to write the foreword of this book.

Recognizing that many colleagues have influenced my practice throughout my years as a nurse, it is with heartfelt gratitude that I would like to acknowledge several groups of colleagues:

- The members of the Pain Management Service at St. Jude, who teach me every day while offering their compassion and skills as we continue to make a difference in the lives of the children who are entrusted to our care.

- The many coworkers at St. Jude, as well as other pain experts I have had the opportunity to network with through the years, who have reviewed and edited one or more chapters of this book, assuring me that my goal of providing the very best in information is finally a reality: Kelley Windsor, MSN, RN-BC, PCNS-BC (Chapters 15 and 18); Doralina Angheslescu, MD (Chapters 1 and 5); Laura Burgoyne, BM, BS, FANZCA (Chapter 4); Roland Kaddoum, MD (Chapters 6 and 7); Valerie Crabtree, PhD (Chapters 4 and 9) ; Deb Ward, PharmD, BCOP (Chapter 3); Becky Wright, MD (Chapter 16); Jane Hankins, MD, MS (Chapter 17); Yvonne Avant, MSN, APRN-BC, CCRN, WCC (Chapter 14); Lama Elbahlawan, MD (Chapter 14); Sandy Merkel, MS, RN (Chapter 14); Kristin Wiese, PT, DPT (Chapter 10); Terese Verklan, PhD, CCNS, RNC (Chapter 2); and Leora Kuttner, PhD (Chapter 9).

- A patient and skilled scientific editor at St. Jude, David Galloway, ELS, who spent countless hours diligently editing each chapter to improve readability.

▓ And others at St. Jude who continually support me professionally, including my director, Robin Mobley, RN, MSN, CNA; and Kelley Windsor, MSN, RN-BC, PCNS-BC, my job partner on the Pain Management Service.

However, no health care provider can remain a healthy and sustained professional without the support of others who keep one grounded during the highs and lows of a long professional career. I am fortunate, indeed, to have many friends who understood the need for me to seclude myself at times to write this book. I want to thank my father, daughters, sons-in-law, and especially my husband of 38 years, Lanny Oakes, all of whom have continued to encourage me to do my very best while often acting as my caregivers. As I complete what my two young granddaughters have named "Nanna's Book," I humbly offer my perspective, along with the best evidence available at this time, so that other health care providers may have more confidence and greater skills to reduce the pain in the children of our future.

Linda L. Oakes, MSN, RN-BC, CCNS

I

Overview of Pain in Infants and Children

1

The Problem of Pain

THE PROBLEM OF PAIN

Pain is defined as "an unpleasant sensory and emotional experience associated with actual or potential tissue damage" (International Association for the Study of Pain [IASP], 1979; Loeser & Treede, 2008). For health care providers, the definition of pain is translated as "whatever the person who is experiencing it says it is" (Pasero, Portenoy, & McCaffery, 1999), which is the basis for effective pain assessment and management. However, health care providers caring for infants and young children have the additional challenge of recognizing how pre-verbal patients report pain in the absence of language skills.

In recent decades, because of basic and clinical research, a heightened awareness of the problem of pain has led to improved measures, at least in the most developed countries, in the prevention, assessment, and treatment of pain in all age groups. Heightened attention from accrediting health care organizations, most notably The Joint Commission (2007) and national professional organizations (American Academy of Pediatrics [AAP], 2001; AAP, Committee on Fetus and Newborn Committee on Drugs, Section on Anesthesiology, Section on Surgery, Canadian Paediatric Society, & Fetus and Newborn Committee, 2000; American Pain Society [APS], 1999, 2005a, 2005b, 2008), has prompted the need for increased knowledge of the physiology of pain and the related pharmacology of analgesics, especially appropriate dosing, as well as incorporating nonpharmacologic techniques into the care of patients (Edwards, 2002; Twycross, 2009). However, even today, the general consensus is that pain is often underrecognized and undertreated (Howard, 2003; Polkki, Pietila, & Vehvilainen-Julkunen, 2003; Twycross, 2007; Van Hulle Vincent & Denyes, 2004), not because health care providers have inadequate human compassion for their patients, but because of the following:

- Incorrect or outdated beliefs about pain (Twycross, 2007),
- Knowledge deficits and decision-making strategies used in pain management (Van Hulle Vincent & Denyes, 2004; Zernikow, Michel, Craig, & Anderson, 2009), and
- An organizational culture regarding the goal of minimizing pain safely and effectively whenever possible (Alley, 2001; Twycross, 2007).

Historically, infants and children have been undertreated for pain because of the now-refuted theory that they neither respond to nor remember painful experiences to the same degree as adults, leading to the erroneous conclusion that optimal pain management is not necessary in this age group (Breau et al., 2006). The ability of children to cope with distress through playing or watching television has led health care providers to conclude that their patients are pain free without asking them, resulting in withholding of appropriate analgesics.

BRIEF REVIEW OF ANATOMY AND PHYSIOLOGY OF PAIN

The transmission and modulation of acute pain is fairly well understood. *Nociception* is the term used to describe normal pain transmission. This process begins in the periphery (i.e., skin, subcutaneous tissue, or visceral or somatic structures), where the sensation of acute pain begins with the activation of nociceptors converting a noxious stimulus (e.g., needle stick) into electrical activity, a process called *transduction*. Sharp pain that is easily localized is typically transmitted along A-delta fibers, but pain transmitted by C fibers is slow, dull, and difficult to localize. Conduction of the impulse occurs via afferent nerves to the dorsal root ganglia of the spinal cord (Edwards, 2002). From the level of the spinal cord, signals travel via the spinothalamic tract to make connections in the thalamus and cerebral cortex, where the pain is ultimately perceived (see Figure 1.1). The cortex also projects impulses to the limbic system, which mediates emotional responses to the pain. The perceptive component is subjective and can be quantified only by the individual.

In addition to receiving and interpreting information from peripheral input, the central nervous system acts as a sensory modulation system that plays a role in enhancing or inhibiting the progression of the pain impulse to the cerebral cortex, a process called *neuromodulation*. Neuromodulators such as endogenous opioids (i.e., endorphins) provide effects similar to those of opioid analgesics in their action on opioid receptors and are responsible for the attenuation of pain signals, resulting in different levels of pain for patients who undergo the same injury or surgical procedure. Spinal nociceptor input is also subject to descending modulatory influences from supraspinal sites.

Actual tissue damage results in the release of local neurotransmitters and neuromodulators, which in turn activate additional local nociceptors. Local neurotransmitters include bradykinins, leukotrienes, histamine, serotonin, and prostaglandins. Activation of these local nociceptors may, in part, be responsible for prolonged pain after acute injury. Neurotransmitters in the spinal cord, such as substance P, amplify pain signals from the periphery. These chemicals facilitate the transmission of the pain impulse from the periphery to the spinal cord, where sensory fibers travel to and converge on cells within the dorsal horn of the spinal cord.

Pain Transmission in the Developing Child

Substantial evidence shows that neonates, even the smallest of preterm infants, perceive and remember pain (Fitzgerald, 2005) and demonstrate specific pain behaviors (e.g, crying and withdrawing

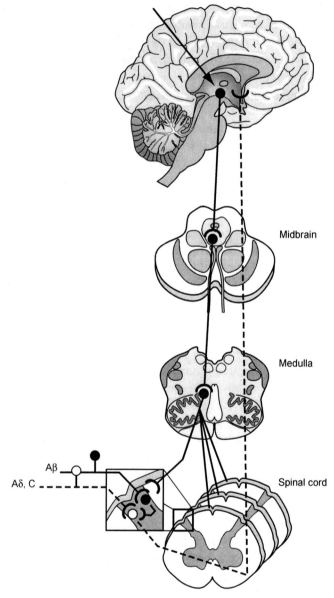

Midbrain

Medulla

Spinal cord

Aβ

Aδ, C

Figure 1.1 ■ Spinal cord nociceptive pathways

limbs), serving as the basis for behavioral pain assessment tools (see Chapter 2). Research confirms that the anatomic structures for pain processing are in place from mid-to-late gestation (AAP, Committee on Fetus and Newborn, Committee on Drugs, Section on Anesthesiology, Section on Surgery, Canadian Paediatric Society, & Fetus and Newborn Committee, 2000; Duhn & Medves, 2004). Peripheral nociceptors remain unmyelinated or thinly myelinated throughout the life cycle from infancy and early childhood. Although incomplete myelination means the transmission of pain impulses is slower, this is offset by the shorter distance the impulse must travel in an infant's central nervous system. Additionally, a lack of neurotransmitters in the descending tract suggests neuromodulating mechanisms are lacking in preterm infants, thereby making them even more sensitive to pain than older children and adults (Anand et al., 2006). Young infants are especially at risk for pain because of lower pain thresholds and enhanced pain sensitivity (Stevens, Anand, & McGrath, 2007).

CLASSIFICATIONS OF PAIN

To determine appropriate interventions for pain, several methods of classifying pain are useful for clinicians. Identifying pain as being either nociceptive or neuropathic in origin is useful when deciding which analgesics are most likely to be effective. Health care providers are to be reminded, however, that classifications may be oversimplifications and that patients can have more than one identifiable type of pain. Nociceptive and neuropathic pain can coexist, making diagnosis and treatment recommendations complex.

Pain in Terms of Injury to Tissues or Nerves

Nociceptive pain is associated with acute tissue injury or acute inflammation, as illustrated in the previous section of this chapter. This type of pain is an expected result of injury, associated with normal nerve transmission processes, and usually resolves with healing.

Nociceptive pain is protective in the sense that it prevents the patient from reinjury and provides an incentive to seek medical attention. This pain will usually respond to nonsteroidal anti-inflammatory drugs (NSAIDs) and opioids.

Neuropathic pain is characterized by altered sensory function often described as burning, electric, prickly, or shooting. Children use words such as "bugs biting" or "pins and needles" to describe such pain. Neuropathic pain is less understood than nociceptive pain. Although many mechanisms have been proposed, the general consensus is that the injury leads to repetitive spontaneous depolarizations, causing excitability within the peripheral nervous system. Neuropathic pain persists well after the injury to the nerve has subsided or the time expected for the injury to resolve has elapsed; it is often associated with motor, sensory, and autonomic deficits and is typically poorly or only partially responsive to opioids. Patients at risk include patients:

- Recovering from surgery involving nerves even within the surgical incision. A specific type of neuropathic pain that is particularly disturbing is that after an amputation of a limb, producing "phantom limb pain."
- Who have disease processes involving or compressing peripheral nerve plexuses, roots, or the spinal cord (e.g., metastatic lesion compressing the spinal cord)
- Who have illnesses associated with nerve damage, such as Guillain-Barré or herpes zoster
- Taking medications associated with nerve damage, such as chemotherapy (e.g., vincristine or cyclosporine)

These sensory abnormalities are further defined as follows:

- *Dysesthesias/paresthesias*—unpleasant abnormal sensations, such as tingling
- *Allodynia*—the sensation of moderate to severe pain from a touch stimulus that is not normally painful (e.g., a bed sheet causing foot pain)
- *Hyperalgesia*—more than the expected pain intensity in response to a stimulus that is normally mildly painful (e.g., severe pain from a pinprick)

The diagnosis is based on clinical examination and the patient's history. Coanalgesic agents, such as anticonvulsants and tricyclic antidepressants, have become the mainstay of treatment (see Chapter 5).

Pain in Terms of Duration and Pattern

Acute pain is an important biological protective mechanism, much like an alarm, notifying the body of harm and prompting a person to avoid further injury. Acute pain is associated with, at least initially, sympathetic autonomic system activity, such as tachycardia, hypertension, diaphoresis, mydriasis, and pallor. Uncomplicated acute pain is self-limiting and brief (lasting only hours to a few days) and generally disappears when the injury heals. A reoccurrence of acute pain may signal a serious problem, such as an abscess.

Chronic pain persists long after the initial acute injury or disease, lasting for as long as 3 to 6 months after the healing has presumed to have occurred (Finley, Kristjánsdóttir, & Forgeron, 2009; Stinson & Bruce, 2009). In other words, the acute phase has moved from a helpful alarm to a syndrome, much like a damaged home alarm ringing out of control (Siddall & Cousins, 2004). In contrast to acute pain, chronic pain is rarely associated with signs of sympathetic nervous system arousal. The lack of objective signs may lead an inexperienced clinician to wrongly conclude that a patient does not have pain (Eccleston, Jordan, & Crombez, 2006). Patients experiencing chronic pain benefit from approaches emphasizing nonpharmacologic interventions and rehabilitation components integrated and tailored to the needs of the patient (Berde & Solodiuk, 2003). For children, most chronic pain complaints are idiopathic in nature (with no known cause), resulting in a cycle of fear and anxiety for both the child and parent, exacerbating the pain (see Chapter 19).

Pain as Somatic or Visceral

Somatic pain arises from stimulation of pain receptors in superficial cutaneous and deeper musculoskeletal structures, usually well localized and described as being sharp, aching, or throbbing. This category includes pain associated with surgical incisions, tissue injury such as mucositis, inflammation, and metastatic lesions.

Visceral pain is caused by infiltration, distension, compression, or distortion of organs within the thorax, abdomen, and pelvis. Typically described as vague, dull discomfort, this type of pain may be difficult to localize, because it may be referred to superficial sites removed from the involved organ (e.g., visceral pain related to hepatomegaly with radiation to the right shoulder).

RESPONSES OF INFANTS AND CHILDREN TO PAIN

Originally, efforts were focused on managing pain by reducing noxious stimuli, such as surgery, but recent advances in our understanding of responses to pain motivate health care providers to provide effective management beyond the obvious humanitarian reasons.

Physiological Effects of Pain on Recovery

Depending on the severity of tissue injury, responses to acute pain may be accompanied by systemic responses that alter hormonal, metabolic, immunologic, and other physiological functions, including the cardiovascular and pulmonary systems (Anand et al., 2006). Cardiovascular effects of pain include elevation in heart rate, blood pressure, afterload, and myocardial oxygen consumption, which can be poorly tolerated in medically fragile children. Negative outcomes of unrelieved pain that affect the recovery of patients from illness and participation in care include the inability to cough or take deep breaths. These conditions increase the risk of atelectasis, pulmonary infection, and nonadherence with treatment regimens such as ambulation and physical therapy (Dowden, 2009). Unrelieved pain can interfere with sleeping and eating and increases the risk of the development of chronic pain (Eccleston et al., 2006).

Multidimensional Nature of the Pain Experience

The expression of pain is multifaceted and is influenced by the child's developmental level, sex, sensory, emotional, cognitive, cultural, and developmental makeup, as well as the context of pain. Further expression and subsequent pain experience are also based on the reception that the child perceives from those around him or her and the social and cultural environment. Experiences of pain can differ even when exposed to the same pain-inducing stimulus. This variation results from differences in personality, learning, expectation, and previous pain experiences. For younger children, the expression of pain will vary greatly, depending on these factors and their cognitive maturation. Therefore, pain can be considered to be a complex and multidimensional experience, incorporating sensory, affective, cognitive, and interpersonal components (see Figure 1.2).

The Developmental Level

The rapid maturation of biological processes during the first years of life and its effects on cognition, language, and behavioral and social competencies influence the meaning of pain and its subsequent expression. See Chapter 2 for further information on developmental level's influence on pain assessment.

Infants may cry intensely and may be inconsolable, draw their knees to the chest, exhibit hypersensitivity or irritability to any stimuli, and be unable to eat or sleep.

Toddlers may be verbally aggressive, cry intensely, exhibit regressive or resistant behavior, and withdraw or guard the painful area but have limited language skills to describe pain further.

Preschool children are very egocentric in their thinking and believe that all events and sensations originate from their internal world. They have little understanding of cause-and-effect relationships, often misunderstanding the meaning and cause of pain. Young children need to be repeatedly reassured that procedures and painful experiences are not punishments for bad behavior or thoughts. Disruptions

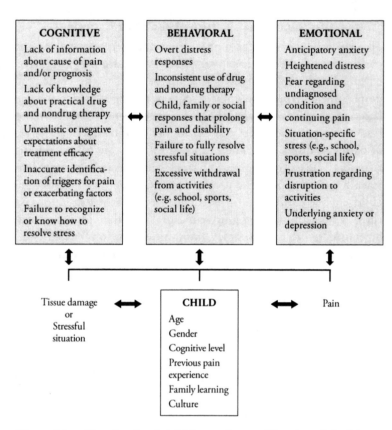

Figure 1.2 ■ Situational and child factors that modify pain and disability. Adapted from "Modifying the Psychologic Factors that Intensify Children's Pain and Prolong Disability," by P. A. McGrath and M. L. Hillier, 2003. In N. L. Schechter, C. B. Berde, & M. Yaster (Eds.), *Pain in Infants, Children, and Adolescents,* 2nd ed., pp. 85–104. Used with permission from Lippincott Williams & Wilkins.

in skin integrity from cuts, abrasions, or incisions are extremely threatening to children because of their fears of bodily injury and mutilation. They may believe that all their body and blood will leak out. Bandages and dressings may hold a special power for children as they "fix the leak" and hold the body in from the environment.

School-age children often resist movement of painful areas and have muscle rigidity, such as clenched fists, gritted teeth, and a wrinkled forehead. Gradually, they become more logical and reasonable in their thinking, gaining greater command over their world and tending to be achievement oriented. Because these children are often organized by rules, they respond well to rituals to cope with painful events. Health care providers need to be aware of these behaviors to gain cooperation during painful procedures.

Adolescents are capable of abstract thinking and have an understanding of "if-then" relationships. Although capable of adult-level problem solving, during stressful situations, adolescents may vacillate between adult-like responses to pain and regression to immature behaviors. How the socialization processes of adolescence affect pain experiences remains understudied in the pain literature, especially the role of their most influential group, their peers. They may deny pain and analgesics in the presence of family or peers because of peer pressure.

Sex

The relationship between the patient's sex and pain varies with the population studied, and most of the work in this area has been done with adults. Whether differences extend to children is less clear, with conclusions that the sex-related differences in sensitivity, experience, and expression are complex, with many situational variables that are also influential in how a child responds to pain (McGrath & Hillier, 2003). However, research for adolescents indicates that the patient's sex did influence anticipatory distress, and girls had higher pain intensity scores, but the studies did not show sex differences in use of opioids after surgery (Logan & Rose, 2004). See Chapter 19 for further information on the influences of a patient's sex on chronic pain.

Culture, Ethnicity, and Influence of the Family

Cultural implications on pain remain elusive with no compelling evidence that culture significantly affects pain perception. Despite an increase in studies examining ethnic and racial differences in pain in adults, with the assumption that children learn pain responses from their adult caretakers, few studies have examined the effect of ethnicity and culture on the experience of pain in children in the United States, suggesting potential cultural differences in how pain is expressed (Bernstein & Pachter, 2003; Jacob, McCarthy, Sambuco, & Hockenberry, 2008).

In the United States, health care providers may interpret their own experiences through the lens of Western medicine and culture, as well as their own cultural background and biases, and when combined, may influence the decision to administer analgesics or withhold them. One study showed that, for children with fractures seen in the emergency department, African American children covered by Medicaid were least likely to receive parenteral analgesia (Hostetler, Auinger, & Szilagyi, 2002), but others found no difference in analgesic administration based on ethnicity for adults (Fuentes, Kohn, & Neighbor, 2002), or adults and children (Yen, Kim, Stremski, & Gorelick, 2003).

Most importantly, children's learning about pain begins at an early age. The feedback parents give by modeling and verbal reinforcement to their young children in response to "everyday" pain influences and shapes how they cope and respond to pain (McGrath & Hillier, 2003). Parents may respond to their younger children who have mild injuries with vigorous attention to every sensation. With older children, especially sons, parents may expect them to "be brave and tough it out" or "be a man," in which the denial of pain is reinforced (McGrath & Hillier, 2003). Family influence can be more profound when one or more of the parents suffer from chronic pain themselves (Saunders, Korff, Leresche, & Mancl, 2007; see Chapter 19).

CONSEQUENCES OF UNTREATED PAIN ON DEVELOPMENT

Besides the initial physical and emotional negative experience of pain itself, growing evidence from both laboratory and clinical studies supports the premise that unrelieved pain has long-term effects on the development of all patients, especially infants. Research has proved that neonates clearly perceive pain, as demonstrated by their behavioral and physiological responses to nociceptive stimulation (Brislin & Rose, 2005). Not only are these sensors fully present at birth, but they also are more sensitive (i.e., having lower thresholds) in infants than in adults (Brislin & Rose, 2005; Fitzgerald & Beggs, 2001; Gibbins & Stevens, 2003). Descending pathways originate in the higher centers of the brain and modulate the output of the nociceptive neurons in the periphery. These descending inhibitory controls are immature at birth and continue to mature until adolescence. Consequently, this important endogenous analgesic system is lacking in infants and young children, and the effects of noxious stimuli on the central nervous system may be more profound in children than in adults (Fitzgerald & Howard, 2003). Yet it is difficult to differentiate between motor reflexes and pain behaviors for infants and young children (Ramelet, Abu-Saad, Rees, & McDonald, 2004).

Long-Term Effects of Unrelieved Pain

Prolonged, untreated pain experienced early in life may have long-lasting effects on nociceptive processing and appear to sensitize infants and young children to subsequent painful experiences (Brislin & Rose, 2005; Fitzgerald & Howard, 2003; Grunau, 2000, 2002; Peters et al., 2005; Plotsky, Bradley, & Anand, 2000; Taddio & Katz, 2005; Taddio, Soin, Schuh, Koren, & Scolnik, 2005). Early work by Taddio, Katz, Ilersich, and Koren (1997) highlighted how painful experiences in early infancy influenced reaction to subsequent pain-generating events. Infants who were circumcised without topical anesthesia showed more behaviors associated with pain during subsequent routine vaccinations at 4 and 6 months of age than uncircumcised infants. In infants who had a eutectic mixture of local anesthetic (EMLA) cream at the site of circumcision, the provision of local anesthetics attenuated the pain response to subsequent vaccinations.

Longitudinal studies have shown that prolonged or repetitive pain at an early age alters the development of the peripheral, spinal, and supraspinal pain systems (Fitzgerald, 2005; Yamada et al., 2008). Relationships between neonatal pain and emotional temperament in infancy or childhood further suggest the widespread distribution of these neurobiologic changes. For example, damage to the peripheral nervous system in the newborn by repetitive pain from heel sticks, leading to hyperinnervation of the affected tissue for a prolonged period, seemed more profound in infants than in adults (Fitzgerald & Beggs, 2001).

In another study, infants who were exposed to repeated heel lance punctures in the first 24 to 36 hours of life exhibited more intense pain response (i.e., they learned to anticipate impending pain) during venipuncture than infants who had not undergone repeated painful procedures (Taddio, Shah, Gilbert-MacLeod, & Katz, 2002). Although the type and extent of the effects of unrelieved acute and repetitive pain during infancy depend on the type of pain stimulus, research suggests that early pain experiences may account for a portion of the variability in the pain thresholds and pain behaviors (both at the site of injury and overall sensitivity) and may influence physiologic, social, and cognitive outcomes (Grunau, Holsti, & Peters, 2006; Stevens et al., 2007). The consensus is that infants are especially vulnerable to the long-term effects, spurring on pain-control efforts in neonatal intensive care units (NICU; Breau et al., 2006).

Development of Hyperalgesia and Chronic Pain

Intense and repeated stimuli from tissue damage or inflammation result in the activation of the *N*-methyl-D-aspartate (NMDA) receptors in the spinal cord, causing the spinal cord neurons to become more responsive to many types of input from damaged or sensitized nociceptors and sensitizing of the area to even minor irritations (Fitzgerald & Howard, 2003). Repeated pain episodes contribute to "rewiring" of neural pathways in the spinal cord and brain, leading to increased and ongoing pain sensitivity. This includes conditioned physiological responses triggered simply by the threat of pain, dissociated from actual nociception, so that chronic pain can become a learned, self-perpetuating behavior. Although the extent to which children recall pain and how early pain experiences significantly affect later development of chronic pain remain yet to be determined, the relationship between temperament and pain reactivity is provocative.

In summary, the need to overcome obstacles in providing effective pain relief is heightened by research that suggests pain experiences during the newborn period may have long-lasting effects on future pain perceptions and behaviors (Fitzgerald, 2005; Goldschneider & Anand, 2003; Grunau, Holsti, & Peters, 2006).

REFERENCES

Alley, L. G. (2001). The influence of an organizational pain management policy on nurses' pain management practices. *Oncology Nursing Forum*, *28*(5), 867–874.

American Academy of Pediatrics. (2001). The assessment and management of acute pain in infants, children, and adolescents. *Pediatrics*, *108*(3), 793–797.

American Academy of Pediatrics, Committee on Fetus and Newborn, Committee on Drugs, Section on Anesthesiology, Section on Surgery, Canadian Paediatric Society, & Fetus and Newborn Committee. (2000). Prevention and management of pain and stress in the neonate. *Pediatrics*, *105*(2), 454–461.

American Pain Society. (1999). *Guideline for management of acute and chronic pain in sickle cell disease*. Glenview, IL: Author.

American Pain Society. (2005a). *Guidelines for the management of cancer pain in adults and children*. Glenview, IL: Author.

American Pain Society. (2005b). *Guideline for the management of fibromyalgia syndrome pain in adults and children*. Glenview, IL: Author.

American Pain Society. (2008). *Principles of analgesic use in the treatment of acute pain and cancer pain*. Glenview, IL: Author.

Anand, K. J., Aranda, J. V., Berde, C. B., Buckman, S., Capparelli, E. V., Carlo, W., . . . Walco, G. A. (2006). Summary proceedings from the neonatal pain-control group. *Pediatrics*, *117*(3), S9–S22.

Berde, C. B., & Solodiuk, J. (2003). Multidisciplinary programs for management of acute and chronic pain in children. In N. L. Schechter, C. B. Berde, & M. Yaster (Eds.), *Pain in infants, children, and adolescents* (2nd ed., pp. 471–486). Philadelphia, PA: Lippincott Williams & Wilkins.

Bernstein, B. A., & Pachter, L. M. (2003). Cultural considerations in children's pain. In N. L. Schechter, C. B. Berde, & M. Yaster (Eds.), *Pain in infants, children, and adolescents* (2nd ed., pp. 142–156). Philadelphia, PA: Lippincott Williams & Wilkins.

Breau, L. M., McGrath, P. J., Stevens, B., Beyene, J., Camfield, C., Finley, G. A., . . . Ohlsson, A. (2006). Judgments of pain in the neonatal intensive care setting: A survey of direct care staffs' perceptions of pain in infants at risk for neurological impairment. *The Clinical Journal of Pain, 22*(2), 122–129.

Brislin, R. P., & Rose, J. B. (2005). Pediatric acute pain management. *Anesthesiology Clinics of North America, 23*(4), 789–814.

Dowden, S. J. (2009). Palliative care in children. In A. Twycross, S. J. Dowden, & E. Bruce (Eds.), *Managing pain in children: A clinical guide* (pp. 171–200). Oxford, UK: Wiley-Blackwell.

Duhn, L. J., & Medves, J. M. (2004). A systematic integrative review of infant pain assessment tools. *Advances in Neonatal Care, 4*(3), 126–140.

Eccleston, C., Jordan, A. L., & Crombez, G. (2006). The impact of chronic pain on adolescents: A review of previously used measures. *Journal of Pediatric Psychology, 31*(7), 684–697.

Edwards, A. (2002). Physiology of pain. In B. St. Marie (Ed.), *Core curriculum for pain management nursing* (pp. 121–145). Philadelphia, PA: Saunders.

Finley, G. A., Kristjánsdóttir, O., & Forgeron, P. A. (2009). Cultural influences on the assessment of children's pain. *Pain Research & Management, 14*(1), 33–37.

Fitzgerald, M. (2005). The development of nociceptive circuits. *Nature Reviews Neuroscience, 6*(7), 507–520.

Fitzgerald, M., & Beggs, S. (2001). The neurobiology of pain: Developmental aspects. *Neuroscientist, 7*(3), 246–257.

Fitzgerald, M., & Howard, R. F. (2003). The neurobiologic basis of pediatric pain. In N. L. Schechter, C. B. Berde, & M. Yaster (Eds.), *Pain in infants, children, and adolescents* (2nd ed., pp. 19–42). Philadelphia, PA: Lippincott Williams & Wilkins.

Fuentes, E. F., Kohn, M. A., & Neighbor, M. L. (2002). Lack of association between patient ethnicity or race and fracture analgesia. *Academic Emergency Medicine, 9*(9), 910–915.

Gibbins, S., & Stevens, B. (2003). The influence of gestational age on the efficacy and short-term safety of sucrose for procedural pain relief. *Advances in Neonatal Care, 3*(5), 241–249.

Goldschneider, K. R., & Anand, K. J. (2003). Long-term consequences of pain in neonates. In N. L. Schechter, C. B. Berde, & M. Yaster (Eds.), *Pain in infants, children, and adolescents* (2nd ed., pp. 58–70). Philadelphia, PA: Lippincott Williams & Wilkins.

Grunau, R. (2000). Long-term consequences of pain in human neonates. In K. J. Anand, B. Stevens, & P. J. McGrath (Eds.), *Pain in infants* (2nd ed., Vol. 10, pp. 55–76). Amsterdam, The Netherlands: Elsevier.

Grunau, R. (2002). Early pain in preterm infants. A model of long-term effects. *Clinics in Perinatology, 29*(3), 373–394.

Grunau, R. E., Holsti, L., & Peters, J. W. (2006). Long-term consequences of pain in human neonates. *Seminars in Fetal Neonatal Medicine, 11*(4), 268–275.

Hostetler, M. A., Auinger, P., & Szilagyi, P. G. (2002). Parenteral analgesic and sedative use among ED patients in the United States: Combined results from the National Hospital Ambulatory Medical Care Survey (NHAMCS) 1992–1997. *American Journal of Emergency Medicine, 20*(3), 139–143.

Howard, R. F. (2003). Current status of pain management in children. *Journal of the American Medical Association, 290*(18), 2464–2469.

International Association for the Study of Pain. (1979). Pain terms: A list with definitions and notes on usage. Recommended by the IASP subcommittee on taxonomy. *Pain, 6*(3), 249.

Jacob, E., McCarthy, K. S., Sambuco, G., & Hockenberry, M. (2008). Intensity, location, and quality of pain in Spanish-speaking children with cancer. *Pediatric Nursing, 34*(1), 45–52.

The Joint Commission. (2007). *2007 hospital accreditation standards.* Oakbrook Terrace, IL: Author.

Loeser, J. D., & Treede, R. D. (2008). The Kyoto protocol of IASP basic pain terminology. *Pain, 137*(3), 473–477.

Logan, D. E., & Rose, J. B. (2004). Gender differences in postoperative pain and patient controlled analgesia use among adolescent surgical patients. *Pain, 109*(3), 481–487.

McGrath, P. A., & Hillier, M. L. (2003). Modifying the psychologic factors that intensify children's pain and prolong disability. In N. L. Schechter, C. B. Berde, & M. Yaster (Eds.), *Pain in infants, children, and adolescents* (2nd ed., pp. 85–104). Philadelphia, PA: Lippincott Williams & Wilkins.

Pasero, C., Portenoy, R. K., & McCaffery, M. (1999). Opioid analgesics. In M. McCaffery & C. Pasero (Eds.), *Pain: Clinical manual* (2nd ed., pp. 161–299). St Louis, MO: Mosby.

Peters, J. W., Schouw, R., Anand, K. J., van Dijk, M., Duivenvoorden, H. J., & Tibboel, D. (2005). Does neonatal surgery lead to increased pain sensitivity in later childhood? *Pain, 114*(3), 444–454.

Plotsky, P. M., Bradley, C. C., & Anand, K. J. (2000). Behavioral and neuroendocrine consequences of neonatal stress. In K. J. Anand, B. Stevens, & P. J. McGrath (Eds.), *Pain in neonates* (2nd ed., Vol. 10, pp. 77–99). Amsterdam, The Netherlands: Elsevier.

Polkki, T., Pietila, A. M., & Vehvilainen-Julkunen, K. (2003). Hospitalized children's descriptions of their experiences with postsurgical pain relieving methods. *International Journal of Nursing Studies, 40*(1), 33–44.

Ramelet, A. S., Abu-Saad, H. H., Rees, N., & McDonald, S. (2004). The challenges of pain measurement in critically ill young children: A comprehensive review. *Australian Critical Care, 17*(1), 33–45.

Saunders, K., Korff, M. V., Leresche, L., & Mancl, L. (2007). Relationship of common pain conditions in mothers and children. *The Clinical Journal Pain, 23*(3), 204–213.

Siddall, P. J., & Cousins, M. J. (2004). Persistent pain as a disease entity: Implications for clinical management. *Anesthesia and Analgesia, 99*(2), 510–520.

Stevens, B., Anand, K. J., & McGrath, P. J. (2007). An overview of pain in neonates and infants. In K. J. Anand, B. Stevens, & P. J. McGrath (Eds.), *Pain research and clinical management. Pain in neonates and infants* (3rd ed., pp. 1–9). Edinburgh, United Kingdom: Elsevier.

Stinson, J., & Bruce, E. (2009). Chronic pain in children. In A. Twycross, S. J. Dowden, & E. Bruce (Eds.), *Managing pain in children: A clinical guide* (pp. 145–170). Oxford, United Kingdom: Wiley-Blackwell.

Taddio, A., & Katz, J. (2005). The effects of early pain experience in neonates on pain responses in infancy and childhood. *Paediatric Drugs, 7*(4), 245–257.

Taddio, A., Katz, J., Ilersich, A. L., & Koren, G. (1997). Effect of neonatal circumcision on pain response during subsequent routine vaccination. *Lancet, 349*(9052), 599–603.

Taddio, A., Shah, V., Gilbert-MacLeod, C., & Katz, J. (2002). Conditioning and hyperalgesia in newborns exposed to repeated heel lances. *The Journal of the American Medical Association, 288*(7), 857–861.

Taddio, A., Soin, H. K., Schuh, S., Koren, G., & Scolnik, D. (2005). Liposomal lidocaine to improve procedural success rates and reduce procedural pain among children: A randomized controlled trial. *Canadian Medical Association Journal, 172*(13), 1691–1695.

Twycross, A. (2007). Children's nurses' postoperative pain management practices: An observational study. *International Journal of Nursing Studies, 44*(6), 869–881.

Twycross, A. (2009). Nondrug methods of pain relief. In A. Twycross, S. J. Dowden, & E. Bruce (Eds.), *Managing pain in children: A clinical guide* (pp. 67–84). Oxford, United Kingdom: Wiley-Blackwell.

Van Hulle Vincent, C., & Denyes, M. J. (2004). Relieving children's pain: Nurses' abilities and analgesic administration practices. *Journal of Pediatric Nursing, 19*(1), 40–50.

Yamada, J., Stinson, J., Lamba, J., Dickson, A., McGrath, P. J., & Stevens, B. (2008). A review of systematic reviews on pain interventions in hospitalized infants. *Pain Research & Management, 13*(5), 413–420.

Yen, K., Kim, M., Stremski, E. S., & Gorelick, M. H. (2003). Effect of ethnicity and race on the use of pain medications in children with long bone fractures in the emergency department. *Annals of Emergency Medicine, 42*(1), 41–47.

Zernikow, B., Michel, E., Craig, F., & Anderson, B. J. (2009). Pediatric palliative care: Use of opioids for the management of pain. *Paediatric Drugs, 11*(2), 129–151.

2

Pain Assessment

Assessment of pain is an essential prerequisite to safe and efficacious pain management. A clear standard of care has emerged requiring routine measurement of pain at regular intervals using consistent and valid pain assessment tools. Successful assessment depends, in part, on a positive relationship between health care providers, children, and their families. Because no objective measure of the presence of pain is available for the neonate or younger child, health care providers must be willing to believe that their patient's pain is real. Older children are able to describe many aspects of their pain. However, fear, confusion, and the severity of illness can hinder their ability to communicate pain to health care providers and parents.

Reliance on children to voluntarily report their pain is likely to lead to underestimations. Children may be reluctant to report pain for fear of unpleasant consequences, such as prompting a diagnostic test, a longer inpatient stay, or, for adolescents, causing their parents to worry (American Pain Society [APS], 2008). Intramuscular administration of analgesics should be eliminated because children instinctively fear needles and may deny the existence of pain to avoid a "shot" (von Baeyer, 2006).

PAIN ASSESSMENT TOOLS

All methods used to assess pain and its intensity in children are subjective for the health care provider because the existence of pain

23

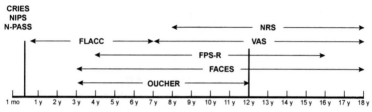

Figure 2.1 ■ Guidelines on age-appropriate one-dimensional pain intensity scales

cannot be proved or disproved (APS, 2008; Herr et al., 2006). The presence of pain is usually determined by the use of pain scales, most of which are one-dimensional (i.e., rating a single aspect, such as intensity). Despite the abundance of reliable, valid, and clinically useful pain assessment tools, no single pain assessment tool is appropriate across all ages of children or all types of pain (Stinson, 2009; von Baeyer & Spagrud, 2007), making it necessary for health care providers to select more than one tool when caring for children of various ages and conditions. See Figure 2.1 for basic guidelines on recommended ages for each pain assessment tool. The successful acceptance of a pain assessment tool by the health care provider depends on how it is valued. Research has shown that tools that incorporate a common metric of 0 to 10 to indicate "no pain" (0) to "worst pain" (10) are by far the most favored (Hicks, von Baeyer, Spafford, van Korlaar, & Goodenough, 2001; von Baeyer, 2009). However, no research has been conducted to determine that a specific rating, such as "5" on a 0–10 scale, means the same pain intensity on another scale.

Clinical Pearl	An ideal pain assessment tool needs to (Stinson, 2009; von Baeyer, 2006):
	■ Have demonstrated reliability (consistent and trustworthy rating regardless of item, setting, or who is administering the measure; extent to which pain measurement is consistent and free from random errors); interrater reliability (consistency or agreement among observers using the same tool).

- Have demonstrated validity (unequivocally measure a specific dimension of pain).
- Be responsive to the symptom being tested (able to detect a change in pain caused by treatment; measures pain and not another symptom).
- Have clinical utility (simple format, easy to use and score after a short training time, easy and efficient to administer and score). *Acceptance in clinical practice is very dependent on the tool requiring minimal burden on the part of the health care provider.*
- Be practical (able to use for different types of pain).
- Be developmentally, culturally, and medically relevant for the patient group; ability to use a single tool in different populations of patients increases its clinical utility.
- Be easily and quickly understood by patients.
- Be well liked by patients, clinicians, and researchers.
- Be inexpensive and easy to obtain, reproduce, and distribute with minimal disinfection between patients.
- Be available in various languages or easily translatable.

Self-Report Method

Self-report has been regarded as the optimal method of determining pain intensity. Age is the best predictor of determining the child's ability to use a self-report scale. The ability of younger children to abstract and quantify their pain is limited by their cognitive development, vocabulary, and pain experiences. Most children older than 4 years of age have some capacity to alert their caregivers that they have pain with progressive ability as they develop to communicate the intensity and characteristics of pain. A preschool child can tell a health care provider about his or her pain as "a little," "some," or "a lot," and, gradually, over the years will develop the ability to use one of more than 30 currently available self-report scales developed for children and adolescents. The detailed ratings of pain intensity may be more complicated for young children, ages 3 to 6 years old, than is commonly believed (Besenski, Forsyth, & von Baeyer, 2007; Stanford, Chambers, & Craig, 2006). Younger children may not be able to understand how to use an age-appropriate self-report tool and tend to answer using only the extreme ends of a pain scale (Stinson, Kavanagh, Yamada, Gill, & Stevens, 2006; von Baeyer, 2009).

Self-report is the gold standard and includes routine questions, verbal scales, numerical scales, and pictorial scales. Optimal results occur if the child is not overtly distressed at the time so that he or she can have an understanding of how to use the tool. If the child cannot self-report, behavioral and physiologic indicators (how the child acts and how the body reacts) need to be used as surrogate markers for self-report of pain. However, behavioral or physiologic indicators are not to replace patient self-report.

Self-Report Method for Older Children and Adolescents

The Numeric Rating Scale (NRS) is often used in determining pain intensity by asking the patient, "If 0 is no pain and 10 is the worst pain you can think of having, how much pain are you having now?" This test can be verbally administered without the use of physical materials such as laminated cards. To be able to use the NRS, the patient must be able to count up to 10 and understand the principle of increasing value of each number, which is generally considered possible for children who are at least 8 years old (APS, 2008; Miro, Castarlenas, & Huguet, 2009; von Baeyer, 2009; von Baeyer & Spagrud, 2007; von Baeyer et al., 2009). However, conceptualizing the "worst pain" they could ever have may be difficult for children who do not have abstract thinking skills (von Baeyer, 2006). Even though this method tends to be the most frequently used pain intensity measure with children in clinical practice (Stinson, 2009), limited research has been conducted in children (von Baeyer et al., 2009). One study showed poor agreement between the NRS, the Wong-Baker FACES Pain Rating Scale, and the Color Analog Scale in children experiencing high levels of pain in an emergency department (Bailey, Bergeron, Gravel, & Daoust, 2007). Children may answer with a number because they have the ability to count but may have not yet developed an understanding of the value and significance of numbers (von Baeyer et al., 2009).

Self-Report Method for Younger Children

One method of having the child self-report using a natural body movement is *The Finger Span Test* (Gaffney, McGrath, & Dick, 2003). The child is asked to put the thumb and forefinger together to indicate "no pain" and as far apart as possible to indicate "worst pain." Then the child is asked to represent his or her current pain intensity by demonstrating the finger distance between the two positions (Merkel, 2002). However, this format is difficult to document clinically for trending the efficacy of pain interventions and is generally not incorporated into routine pain practices for institutions.

Many tools have been developed to help younger children provide a numerical score of pain intensity. Although it has been suggested that children as young as 3 years old can use some of these scales, validation is most consistent with children who are 5 years or older (Stinson et al., 2006). One way to determine whether a child has the ability to use a self-report scale is to first ask, "How much does it hurt when you eat lunch?" and "How much does it hurt when you have an operation in the hospital?" (Besenski et al., 2007).

Faces pain scales tend to be favored over other measurement tools by pediatric patients, caregivers, and nurses (von Baeyer, 2006) and consist of stylized drawings (Hicks et al., 2001; Hockenberry & Wilson, 2009) or photographic series of faces (Beyer, Denyes, & Villarruel, 1992) with increasing signs of distress. Each face is assigned with a numerical value reflecting its order within a series of facial expressions. Faces pain scales with neutral expressions for no pain (Hicks et al., 2001) are generally recommended as some researchers question the added detail of a face that is smiling (von Baeyer, 2006) or scales with tears, which may skew children's abilities to differentiate pain from other emotions (Stinson, 2009). Most facial scales are shown to reflect pain effect, not just pain intensity. In other words, the face chosen by a child while sitting on his or her mother's lap may be higher than when the mother is out of the room. More research is needed in determining when a child can use a self-report scale, especially when he or she is experiencing chronic pain (Stanford et al., 2006).

The Faces Pain Scale-Revised (FPS-R). The FPS-R (Hicks et al., 2001) was adapted from the Bieri Pain Scale (Bieri, Reeve, Champion, Addicoat, & Ziegler, 1990; see Figure 2.2). This scale is intended for use in children 4 to 12 years old with well-established evidence of reliability, validity, and high clinical utility. It has been translated into more than 35 languages and is readily available and easily reproduced or downloaded at no cost (see Appendix). However, mixed findings have been reported concerning the acceptability of the scale with children and their adult caretakers because of the faces being seen as "scary" (Stinson, 2009; von Baeyer, 2009). This scale has the advantage of having neutral faces (not smiling) and is the most psychometrically sound measure for use in school-aged children (Stinson et al., 2006).

The Wong-Baker FACES Pain Rating Scale. The FACES Pain Rating Scale is intended for use with children 3 years and older (Hockenberry & Wilson, 2009; see Figure 2.3). This scale has well-established

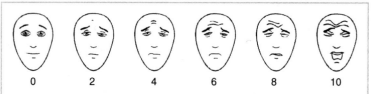

0	2	4	6	8	10

Instructions: Say "hurt" or "pain", whichever seems right for a particular child. "These faces show how much something can hurt. This face [point to left-most face] shows no pain. The faces show more and more pain [point to each from left to right] up to this one [point to right-most face]—it shows very much pain. Point to the face that shows how much you hurt [right now]. Score the chosen face 0, 2, 4, 6, 8, 10, counting left to right, so 0 = no pain and 10 = very much pain. Do not use words like "happy" and "sad." This scale is intended to measure how children feel inside, not how their face looks.

Note. From "The Faces Pain Scale-Revised: Toward a common metric in pediatric pain measurement," by C. L. Hicks, C. L. von Baeyer, P. A. Spafford, I. van Korlaar, & B. Goodenough, 2001, *Pain, 93*, pp. 173–183. Copyright 2001 by the International Association for the Study of Pain (IASP). Used with permission.

Figure 2.2 ■ Faces Pain Scale-Revised (FPS-R)

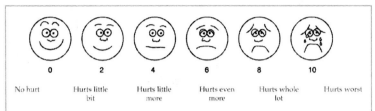

Instructions: Explain to the person that each face is for a person who feels happy because he has no pain (hurt) or sad because he has some or a lot of pain. Face 0 is very happy because he does not hurt at all. Face 2 hurts just a little bit. Face 4 hurts a little more. Face 6 hurts even more. Face 8 hurts a whole lot. Face 10 hurts as much as you can imagine, although you do not have to be crying to feel this bad. Ask the person to choose the face that best describes how he is feeling.

Note. From *Wong's Essentials of Pediatric Nursing*, by M. Hockenberry and D. Wilson (Eds.), 2009. St. Louis, MO: Elsevier Mosby. Copyright 2009 by Elsevier. Used with permission.

Figure 2.3 ▓ Wong-Baker FACES Pain Rating Scale

evidence of reliability, validity, and the ability to detect changes in pain intensity. It has high clinical utility and acceptability, has been translated into 10 languages, and is readily available and easily reproduced or downloaded at no cost (see Appendix). However, concerns have been noted about the scale for having a face with a smile for "no pain" as well as a face with tears representing "most pain" (Stinson, 2009), which may lead to an overestimation of pain for children who are reluctant to report no pain when they do not feel well enough to smile or severe pain if they are not crying. Health care providers are cautioned to direct the child to not confuse rankings of happiness or well-being with that of the intensity of pain when using such tools.

The Oucher Photographic Scale. The Oucher consists of two scales: the six photographs of children with numerical ratings and the 0- to 100-mm vertical numerical rating scale (Beyer et al., 1992; see Figure 2.4). This scale is intended for children 3 to 12 years old with well-established evidence of reliability, validity, and the ability to

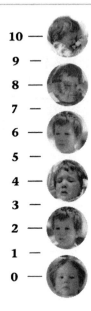

Once children select a picture, their selection is changed to a number score from 0–10. The Caucasian version of the Oucher was developed and copyrighted in 1983 by Judith E. Beyer, PhD, RN (University of Missouri-Kansas City School of Nursing), USA.

Instructions: This is a poster called the Oucher. It helps children tell others how much hurt they have. (For younger children, it may be useful to ask: "Do you know what I mean by hurt?" If the child is not sure, then an explanation should be provided). Here is how this works. This picture shows no hurt (point to the bottom picture), this picture shows just a little bit of hurt (point to the second picture), this picture shows a little more hurt (point to the third picture), this picture shows even more hurt (point to the fourth picture), this picture shows a lot of hurt (point to the fifth picture), and this picture shows the biggest hurt you could ever have (point to the sixth picture). Can you point to the picture that shows how much hurt you are having right now?

Note. From "The Creation, Validation, and Continuing Development of the Oucher: A measure of Pain Intensity in Children," by J. E. Beyer, M. J. Denyes, and A. M. Villarruel, 1992, *Journal for Pediatric Nursing, 7,* pp. 335–346. Used with permission.

Figure 2.4 ▦ Oucher Pain Scale

detect changes (von Baeyer, 2009) as well as having moderate clinical utility. However, it has mixed acceptability from children that may be related to the photographs not being sex-neutral, illustrating children in acute pain expressions. Other disadvantages include the cost to purchase these scales and the need to disinfect each copy between patients. A unique feature of the Oucher is the availability of multiple ethnicity versions for Caucasian, African American, Asian, and Hispanic patients (Beyer et al., 2005; Yeh, 2005). However, African American children preferred the FACES scale over the culturally specific African American Oucher version (Beyer et al., 2005; Luffy & Grove, 2003; Yeh, 2005). There is no research indicating that culturally specific scales are superior to generic versions or those with images of Caucasian children (Finley, Kristjansdottir, & Forgeron, 2009).

Visual Analog Scale (VAS). The VAS is used by asking the child to make a mark on a horizontal line, usually 100 mm long, indicating pain intensity (see Figure 2.5). Some versions have word anchors, such as "no pain" and "pain as bad as it could be," along the line to indicate the intensity of pain (Luffy & Grove, 2003). Although the VAS is easy to reproduce, the requirement of the extra step to measure the line to determine the pain intensity score makes it more burdensome and less appealing to health care providers (Stinson, 2009). The VAS is also thought to be less reliable for children younger than 7 years old (Shields, Palermo, Powers, Grewe, & Smith, 2003; Stinson et al., 2006).

Multidimensional Self-Report Tools

By including more than the intensity of pain and asking the child about how the pain feels and interferes with aspects of daily life, multidimensional self-report scales are more useful, especially for children with chronic pain (Stinson, 2009). All three of the following

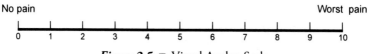

Figure 2.5 ■ Visual Analog Scale

tools have well-established evidence of reliability and validity with some evidence of ability to detect change, require minimal training for the health care provider, and require an administration time of 3 to 15 minutes (Stinson, 2009).

The Adolescent Pediatric Pain Tool (APPT). The APPT (Crandall & Savedra, 2005) was originally developed for children and adolescents 8 to 17 years old who are recovering from surgery, and a Spanish translation has been used in children with arthritis (Stinson, 2009), sickle-cell disease, and cancer (Jacob, McCarthy, Sambuco, & Hockenberry, 2008). The components of this scale include a 0- to 100-mm word graphic rating scale, a body outline to describe the location of the pain, and 56 word descriptors of the pain.

The Pediatric Pain Adolescent Tool (PPT). The PPT (Abu-Saad, Kroonen, & Halfens, 1990) is also useful for adolescents with acute medical and surgical pain and has been used with both recurrent pain (headaches) and chronic pain (arthritis) (Stinson, 2009). The components of this scale include a VAS, a body outline for marking the sites of pain, and a list of 32 words to describe the pain.

The Pediatric Pain Questionnaire (PPQ). The PPQ (Varni, Thompson, & Hanson, 1987) was developed specifically for children and adolescents with chronic pain, such as arthritis (Anthony & Schanberg, 2007; Rapoff, 2003). The components of this scale include a 0- to 10-cm VAS anchored with happy and sad faces, a body outline to describe the location of the pain, including a coloring scale, and 46 word descriptors of the pain. Varni, Seid, and Kurtin (2001) recently developed a quality-of-life inventory (PedsQL) to assess pain and its impact on the child's physical function in various pediatric chronic health conditions.

Behavioral Indicators of Pain for Infants and Children

Because young children lack the verbal and cognitive abilities to self-report their pain, indirect methods of determining the presence of pain and estimating its intensity are necessary. Rather than watching a child for any signs of pain with no specific set of indicators, a specific tool providing a consistent systematic means of assessing behaviors and changes in physiologic indicators associated with pain is recommended. Over the past 3 decades, a rapid proliferation of measurement tools with varying degrees of psychometric testing, feasibility, and clinical utility have been developed. However, some of these tools are not clinically practical because of excessive administrative time at the bedside. Most pain assessment tools have been designed and tested for Caucasian children. Culturally sensitive studies to document validity, reliability, or preference of non-Caucasian children have been infrequently reported. Psychometric testing of measurement tools is a dynamic and ongoing process. As the body of evidence supporting the properties of pain intensity measurement tools increases, any recommendations regarding use of pain assessment tools will undoubtedly change.

Clinical Pearl	When using observational pain measurement methods, health care providers need to be aware of the limitations of these methods of pain assessment (Anthony & Schanberg, 2007; Finley et al., 2009; Gaffney et al., 2003):

- Pain is always stressful, but stress is not necessarily painful. The inability to always differentiate pain from distress arising from related conditions such as fear, anxiety, agitation, fatigue, hunger, thirst, and hypoxia needs to be recognized. All conditions require assessment, evaluation, and treatment.
- Except for the initial response to acute pain, such as immediately after a needle procedure, discordance was found in validity testing between behavioral indicators and self-report for acute pain for children who could self-report.
- Although self-report scales appear to be transferrable between cultural groups and countries, the use of behavioral scoring methods are not universal, because socialization influences crying and limb withdrawal at very young ages, and Western-based identified behaviors indicating pain may be very different from those of other cultures.

(Continued)

(Continued)

▓ Although several tools exist to assess pain in the acute setting, no behavioral assessment tools have been developed specifically for use in children with chronic pain. Clinicians are to be reminded that the behaviors seen as indicative of acute pain are not likely to be present for children with chronic pain, even when they have a flare-up of their pain, because they have habituated to their pain.

▓ A behavioral pain assessment tool is not to be used to refute a patient's self-report of pain.

A behavioral pain assessment tool provides a framework in the form of a checklist assigning numerical values to common behaviors associated with pain, including crying and other vocalizations, specific facial expressions, and gross body movements or positioning that can range from rigidity to thrashing (Bringuier et al., 2009; Crellin, Sullivan, Babl, O'Sullivan, & Hutchinson, 2007; Johnston, Stevens, Boyer, & Porter, 2003; Stevens, Pillai-Riddell, Oberlander, & Gibbins, 2007; von Baeyer & Spagrud, 2007). Almost all behavioral pain tools require scoring within categories of behaviors, usually with each behavior having 2 to 6 gradations. The subscores are then totaled to produce a composite pain score with the assumption that a higher score indicates a greater probability that the child is experiencing pain.

Observational Tools for Children

The FLACC. The name of this scale is an acronym for the components of the scale, specifically the facial expressions, leg position, generalized activity, type of cry, and ease in consoling, with subscales yielding a total score from 0 to 10, similar to many other self-report pediatric scales (see Table 2.1). Initial interrater reliability and validity for scoring postoperative pain in children ages 2 months to 7 years (Merkel, Voepel-Lewis, Shayevitz, & Malviya, 1997) were expanded recently with further validation for children receiving analgesics (Willis, Merkel, Voepel-Lewis, & Malviya, 2003), children

Table 2.1 ▓ *FLACC Behavioral Pain Scale*

Categories	Scoring		
	0	*1*	*2*
Face	No particular expression or smile	Occasional grimace or frown; withdrawn, disinterested	Frequent to constant frown, clenched jaw, quivering chin
Legs	Normal position or relaxed	Uneasy, restless, tense	Kicking, or legs drawn up
Activity	Lying quietly, normal position, moves easily	Squirming, shifting back and forth, tense	Arched, rigid, or jerking
Crying	No crying (awake or asleep)	Moans or whimpers, occasional complaint	Crying steadily, screams or sobs, frequent complaints
Consolability	Content, relaxed	Reassured by occasional touching, hugging, or being talked to, distractible	Difficult to console or comfort

Instructions: Each of the five categories is scored from 0–2, resulting in a total score between 0–10.

Abbreviations: FLACC, face, legs, activity, cry, and consolability.
Source: From "The FLACC: A Behavioral Scale for Scoring Postoperative Pain in Young Children," by S. I. Merkel, T. Voepel-Lewis, J. R. Shayevitz, & S. Malviya, 1997, *Pediatric Nursing, 23,* pp. 293–297. Copyright 2002 by The Regents of the University of Michigan. Used with permission.

in hematology/oncology units (Manworren & Hynan, 2003), and critically ill adults and children (Voepel-Lewis, Zanotti, Dammeyer, & Merkel, 2010). FLACC is simple to use, score, and interpret; it is widely recognized in the United States; and it has been translated into several other languages, including French, Chinese, Portuguese, Swedish, and Italian (Voepel-Lewis et al., 2010).

The Children's Hospital of Eastern Ontario Pain Scale (CHEOPS). The CHEOPS was one of the first to be developed by health care providers for the assessment of procedural and postoperative pain in children younger than 5 years (McGrath, 1998). Although the CHEOPS has well-established evidence of reliability, validity, and the ability to detect change (von Baeyer & Spagrud, 2007), the number of subscales requires a longer administration time and a more complicated scoring system, making it less appealing for clinical practice (Stinson, 2009).

The COMFORT Scale. This scale is most often used for assessment of children who are critically ill (Ambuel, Hamlett, Marx, & Blumer, 1992; see Chapter 14, Critical Illness).

Observational Tools for Infants

The ability to assess pain in infants has greatly expanded in the past 20 years in response to increasing recognition that pain is often under treated in this vulnerable population (American Academy of Pediatrics and Canadian Pediatric Society, 2000; Anand et al., 2006; Duhn & Medves, 2004; Stevens, 2007). Certain facial expressions are indicative of pain in infants: bulged brow, eyes squeezed tightly shut, eyebrows drawn lower and together, and open lips and mouth stretched vertically and horizontally with a taut tongue (Stinson, 2009). See Figure 2.6. A systematic review of infant pain assessment measures indicates varying degrees of evidence for reliability and

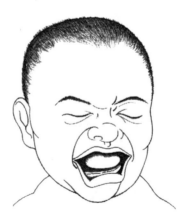

Figure 2.6 ■ Infant face in pain.

validity (Duhn & Medves, 2004; Pillai Riddell et al., 2009), with no single simple and widely accepted technique to define pain in neonates.

The CRIES Scale. CRIES is an acronym of the scale's pain indicators, specifically crying, requiring oxygen, increased vital signs, expression, and sleeplessness (see Table 2.2). This scale has been shown to have reliability and validity for assessment of postoperative pain

Table 2.2 ▩ *CRIES Neonatal Pain Postoperative Assessment Tool*

	Scoring		
Category	*0*	*1*	*2*
Crying	No	High pitched	Inconsolable
Requires O₂ sat <95%	No	<30%	>30%
Increased vital signs	HR and BP ≤ Preop	HR or BP increased <20% of Preop	HR or BP increased >20% of Preop
Expression	None	Grimace	Grimace/Grunt
Sleepless	No	Wakes at frequent intervals	Constantly Awake

Scoring Tips
- Crying: Characteristic cry of pain is *high pitched.*
- O₂ saturation: Consider other causes of changes, such as atelectasis, pneumothorax, oversedation.
- Increased vital signs: Use baseline from preop parameters from a nonstressed period; use mean BP; Take BP last, as this may wake the child causing difficulty in scoring other assessments.
- Expression: Grimace is characterized by brow lowering, eyes squeezed shut, deepening of the nasolabial furrow, and open lips and mouth.
- Sleepless: Score is based on the infant's state during the hour preceding the current score.

Abbreviations: BP, blood pressure; HR, heart rate; O₂ sat, oxygen saturation; preop, preoperative.
Source: From "CRIES: A New Neonatal Postoperative Pain Measurement Score. Initial Testing of Validity and Reliability," by S. W. Krechel & J. Bildner, 1995, *Paediatric Anaesthesia, 5,* pp. 53–61. Copyright 1995 by John Wiley and Sons, Blackwell Publishing. Used with permission.

in infants with a gestational age of at least 32 weeks (Krechel & Bildner, 1995; Suraseranivongse et al., 2006). Although this tool is easy to use, it is difficult to interpret, because the oxygenation measure can be influenced by conditions other than pain. In addition, measuring the blood pressure noninvasively requires disturbing the infant (Stinson, 2009).

The Neonatal Infant Pain Scale. The Neonatal Infant Pain Scale (NIPS) was developed for neonates 24 to 40 weeks gestational age. This tool is used by observing facial expression, cry, breathing pattern, arms, legs, and state of arousal to determine a pain score and has shown evidence of interrater reliability and validity (Duhn & Medves, 2004; Lawrence et al., 1993; Suraseranivongse et al., 2006; see Table 2.3). NIPS has been used to evaluate pain during minor procedures (Bellieni et al., 2007). However, difficulty in remembering the scoring system has led to limited clinical utility (Stinson, 2009).

The Neonatal Pain, Agitation, Sedation Scale (N-PASS). The N-PASS was developed in response to the need for a tool to assess infant pain as well as sedation level for infants cared for in neonatal intensive care units. N-PASS has shown evidence of reliability and validity in infants who are 30 days old, 23 to 40 weeks gestational age, with prolonged pain, including postoperative pain and conditions such as necrotizing enterocolitis or mechanical ventilation (Hummel, Lawlor-Klean, & Weiss, 2010). Requiring an observation period of 5 to 10 minutes, the health care provider is to assess crying/irritability, behavioral state, facial expression, extremities/tone, heart rate, respiratory rate, blood pressure, and oxygen saturation, which may not be practical for the health care provider (see Appendix).

Physiologic Signs

Although appealing as concrete markers, physiologic indicators, such as blood pressure, heart rate, respiratory rate, and oxygen saturation, are often not sensitive for distress of a prolonged nature for a

Table 2.3 ■ *Neonatal Infant Pain Scale (NIPS)*

Parameter	Finding	Points
Facial expression	Relaxed	0
	Grimace	1
Crying	No crying	0
	Whimper	1
	Vigorous cry	2
Breathing patterns	Relaxed	0
	Change in breathing	1
Arms	Restrained	0
	Relaxed	0
	Flexed	1
	Extended	1
Legs	Restrained	0
	Relaxed	0
	Flexed	1
	Extended	1
State of arousal	Sleeping	0
	Awake	0
	Fussy	1

Scoring Tips

■ Facial expression, relaxed muscles: restful face, neutral expression; grimace: tight facial muscles, furrowed brow, negative facial expression.

■ Cry, vigorous: loud scream, rising, shrill, continuous (Note: Silent cry may be scored if infant is intubated as evidenced by obvious mouth, facial movements).

■ Breathing patterns: relaxed is a usual pattern for infants; change in breathing is irregular, faster than usual, gagging, and breath holding

■ Arms and legs: relaxed/restrained: no muscular rigidity, occasional random movements of limb; flexed or extended is tense straight rigid and/or rapid extension flexion

■ State of arousal: sleeping is quiet peaceful sleeping; awake is alert and settled; fussy is alert but restless and/or thrashing

Source: From "The Development of a Tool to Assess Neonatal Pain," by J. Lawrence, D. Alcock, P. McGrath, J. Kay, S. B. MacMurray, & C. Dulberg, 1993, *Neonatal Network*, *12*, pp. 59–66. Used with permission from Children's Hospital of Eastern Ontario.

child of any age. Children may have increases in heart rate, respiratory rate, and blood pressure at least initially when they are experiencing acute pain. These responses are a result of the release of catecholamines from the adrenal medulla in the body's preparation for "fight or flight." However, the body cannot sustain the stress response for extended periods. Physiologic adaptation will occur, sometimes within minutes of the stimulus. Vital signs will then return to normal, and other physical parameters associated with acute pain, such as sweating and papillary dilation, will cease. In the neonate, the vital signs may "reset" at a higher resting baseline. A nurse assessing a child for pain may be misled by the presence of "normal" physiologic parameters. Therefore, on their own, physiologic indicators do not constitute a valid clinical pain measure for children, as evidenced by studies in older children who were able to self-report, and physiologic signs may be only loosely correlated with pain intensity scores (Stinson, 2009).

Although some tools incorporate physiologic biomarkers of pain, such as skin conductance fluctuations (Gjerstad, Wagner, Henrichsen, & Storm, 2008) and hair cortisol (Yamada et al., 2007) or saliva cortisol levels (Hunt et al., 2007), such measurements really are not seen as practical at the bedside. However, biomarkers are useful in developing and validating observational tools in children who cannot self-report.

PAIN ASSESSMENT: MORE THAN A PAIN INTENSITY SCORE

A complete physical examination, especially of the neurologic and musculoskeletal systems, is essential to determine all causes of pain even when the source may appear obvious. Establishing a diagnosis is a priority when the cause of pain is uncertain, but clinicians should initiate symptomatic pain treatment while the investigation proceeds. It rarely is justifiable to defer analgesia until a diagnosis is made (APS, 2008; Finley et al., 2009). A comfortable patient is better able to cooperate with diagnostic procedures.

Pain Assessment in Preschool and School-Age Children and Adolescents

Collapsing the pain assessment into a single number, such as a pain intensity score, does not represent pain assessment. Nurses are to use judgment in fitting the pain intensity score into the assessment process, including obtaining a history about the pain, especially for young children who have limited verbal skill, including questions to the child (or parent) such as (Stinson, 2009):

- What word do you use for pain?
- Where is your pain? Does it spread to another area?
- What words can you tell me that describe your pain (i.e., sharp, burning)?
- When did it start? Is the pain there more in the daytime or nighttime?
- How often does the pain occur? Is it always there (constant), or does it go away and come back?
- If it is not constant, how many times does it occur each day? How long does the pain last? Are there certain times of day you feel pain more frequently? What makes the pain go away? What makes it worse?
- What medicines have you taken before to help with your pain? Did it help? Did you have any side effects? Do you use any complementary or over-the-counter therapies?
- Over the past week (or day for younger children), what is the least amount of pain you have had? Worst? How much pain do you have now? What is the usual level of pain?
- Does it keep you from eating? Playing?
- Does it wake you up at night?
- Are there other symptoms that happen at the same time, such as nausea?
- Is there anything special you want me to know about your pain?

Parents play a role in knowing their child's pain cues and thus are in a unique position to advocate for appropriate pain management for their children. Parents should be an integral part of the process, providing pain-relevant information, including specific words their children use for pain such as "boo-boo" or "owie." However, having parents determine the pain intensity score for their children often leads to a underestimation or overestimation of the pain in their children (Boldingh, Jacobs-van der Bruggen, Lankhorst, & Bouter, 2004; Kelly, Powell, & Williams, 2002; Nader, Oberlander, Chambers, & Craig, 2004; Voepel-Lewis, Malviya, & Tait, 2005).

Pain Assessment in Infants and Toddlers

For infants and toddlers, many of the preceding questions will not be answerable, and the assessment is enhanced by the health care provider considering the following questions:

- Given the infant's diagnosis and treatments, is it reasonable to infer that this child is experiencing pain?
- Do the infant's behavioral changes respond to analgesics?
- Could other factors be contributing to the infant's behaviors, such as hunger or needing a diaper change?

Although newborns are initially highly reactive to painful stimuli, over time or if the severity of the illness depletes their reserves, their response to pain becomes less vigorous to conserve energy. The presence of pain is reflected instead in how the infant responds to caregivers by either hyperarousal or withdrawal as well as changes in sleeping and eating patterns (Pillai Riddell et al., 2009).

The Use of Pain Diaries

Pain levels may fluctuate throughout the day. A pain diary to write pain scores, precipitating factors, and responses to analgesics or non-pharmacologic interventions can be a useful method of identifying patterns of pain and potential treatment strategies. Having the child take some ownership in completing the diary has been shown to be useful for children with sickle-cell disease, juvenile arthritis, and headaches (Anthony & Schanberg, 2007; McClish et al., 2009). Recently, electronic hand-held diaries have been developed for children with recurrent and chronic pain, recording pain intensity and its interference with activities of daily living (Anthony & Schanberg, 2007; Palermo, Valenzuela, & Stork, 2004; Stinson et al., 2008).

The Limitations of Pain Assessment Tools

Because many of these instruments were developed and tested in children with acute and self-limiting illnesses or injuries, they may be less useful for chronic pain and for children who are developmentally or cognitively delayed, very ill, or dying. Initially, pain induces behaviors often associated with noxious stimuli (i.e., crying, withdrawing from stimuli, flailing of limbs, and grimacing). As pain continues, the behavioral responses are progressively blunted. Children with long-term pain may appear depressed and withdrawn.

Children with unrelieved acute pain frequently will lie immobile in bed, not because they are comfortable, but because of severe incidental pain related to movement. Conversely, behavioral scales may overrate procedural pain by reflecting fear and distress in addition to pain (Ljungman, Kreuger, Gordh, & Sorensen, 2006). With their vivid imaginations and interest at playing, children can make efforts at distracting themselves to help relieve their discomfort, especially of ongoing pain. Children who are experiencing persistent or chronic pain often participate in age-appropriate normal activities such as playing or watching television despite feeling some level of pain. Consequently, clinicians may underrate pain intensity and erroneously conclude that the child is not in pain.

ASSESSMENT OF PAIN IN PHYSICALLY AND COGNITIVELY IMPAIRED CHILDREN

Recently, more attention has been focused on assessing pain in children with a range of significant disabilities (Breau, Camfield, McGrath, & Finley, 2004) such as autism (Nader et al., 2004), cerebral palsy (Boldingh et al., 2004; Hadden & von Baeyer, 2002), developmental delay (Stinson, 2009), or Down syndrome (Hennequin, Faulks, & Allison, 2003). Children who are physically or cognitively impaired by stroke associated with sickle-cell disease, for example, present additional pain assessment challenges involving parental input in regard to specific questions related to their child's responses to pain (Breau, Finley, et al., 2002; Solodiuk & Curley,

2003). These children are at increased risk for pain due to multiple medical problems either causing pain itself or requiring frequent procedures that are often painful. The inability of cognitively impaired children and adolescents to communicate information about their pain places them at high risk for inadequate pain relief (APS, 2008). If idiosyncratic behaviors, such as vocal abnormalities (e.g., moaning and grunting), or more confusing idiosyncratic behaviors, such as laughing, are present, pain is often underestimated or overestimated by their caretakers. Recommended strategies to assess pain are the following:

- Ask the patient; many patients who appear cognitively impaired may still be able to provide useful information concerning pain.
- Interview their parents about patterns of particular behaviors that may indicate pain (e.g., placing a hand on the forehead for headache).
- Review the medical record for known potentially pain-inducing conditions such as chemotherapy, which is known to cause pain (e.g., vincristine).
- Complete a physical examination and directed laboratory and diagnostic imaging studies to assess common pain-inducing problems, such as urinary tract infections.

Assessment Tools for Physically and Cognitively Impaired Children

Research is ongoing in the development of formal tools with varying degrees of reliability and validity, but the following may be useful:

The Non-Communicating Children's Pain Checklist-Revised

The Non-Communicating Children's Pain Checklist-Revised (NCCPC-R) is a tool specifically designed for children with cognitive impairments who are unable to communicate verbally for both chronic and acute pain. This tool uses a list of 30 items divided into seven subscales: vocal, eating/sleeping, social, facial, activity, body/limb, and physiologic signs (Breau, McGrath, et al., 2002;

see Appendix). This tool was further revised into a 27-item checklist as the Non-Communicating Children's Pain Checklist-Postoperative Version (NCCPC-PV) to make it more specific to children recovering from surgery (Breau et al., 2002).

The Pediatric Pain Profile

This tool is a 20-item behavior rating scale for assessing pain in children with severe neurologic disabilities who are unable to communicate through speech or augmentative communication (Hunt et al., 2004).

The FLACC

This tool has recently been offered as an alternative for pain assessment in children with cognitive impairment. It has overall more clinical utility than the NCCPC-PV because of health care provider familiarity with its use for unimpaired children and only 5 versus 27 items to be scored from 0 to 3 (Malviya, Voepel-Lewis, Burke, Merkel, & Tait, 2006; Voepel-Lewis et al., 2008). By adding specific behavioral descriptors under the relevant r-FLACC categories, the reliability of this tool for pain assessment was improved.

PLACEBOS AS AN UNACCEPTABLE ASSESSMENT METHOD

The use of placebos to discredit a patient's self-report of pain intensity is considered unethical and deceptive and not an appropriate pain assessment method for any person, regardless of age or diagnosis (APS, 2008; American Society of Pain Management Nursing [ASPMN], 2004). Many patients have temporary relief from the "placebo response" that is associated with the belief that a health care provider has provided a pain-relieving intervention. Whether with good intentions or as a means to discredit a patient's pain report, placebo use without consent compromises the trusting and therapeutic relationship between clinicians and patients.

FITTING ASSESSMENT INTO OVERALL
TREATMENT PLAN FOR PAIN

Health care providers assess children's pain on admission to the hospital and when they visit the emergency department or an ambulatory clinic. Generally, for inpatients, the pain intensity score is reassessed at least once a shift to determine whether pain is present and more frequently if the patient has a known painful medical condition, such as surgery or cancer (Stinson, 2009). Treatment plan adjustments are based on careful evaluation of a child's responses to pharmacologic and nonpharmacologic interventions. The severity of a disease and injury is often dynamic, fluctuating as the disease progresses or the injury heals and as various therapies are administered. Although many health care providers are involved and share responsibility in assessing pain, it is the nurse who is best positioned to identify children who are in pain, to appropriately assess the pain and its impact on the child and family, to apply appropriate interventions found useful in the reduction of pain, and to determine the effectiveness of the intervention to reassess the treatment plan for pain. Understanding how a child is rating pain intensity over a continuum of time and activities gives more information about the child's experience.

Determining the Effectiveness of the Pain Treatment Plan

The frequency of reassessment of the plan will depend on the severity of the pain condition, the onset of action of the intervention, and the risk for adverse effects if analgesics have been administered. For hospitalized children, along with the pain intensity score, reassessment needs to include how well the child is able to:

- Rest and sleep
- Move and turn in the bed and ambulate
- Take a deep breath and cough
- Comply with the rehabilitation plan

When a child is an outpatient, additional components of reassessment of the pain treatment include how well the child is able to play, go to school, and, in general, return to a normal routine.

The clinical significance of any reduction in pain scores should be interpreted in terms of the patient (von Baeyer, 2006). The smallest meaningful improvement, meaning a reduction in pain intensity, seems to be in the 10 to 20 percentage point range for children (Anand et al., 2006; Bijur, Latimer, & Gallagher, 2003; Powell, Kelly, & Williams, 2001) and for adults (Bijur et al., 2003) treated in an emergency department. These findings cannot be generalized to children with chronic pain.

One approach to determining the effectiveness of a pain management plan is by establishing a number on the pain intensity scale as a treatment target, often called a *pain goal*, defined by the patient as the threshold above which interventions (pharmacologic or nonpharmacologic) are considered. Ask the child, "What level would the pain need to be so that you could do all your normal activities?" (Stinson, 2009).

Promising children that all pain will be treated to a pain intensity goal of 0 out of 10 is misguided, especially for chronic pain. Evaluating treatment of chronic pain is often more realistic in terms of restoring function and improving quality of life, including a child's ability to return to normal activities, such as play, school, or sleep, while controlling pain intensity (Jacob et al., 2006).

In summary, mechanisms need to be in place for health care providers to be able to provide age-appropriate pain assessment tools imbedded within a comprehensive pain assessment process. Documentation mechanisms need to be in place that are as uncomplicated and effortless as possible for health care providers, including the reassessment of pain to determine how the patient has responded to interventions, especially with the current movement into electronic entry.

REFERENCES

Abu-Saad, H. H., Kroonen, E., & Halfens, R. (1990). On the development of a multidimensional Dutch pain assessment tool for children. *Pain*, *43*(2), 249–256.

Ambuel, B., Hamlett, K. W., Marx, C. M., & Blumer, J. L. (1992). Assessing distress in pediatric intensive care environments: The COMFORT scale. *Journal of Pediatric Psychology*, *17*(1), 95–109.

American Academy of Pediatrics and Canadian Pediatric Society. (2000). Prevention and management of pain and stress in the neonate. American Academy of Pediatrics. Committee on Fetus and Newborn, Committee on Drugs, Section on Anesthesiology, Section on Surgery. Canadian Paediatric Society, Fetus and Newborn Committee. *Pediatrics, 105*(2), 454–461.

American Pain Society. (2008). *Principles of analgesic use in the treatment of acute pain and cancer pain.* Glenview, IL: Author.

American Society of Pain Management Nursing. (2004). *Position statement on use of placebos in pain management.* Retrieved from www.aspmn.org

Anand, K. J., Aranda, J. V., Berde, C. B., Buckman, S., Capparelli, E. V., Carlo, W., . . . Walco, G. A. (2006). Summary proceedings from the neonatal pain-control group. *Pediatrics, 117*(3, Pt. 2), S9–S22.

Anthony, K. K., & Schanberg, L. E. (2007). Assessment and management of pain syndromes and arthritis pain in children and adolescents. *Rheumatic Diseases Clinics of North America, 33*(3), 625–660.

Bailey, B., Bergeron, S., Gravel, J., & Daoust, R. (2007). Comparison of four pain scales in children with acute abdominal pain in a pediatric emergency department. *Annals of Emergency Medicine, 50*(4), 379–383.

Bellieni, C. V., Cordelli, D. M., Caliani, C., Palazzi, C., Franci, N., Perrone, S., . . . Buonocore, G. (2007). Inter-observer reliability of two pain scales for newborns. *Early Human Development, 83*(8), 549–552.

Besenski, L. J., Forsyth, S. J., & von Baeyer, C. L. (2007). Commentary: Screening young children for their ability to use self-report pain scales. *Pediatric Pain Letter.* Retrieved from www.pediatric-pain.ca/ppl

Beyer, J. E., Denyes, M. J., & Villarruel, A. M. (1992). The creation, validation, and continuing development of the Oucher: A measure of pain intensity in children. *Journal for Pediatric Nursing, 7*(5), 335–346.

Beyer, J. E., Turner, S. B., Jones, L., Young, L., Onikul, R., & Bohaty, B. (2005). The alternate forms reliability of the Oucher pain scale. *Pain Management Nursing, 6*(1), 10–17.

Bieri, D., Reeve, R. A., Champion, G. D., Addicoat, L., & Ziegler, J. B. (1990). The Faces Pain Scale for the self-assessment of the severity of pain experienced by children: Development, initial validation, and preliminary investigation for ratio scale properties. *Pain, 41*(2), 139–150.

Bijur, P. E., Latimer, C. T., & Gallagher, E. J. (2003). Validation of a verbally administered numerical rating scale of acute pain for use in the emergency department. *Academic Emergency Medicine, 10*(4), 390–392.

Boldingh, E. J., Jacobs-van der Bruggen, M. A., Lankhorst, G. J., & Bouter, L. M. (2004). Assessing pain in patients with severe cerebral palsy: Development, reliability, and validity of a pain assessment instrument for cerebral palsy. *Archives of Physical Medicine and Rehabilitation, 85*(5), 758–766.

Breau, L. M., Camfield, C. S., McGrath, P. J., & Finley, G. A. (2004). Risk factors for pain in children with severe cognitive impairments. *Developmental Medicine and Child Neurology, 46*(6), 364–371.

Breau, L. M., Finley, G. A., McGrath, P. J., & Camfield, C. S. (2002). Validation of the Non-communicating Children's Pain Checklist-Postoperative Version. *Anesthesiology, 96*(3), 528–535.

Breau, L. M., McGrath, P. J., Camfield, C. S., & Finley, G. A. (2002). Psychometric properties of the non-communicating children's pain checklist-revised. *Pain, 99*, 349–357.

Bringuier, S., Picot, M. C., Dadure, C., Rochette, A., Raux, O., Boulhais, M., & Capdevila, X. (2009). A prospective comparison of post-surgical behavioral pain scales in preschoolers highlighting the risk of false evaluations. *Pain, 145*, 60–68.

Crandall, M., & Savedra, M. (2005). Multidimensional assessment using the adolescent pediatric pain tool: A case report. *Journal of Specialists in Pediatric Nursing, 10*(3), 115–123.

Crellin, D., Sullivan, T. P., Babl, F. E., O'Sullivan, R., & Hutchinson, A. (2007). Analysis of the validation of existing behavioral pain and distress scales for use in the procedural setting. *Paediatric Anaesthesiology, 17*(8), 720–733.

Duhn, L. J., & Medves, J. M. (2004). A systematic integrative review of infant pain assessment tools. *Advances in Neonatal Care, 4*(3), 126–140.

Finley, G. A., Kristjansdottir, O., & Forgeron, P. A. (2009). Cultural influences on the assessment of children's pain. *Pain Research and Management, 14*(1), 33–37.

Gaffney, A., McGrath, P., & Dick, B. (2003). Measuring pain in children: Developmental and instrument issues. In N. L. Schechter, C. B. Berde, & M. Yaster (Eds.), *Pain in infants, children, and adolescents* (2nd ed., pp. 128–141). Philadelphia, PA: Lippincott, Williams, & Wilkins.

Gjerstad, A. C., Wagner, K., Henrichsen, T., & Storm, H. (2008). Skin conductance versus the modified COMFORT sedation score as a measure of discomfort in artificially ventilated children. *Pediatrics, 122*(4), e848–e853.

Hadden, K. L., & von Baeyer, C. L. (2002). Pain in children with cerebral palsy: Common triggers and expressive behaviors. *Pain, 99*, 281–288.

Hennequin, M., Faulks, D., & Allison, P. J. (2003). Parents' ability to perceive pain experienced by their child with Down syndrome. *Journal of Orofacial Pain, 17*(4), 347–353.

Herr, K., Coyne, P. J., Key, T., Manworren, R., McCaffery, M., Merkel, S., . . . Wild, L. (2006). Pain assessment in the nonverbal patient: Position statement with clinical practice recommendations. *Pain Management Nursing, 7*(2), 44–52.

Hicks, C. L., von Baeyer, C. L., Spafford, P. A., van Korlaar, I., & Goodenough, B. (2001). The Faces Pain Scale-Revised: Toward a common metric in pediatric pain measurement. *Pain, 93*(2), 173–183.

Hockenberry, M., & Wilson, D. (2009). Wong's essentials of pediatric nursing. In M. Hockenberry & D. Wilson (Eds.), *Wong's essentials of pediatric nursing*. St. Louis, MO: Elsevier Mosby.

Hummel, P., Lawlor-Klean, P., & Weiss, M. G. (2010). Validity and reliability of the N-PASS assessment tool with acute pain. *Journal of Perinatology, 30*(7), 474–478.

Hunt, A., Goldman, A., Seers, K., Crichton, N., Mastroyannopoulou, K., Moffat, V., . . . Brady, M. (2004). Clinical validation of the paediatric pain profile. *Developmental Medicine and Child Neurology, 46*(1), 9–18.

Hunt, A., Wisbeach, A., Seers, K., Goldman, A., Crichton, N., Perry, L., & Mastroyannopoulou, K. (2007). Development of the paediatric pain profile: Role of video analysis and saliva cortisol in validating a tool to assess pain in children with severe neurological disability. *Journal of Pain and Symptom Management, 33*(3), 276–289.

Jacob, E., McCarthy, K. S., Sambuco, G., & Hockenberry, M. (2008). Intensity, location, and quality of pain in Spanish-speaking children with cancer. *Pediatric Nursing, 34*(1), 45–52.

Jacob, E., Miaskowski, C., Savedra, M., Beyer, J. E., Treadwell, M., & Styles, L. (2006). Changes in sleep, food intake, and activity levels during acute painful episodes in children with sickle cell disease. *Journal of Pediatric Nursing, 21*(1), 23–34.

Johnston, C. C., Stevens, B., Boyer, K., & Porter, F. L. (2003). Development of psychologic responses to pain and assessment of pain in infants and toddlers. In N. L. Schechter, C. B. Berde, & M. Yaster (Eds.), *Pain in infants, children, and adolescents* (2nd ed., pp. 105–127). Philadelphia, PA: Lippincott, Williams, & Wilkins.

Kelly, A. M., Powell, C. V., & Williams, A. (2002). Parent visual analogue scale ratings of children's pain do not reliably reflect pain reported by child. *Pediatric Emergency Care, 18*(3), 159–162.

Krechel, S. W., & Bildner, J. (1995). CRIES: A new neonatal postoperative pain measurement score. Initial testing of validity and reliability. *Paediatric Anaesthesia, 5*(1), 53–61.

Lawrence, J., Alcock, D., McGrath, P., Kay, J., MacMurray, S. B., & Dulberg, C. (1993). The development of a tool to assess neonatal pain. *Neonatal Network, 12*(6), 59–66.

Ljungman, G., Kreuger, A., Gordh, T., & Sorensen, S. (2006). Pain in pediatric oncology: Do the experiences of children and parents differ from those of nurses and physicians? *Upsala Journal of Medical Sciences, 111*(1), 87–95.

Luffy, R., & Grove, S. K. (2003). Examining the validity, reliability, and preference of three pediatric pain measurement tools in African-American children. *Pediatric Nursing, 29*(1), 54–59.

Malviya, S., Voepel-Lewis, T., Burke, C., Merkel, S., & Tait, A. R. (2006). The revised FLACC observational pain tool: Improved reliability and validity for pain assessment in children with cognitive impairment. *Paediatric Anaesthesia, 16*(3), 258–265.

Manworren, R. C., & Hynan, L. S. (2003). Clinical validation of FLACC: Preverbal patient pain scale. *Pediatric Nursing, 29*(2), 140–146.

McClish, D. K., Smith, W. R., Dahman, B. A., Levenson, J. L., Roberts, J. D., Penberthy, L. T., . . . Bovbjerg, V. E. (2009). Pain site frequency and location in sickle cell disease: The PiSCES project. *Pain, 145*, 246–251.

McGrath, P. J. (1998). Behavioral measures of pain. In G. A. Finley & P. J. McGrath (Eds.), *Measurements of pain in infants and children: Progress in pain research and management* (Vol. 12, p. 91). Seattle, WA: IASP Press.

Merkel, S. (2002). Pain assessment in infants and young children: The Finger Span Scale. *American Journal of Nursing, 102*(11), 55–56.

Merkel, S. I., Voepel-Lewis, T., Shayevitz, J. R., & Malviya, S. (1997). The FLACC: A behavioral scale for scoring postoperative pain in young children. *Pediatric Nursing, 23*(3), 293–297.

Miro, J., Castarlenas, E., & Huguet, A. (2009). Evidence for the use of a numerical rating scale to assess the intensity of pediatric pain. *European Journal of Pain, 13*(10), 1089–1095.

Nader, R., Oberlander, T. F., Chambers, C. T., & Craig, K. D. (2004). Expression of pain in children with autism. *The Clinical Journal of Pain, 20*(2), 88–97.

Palermo, T. M., Valenzuela, D., & Stork, P. P. (2004). A randomized trial of electronic versus paper pain diaries in children: Impact on compliance, accuracy, and acceptability. *Pain, 107*(3), 213–219.

Pillai Riddell, R. R., Stevens, B. J., McKeever, P., Gibbins, S., Asztalos, L., Katz, J., . . . Din, L. (2009). Chronic pain in hospitalized infants: Health professionals' perspectives. *The Journal of Pain, 10*(12), 1217–1225.

Powell, C. V., Kelly, A. M., & Williams, A. (2001). Determining the minimum clinically significant difference in visual analog pain score for children. *Annals of Emergency Medicine, 37*(1), 28–31.

Rapoff, M. A. (2003). Pediatric measures of pain: The pain behavior observation method, Pain Coping Questionnaire (PCQ), and Pediatric Pain Questionnaire (PPQ). *Arthritis & Rheumatism, 49*(5S), S90–S95.

Shields, B. J., Palermo, T. M., Powers, J. D., Grewe, S. D., & Smith, G. A. (2003). Predictors of a child's ability to use a visual analogue scale. *Child Care Health Development, 29*(4), 281–290.

Solodiuk, J., & Curley, M. A. (2003). Pain assessment in nonverbal children with severe cognitive impairments: The Individualized Numeric Rating Scale (INRS). *Journal of Pediatric Nursing, 18*(4), 295–299.

Stanford, E. A., Chambers, C. T., & Craig, K. D. (2006). The role of developmental factors in predicting young children's use of a self-report scale for pain. *Pain, 120*, 16–23.

Stevens, B. (2007). Pain assessment and management in infants with cancer. *Pediatric Blood and Cancer, 49*(7 Suppl.), 1097–1101.

Stevens, B., Pillai-Riddell, R., Oberlander, T. F., & Gibbins, S. (2007). Assessment of pain in neonates and infants. In K. J. Anand, B. Stevens, & P. J. McGrath (Eds.), *Pain in neonates and infants* (3rd ed., pp. 67–90). Philadelphia, PA: Elsevier.

Stinson, J. N. (2009). Pain assessment. In A. Twycross, S. J. Dowden, & E. Bruce (Eds.), *Managing pain in children: A clinical guide* (pp. 85–108). Oxford, United Kingdom: Wiley-Blackwell.

Stinson, J. N., Kavanagh, T., Yamada, J., Gill, N., & Stevens, B. (2006). Systematic review of the psychometric properties, interpretability and feasibility of self-report pain intensity measures for use in clinical trials in children and adolescents. *Pain*, *125*, 143–157.

Stinson, J. N., Stevens, B. J., Feldman, B. M., Streiner, D., McGrath, P. J., Dupuis, A., . . . Petroz, G. C. (2008). Construct validity of a multidimensional electronic pain diary for adolescents with arthritis. *Pain*, *136*(3), 281–292.

Suraseranivongse, S., Kaosaard, R., Intakong, P., Pornsiriprasert, S., Karnchana, Y., Kaopinpruck, J., & Sangjeen, K. (2006). A comparison of postoperative pain scales in neonates. *British Journal of Anaesthesiology*, *97*(4), 540–544.

Varni, J. W., Seid, M., & Kurtin, P. S. (2001). PedsQL 4.0: Reliability and validity of the Pediatric Quality of Life Inventory version 4.0 generic core scales in healthy and patient populations. *Medical Care*, *39*(8), 800–812.

Varni, J. W., Thompson, K. L., & Hanson, V. (1987). The Varni/Thompson Pediatric Pain Questionnaire. I. Chronic musculoskeletal pain in juvenile rheumatoid arthritis. *Pain*, *28*(1), 27–38.

Voepel-Lewis, T., Malviya, S., & Tait, A. R. (2005). Validity of parent ratings as proxy measures of pain in children with cognitive impairment. *Pain Management Nursing*, *6*(4), 168–174.

Voepel-Lewis, T., Malviya, S., Tait, A. R., Merkel, S., Foster, R., Krane, E. J., & Davis, P. J. (2008). A comparison of the clinical utility of pain assessment tools for children with cognitive impairment. *Anesthesia and Analgesia*, *106*(1), 72–78.

Voepel-Lewis, T., Zanotti, J., Dammeyer, J. A., & Merkel, S. (2010). Reliability and validity of the face, legs, activity, cry, consolability behavioral tool in assessing acute pain in critically ill patients. *American Journal of Critical Care*, *19*(1), 55–61.

von Baeyer, C. L. (2006). Children's self-reports of pain intensity: Scale selection, limitations and interpretation. *Pain Research and Management*, *11*(3), 157–162.

von Baeyer, C. L. (2009). Children's self-report of pain intensity: What we know, where we are headed. *Pain Research and Management*, *14*(1), 39–45.

von Baeyer, C. L., & Spagrud, L. J. (2007). Systematic review of observational (behavioral) measures of pain for children and adolescents aged 3 to 18 years. *Pain*, *127*, 140–150.

von Baeyer, C. L., Spagrud, L. J., McCormick, J. C., Choo, E., Neville, K., & Connelly, M. A. (2009). Three new datasets supporting use of the

Numerical Rating Scale (NRS-11) for children's self-reports of pain intensity. *Pain, 143*(3), 223–227.

Willis, M. H., Merkel, S. I., Voepel-Lewis, T., & Malviya, S. (2003). FLACC Behavioral Pain Assessment Scale: A comparison with the child's self-report. *Pediatric Nursing, 29*(3), 195–198.

Yamada, J., Stevens, B., de Silva, N., Gibbins, S., Beyene, J., Taddio, A., . . . Koren, G. (2007). Hair cortisol as a potential biologic marker of chronic stress in hospitalized neonates. *Neonatology, 92*(1), 42–49.

Yeh, C. H. (2005). Development and validation of the Asian version of the Oucher: A pain intensity scale for children. *The Journal of Pain, 6*(8), 526–534.

II

Common Medications for Managing Acute and Chronic Pain

3

General Principles and Nonopioids

GENERAL PRINCIPLES FOR PHARMACOLOGIC MANAGEMENT

Drug therapy is the mainstay of acute pain management for all age groups, including neonates, and is complemented by nonpharmacologic approaches to ensure optimal pain relief. General guidelines that are periodically updated and republished are available to health care providers (American Academy of Pediatrics, 2001; American Academy of Pediatrics Subcommittee on Chronic Abdominal Pain, & North American Society for Pediatric Gastroenterology, Hepatology, and Nutrition, 2005; American Pain Society [APS], 2008; World Health Organization [WHO], 1998; Zempsky & Cravero, 2004). As with all medications, health care providers need to consider and discuss with their patients the need to balance the potential benefits and risks of a particular analgesic.

Selection of Analgesics

Factors to consider when individualizing the selection of an analgesic (APS, 2008) are the following:

- The cause of the patient's pain
- The patient's age and general health, as well as the presence of comorbidities

▨ The potential for adverse outcomes associated with medication-related adverse effects
▨ The patient's history of reactions to medicines; if an allergy is reported, the medicine and any other medicines within the class of the offending medicine is to be considered contraindicated until otherwise determined that it is safe to administer
▨ Potential drug interactions
▨ What has been effective in the past medical treatment
▨ What has not been effective (inquire about dose and schedule in the past to determine if an effective treatment regimen was administered)

Scheduling Doses of Analgesics

Acute pain should be treated by medications prescribed at appropriate doses to control pain and by closely monitored titration of the medications in response to the child's needs. The pattern of pain can be the following:

▨ *Intermittent*, such as a headache with the need for medications in response to early signs of pain, administered on an "as-needed" basis, commonly known as *pro re nata* (PRN), useful only when pain is intermittent (i.e., separated by long pain-free intervals) or unpredictable. To use these regimens, children must have the ability to communicate the presence of pain and be able to ask nurses or parents to administer the ordered dose. Children may then reexperience pain before the next dose of PRN medication is scheduled to be administered, potentially leading to cycles of undermedication and pain, alternating with the risk of periods of overmedication and drug toxicity.
▨ *Persistent* or *continuous* throughout day and night, prompting the need for medications to be prescribed around-the-clock (ATC) or in controlled-release formulations. When indicated, acute or chronic pain is also treated with ATC medicines.
▨ *Breakthrough pain* or episodic pain that "breaks through" analgesia that previously controlled the pain with a transitory flare-up of moderate to severe pain (APS, 2008) seen as negatively affecting patient function and quality of life from the following:
  ● Precipitated or associated with an identifiable stimulus, such as physical activity or sudden movement

- Idiopathic, occurring independently of an identifiable cause
- End-of-dose failure, occurring regularly before the next dose of a controlled-release pain medication

---

Clinical Pearl

Analgesic administration needs to:

- Match the analgesic order to the pattern of pain
- Avoid the intramuscular and rectal routes for children
- Anticipate the need for breakthrough doses for activities or treatments that are likely to temporarily increase pain, such as dressing changes, physical therapy, or movement in bed
- Include nonpharmacologic techniques that "make the pain medicines work better," such as relaxation or application of warm pads
- Be followed by ongoing assessments to evaluate the efficacy of treatment
- Anticipate, recognize, and treat adverse effects
- Have an adequate trial of an analgesic before changing to another analgesic

---

Optimizing Safety

Safe and effective use of analgesics require a thorough understanding of various developmental aspects of drug disposition and metabolism. Clearance of medicines can be slower in younger infants than in adults and older children. This can be attributed to both the immaturity of renal function and a lower capacity of drug-metabolizing enzymes (Kearns et al., 2003; McCarver & Hines, 2002). Developmental differences that affect the pharmacokinetics and pharmacodynamics of analgesics have been well summarized elsewhere (Berde & Sethna, 2002; Yaster, Tobin, & Kost-Byerly, 2003). However, much of the information about analgesics given to children is based on data extrapolated from adult studies, including equianalgesic dose conversions.

> *Clinical Pearl*
>
> Multimodal therapy is the combined use of several types of analgesic drugs with different mechanisms of action to optimize the analgesic effect, which are as follows:
>
> ▪ Allows for lower drug doses, thus minimizing the adverse effects of analgesics i.e., adding a nonsteroidal anti-inflammatory drug [NSAID] to an opioid to decrease the opioid dose, referred to as "opioid sparing," thus potentially decreasing the risk of opioid-induced respiratory depression.
> ▪ Uses various receptors that balance analgesia and target the pain at different points on the pain pathway.

NONOPIOIDS

Nonopioids are a heterogeneous group of medications that share common antipyretic, analgesic, and anti-inflammatory effects. The group includes acetaminophen, NSAIDs, and salicylates, which are useful for mild to moderate nociceptive pain either alone or in combination with opioids. For severe pain, opioids are often added because NSAIDs have a "ceiling effect" (i.e., higher than recommended doses do not provide additional analgesia, but add a risk of significant toxicity).

▪ *Acetaminophen (Tylenol)*

Indications: Acetaminophen is the most widely used analgesic for mild to moderate pain in infants, including newborns, and children, with a good safety margin if used as directed (Greco & Berde, 2005). By selectively inhibiting prostaglandin synthesis, which is thought to be by inhibiting cyclooxygenase (COX)-3 in the central nervous system, acetaminophen has antipyretic and analgesic effects but minimal anti-inflammatory effects (Berde et al., 2005; Remy, Marret, & Bonnet, 2006).

Dosage: Recommended dosage information is listed in Table 3.1. Various forms can be given, such as capsules, tablets, suspensions, and suppositories. Health care providers are to carefully consider the formulation when choosing a dose. For example, the infant drops are more concentrated (80 mg in 0.8 ml) than the pediatric suspensions (160 mg in 5 ml).

Table 3.1 ▪ *Dosing Guidelines for Nonopioid Analgesics*

Drug	Pediatric Dosage (<12 years old)	Maximum Dose/kg/day	Adult Dosage (>12 years old)	Maximum/ Day
Acetaminophen	10–15 mg/kg q 4–6 h PO	75 mg	325–1,000 mg q 4–6 h PO	4,000 mg
Choline magnesium trisalicylate	10–15 mg/kg q 8–12 h PO	Total salicylate content 1,000 mg/dose or 3,000 mg/day	1,000–1,500 mg q 12 h PO	3,000 mg
Ibuprofen	5–10 mg/kg q 6 to 8 h PO (maximum 600 mg/dose)	30 mg/kg/day	400–800 mg q 6 h PO	3,200 mg
Naproxen	5–20 mg/kg q 12 h PO	20 mg/kg/day (no safety data on newborns or infants)	250–550 mg q 12 h PO	1,250 mg
Indomethacin	1–2 mg/kg q 6–12 h	4 mg/kg/day	25–50 mg q 8 h PO	200 mg
Diclofenac potassium	0.5–0.75 mg/kg q 6–12 h PO	3 mg/kg/day	50 mg q 8 h	200 mg
Ketorolac	0.2–0.5 mg/kg q 6–8 h IV (maximum 30 mg/dose)	Give no more than 5 days with limited safety data for infants	15–30 mg q 6–8 h IV	120 mg; give no more than 5 days
Celecoxib (COX-2 inhibitor)	10–25 kg: 50 mg bid >25 kg: 100 mg bid	No data reported	200–400 mg q 12–24 h PO	400 mg

Abbreviations: bid, two times a day; COX, cyclooxygenase; IV, intravenous; PO, by mouth.
Source: From American Pain Society, 2005, 2008; Anghelescu, Oakes, & Popenhagan, 2006; Berde et al., 2005; Brislin & Rose, 2005; Dowden, 2009; Greco & Berde, 2005; Kraemer & Rose, 2009; Litalien & Jacqz-Aigrain, 2001; Maunuksela & Olkkola, 2003.

Chewable tablets are available in both 80 mg and 160 mg, and the simple tablet is available in either 325 mg or 500 mg. Various rectal formulations exist as well. Many over-the-counter medicines as well as certain opioids, such as oxycodone and codeine, are available alone or compounded with acetaminophen. However, in the United States, hydrocodone is available only in combination with acetaminophen. The use of such opioids should not exceed the recommended maximum dose of acetaminophen per day.

Adverse Effects: Although lacking the troublesome adverse effects of NSAIDs, hepatic and renal injury are possible if the dose exceeds the recommended limits per day (see Table 3.1). In fact, hepatotoxicity may result for children taking doses within the recommended limits, especially when they are taken with other medications associated with hepatic toxicity (APS, 2008).

Salicylates

▣ *Acetylsalicylic Acid (Aspirin)*

Indications: Aspirin is a useful analgesic for mild to moderate pain. It is also useful as an antipyretic, anti-inflammatory, and prophylactic thrombotic event agent. However, it is recommended to be used only for adolescents and has largely been replaced by various NSAIDs available for analgesia.

Dosage: When used in adolescents, the dosage is 10 to 15 mg/kg orally administered every 4 to 6 hours with a maximum dose of 90 mg/kg/day or 4,000 mg/day (Kraemer & Rose, 2009).

Contraindications: Aspirin is no longer recommended for use in infants and children because of its association with Reye's syndrome, a potentially fatal disease in younger children and infants (APS, 2008), affecting all organs of the body but most harmful to the brain and the liver, causing an acute increase of pressure within the brain and, often, massive accumulations of fat in the liver and other organs. The availability of newer NSAIDs has further limited the need for aspirin.

Adverse Effects: Gastrointestinal (GI) irritation, ulceration, and bleeding; inhibition of platelet aggregation, leading to a risk of bleeding.

▓ *Choline Magnesium Trisalicylate (Trilisate)*

Indications: Trisalicylate is useful as an antipyretic agent and analgesic for mild to moderate pain, especially for inflammatory or bone pain. As a newer salicylate, few trials have been conducted regarding safety and efficacy, but unlike aspirin and other nonselective NSAIDs, if used in therapeutic doses, bleeding time and platelet aggregation are not affected (APS, 2008). Therefore, health care providers can consider this as an option for patients with moderate thrombocytopenia.

Dosage: Recommended dosage information is noted in Table 3.1. Trisalicylate is available in a tablet and liquid form.

Contraindications: Data are insufficient for use in patients with severe clotting abnormalities (APS, 2008).

Adverse Effects: Gastric irritation and renal dysfunction.

NONSTEROIDAL ANTI-INFLAMMATORY DRUGS

NSAIDs provide analgesia through the inhibition of COX, an enzyme that contributes to the production of prostaglandins and thromboxanes that, in turn, sensitize peripheral nerve endings and vasodilate vessels, causing pain, erythema, and inflammation (APS, 2008; Litalien & Jacqz-Aigrain, 2001). In fact, NSAIDs are superior to opioids for reducing pain from inflammation (Kraemer & Rose, 2009). Several COX isoenzymes have been identified. COX-1 is present throughout the body and plays a role in protecting the gastric mucosa, regulating renal blood flow, and promoting platelet aggregation. COX-2 is another isoform that is induced by inflammatory mediators in traumatized cells. NSAIDs that block COX-1 and COX-2, called nonselective COX inhibitors, are generally well tolerated but can have adverse effects on protective mechanisms leading to gastric irritation and potential ulceration, impaired renal function, and bleeding (Litalien & Jacqz-Aigrain, 2001). Topical formulations of NSAIDs have been developed recently to provide analgesia similar to their oral counterparts with less systemic exposure and potentially fewer serious adverse effects without a loss of efficacy.

Indications: All NSAIDs are useful for their antipyretic effects, anti-inflammatory activities, and analgesic effects, especially for reducing bone or muscle pain. NSAIDs are effective for mild to moderate intermittent pain as well as postoperative pain, although most studies have been conducted in children older than 1 year undergoing minor surgeries (Litalien & Jacqz-Aigrain, 2001). The margin of safety for children is at least equal to that of adults. The opioid-sparing effects of NSAIDs serve as a valuable addition in multimodal therapy, resulting in improved pain relief with less risk of respiratory depression.

Dosage: Recommended dosage information for specific oral and parenteral NSAIDs is available in Table 3.1.

Drug Interactions: Concomitant administration of aspirin and an NSAID is not recommended because of an increased risk of adverse NSAID effects. An increase in bleeding risk is possible with concomitant anticoagulant administration.

Contraindications: NSAIDs should be avoided or used with caution in children with bleeding disorders or at risk for hemorrhage, renal or hepatic impairment, or dehydration; a history of GI ulcerations or bleeding; and in the setting of coronary artery bypass graft surgery (Litalien & Jacqz-Aigrain, 2001). Because of concerns about NSAIDs interfering with bone healing or coagulation, administration after fractures, surgery to correct scoliosis, or tonsillectomy is controversial (Greco & Berde, 2005; Maunuksela & Olkkola, 2003). Children with asthma should be given NSAIDs with caution. Aspirin- or NSAID-induced asthma and bronchospasms are rare but potentially fatal (Maunuksela & Olkkola, 2003).

Adverse Effects: Adverse effects can occur with all routes of administration, not just when taken orally, but usually are infrequent if used for a minimal duration unless the child has a preexisting organ dysfunction. However, neonates are at particular risk for such adverse effects (Kraemer & Rose, 2009).

Gastrointestinal Effects: Minor complaints of dyspepsia can occur with NSAIDs, even if they are taken with food to minimize local irritation of the gastric mucosa. Serious upper GI problems, such as ulceration and bleeding, can occur at any time, most commonly without warning (APS, 2008). Patients with a history of GI tract bleeding or concurrent corticosteroid use should be evaluated before NSAIDs are administered because the risk of GI bleeding is increased fivefold when steroids and NSAIDs are given together (APS, 2008). To minimize the risk of GI complications, NSAIDs should be used at the lowest effective dose for the shortest duration for which they are needed (APS, 2008), and histamine-2 receptor antagonists (i.e., ranitidine [Zantac]) or protein-pump inhibitors (i.e., omeprazole [Prilosec]) should be provided (APS, 2008). NSAIDs and aspirin can produce liver damage, prompting the need to periodically monitor liver enzymes and bilirubin if NSAIDs are a part of chronic therapy (APS, 2008).

Renal Effects: Both nonselective and selective NSAIDs can cause renal insufficiency. Patients at highest risk for renal complications include those with preexisting renal conditions, hepatic dysfunction, or concomitant therapy with other nephrotoxic medications, such as diuretics, chemotherapy (e.g., cisplatin), aminoglycosides, and amphotericin B. Inhibition of prostaglandin-mediated intrarenal vasodilation during hypovolemia or reduced renal blood flow further increases the risk of renal toxicity but is usually reversible if the NSAID is withheld. Appropriate hydration is essential, especially with parenteral ketorolac (Toradol). Caution should be taken when giving NSAIDs to a patient with preexisting renal insufficiency or who also requires diuretics. Parents are to be informed of the need to ensure their children have adequate oral intake of fluids.

Platelet Effects: All NSAIDs inhibit platelet aggregation by reversibly inhibiting COX-1, leading to a slightly increased bleeding time but within normal limits in children with normal coagulation function (Anderson & Palmer, 2006). However, NSAIDs remain contraindicated in children with coagulopathies or otherwise at risk for bleeding, such as those with chemotherapy-induced thrombocytopenia or who have undergone recent cardiovascular events or cardiovascular surgery (APS, 2008).

Selective Nonsteroidal Anti-Inflammatory Drugs (COX-2 Inhibitors)

To reduce the adverse effects of NSAIDs, new forms have been developed to selectively block only the COX-2 system. These agents spare the inhibition of COX-1, which protects the GI system, provides renal blood flow regulation, and promotes platelet aggregation. Health care providers can use these selective NSAIDs with the goal of decreasing pain with less toxicity. COX-2 inhibitors do seem to lessen the risk of serious GI effects occurring within at least the first 6 months of use, as well as having minimal effects on platelet function (APS, 2008). Unfortunately, many COX-2 inhibitors were removed from the market because of the increased incidence of cardiovascular and cerebrovascular complications during prolonged use.

▨ *Celecoxib (Celebrex)*

Celecoxib remains available and approved for use in children older than 2 years with juvenile rheumatoid arthritis (Kraemer & Rose, 2009). Recommended dosage information is available in Table 3.1.

Nonselective Nonsteroidal Anti-Inflammatory Drugs

No NSAID is known to be more effective than any other in the general population (McNicol, Strassels, Goudas, Lau, & Carr, 2004; Zernikow et al., 2006). However, intrapatient variability in response to a specific NSAID occurs for reasons that are not completely understood but seems to be related to genetic polymorphisms involved in prostaglandin production (Anderson & Palmer, 2006; APS, 2008; Kraemer & Rose, 2009). Therefore, if a patient does not benefit from one NSAID, it is worthwhile to consider the use of another. The use of more than one NSAID simultaneously is not recommended, because of the additive risk of toxicity without the additional benefit of increased analgesia. Clearance of NSAIDs improves with age, and dosing should take into account the weight and age of the patient.

▨ *Ibuprofen (Motrin)*

Ibuprofen is the most common NSAID used in pediatrics (Brislin & Rose, 2005).

Forms: Ibuprofen is available as oral drops (40 mg/ml), suspension/elixir (100 mg in 5 ml), chewable tablets (50 mg and 100 mg), and various regular tablet strengths. The administration regimen should be explained carefully to caregivers because many different forms and strengths exist.

▒ *Naproxen (Naprosyn)*

Naproxen has a longer half-life than ibuprofen, offering the convenience of only twice-a-day dosing.

Forms: Naproxen is available as an elixir (125 mg in 5 ml) and various strengths in nonchewable tablets.

Adverse Effects: All children should be monitored for pseudoporphyria (bullae and increased fragility of the skin over the nasal bridge) seen in 12% of fair-skinned children. It usually disappears after naproxen is discontinued (Maunuksela & Olkkola, 2003).

▒ *Indomethacin (Indocin)*

Indomethacin is an effective anti-inflammatory agent and can be used in infants for closure of patent ductus arteriosus. It is used less frequently for analgesia because of a higher incidence of adverse GI effects than with other NSAIDs.

Forms: Indomethacin is available as an elixir (25 mg in 5 ml), capsules (25 or 50 mg), extended-release capsules (75 mg), and rectal suppositories (50 mg).

▒ *Diclofenac Potassium (Cambia)*

Diclofenac is another NSAID useful in reducing chronic pain.

Forms: Diclofenac is available in several oral preparations and in rectal suppositories.

▒ *Diclofenac Sodium 1% (Voltaren Gel)*

Diclofenac is also available as a topical NSAID approved for use in adults and, therefore, may be considered in older adolescents. However, safety and efficacy in pediatric patients have not been established.

Indications: The gel is recommended for treatment of osteoarthritis pain in joints amenable to topical applications, such as the knees or hands, as well as for soft tissue injuries (Banning, 2008). The package insert information cautions that the gel has not been evaluated for use on joints of the spine, hip, or shoulder (Endo-Pharmaceutical, 2009).

Drug Interactions: Use of topical NSAIDs while systemic NSAIDs are also being administered is not recommended.

Form: A 100 g tube is supplied with a dosing card that aids in the measurement of the appropriate amount of gel, depending on the area being treated.

Dosage: The dosage for adult/older adolescent is 2 to 4 g up to 4 times per day (Banning, 2008; Kienzler, Gold, & Nollevaux, 2010). Patients are to be instructed to gently massage the dose of gel into the skin, ensuring application to the entire affected joint. Avoid bathing the treated area for at least 1 hour after application. Avoid concomitant use with other topical products on the same skin sites.

Adverse Effects: The most common adverse effects observed are skin reactions to the application site, including dermatitis, pruritus, erythema, paresthesia, dryness, vesicles, and papules (Banning, 2008). The amount of diclofenac sodium systemically absorbed from Voltaren gel is on average 6% of the systemic exposure from oral diclofenac sodium (Banning, 2008). Thus, risks traditionally associated with NSAIDs should be minimized with topical diclofenac sodium gel.

Diclofenac Epolamine 1.3% (Flector)

This is another topical NSAID approved for adult use. No studies have been conducted in children.

Indications: The patch is to be used on muscle strains, sprains, and contusions (APS, 2008; King Pharmaceuticals, 2009).

Drug Interactions: Use of topical NSAIDs while systemic NSAIDs are also being administered is not recommended.

Form: Diclofenac epolamine is available as a patch.

Dosage: The adult dosage is one patch applied to the most painful area twice a day. However, the patch is not to be placed on damaged or nonintact skin and should not be worn while bathing or showering. The patch is not recommended in patients with advanced renal disease or significant renal impairment.

Adverse Effects: Minor skin reactions and minor GI symptoms have been reported (Rainsford, Kean, & Ehrlich, 2008).

▓ *Ketorolac (Toradol)*

Ketorolac is the only parenteral NSAID available and is used primarily for postoperative pain with evidence that adding this to morphine patient-controlled analgesia provides excellent pain relief with opioid-sparing side effects (Litalien & Jacqz-Aigrain, 2001). Hypersensitivity reactions in children have been reported (Kraemer & Rose, 2009). In a prospective study with single doses for postoperative pain in infants and toddlers between 6 and 18 months of age, no adverse effects on renal or hepatic function were found (Lynn et al., 2007). A retrospective chart review for infants younger than 6 months showed that ketorolac was used safely in neonates and infants who had cardiac surgery without adverse hematologic or renal effects (Moffett, Wann, Carberry, & Mott, 2006).

Forms: Both oral and parenteral forms are available.

In summary, acetaminophen, salicylates, and NSAIDs serve as useful analgesics for mild to moderate pain from various etiologies and are a valuable part of multimodal therapy for more severe and complex pain syndromes. However, health care providers need to be aware of the associated adverse effects that limit their use.

REFERENCES

American Academy of Pediatrics. (2001). The assessment and management of acute pain in infants, children and adolescents. *Pediatrics, 108*(3), 793–797.

American Academy of Pediatrics Subcommittee on Chronic Abdominal Pain, & North American Society for Pediatric Gastroenterology, Hepatology, and Nutrition. (2005). Chronic abdominal pain in children. *Pediatrics, 115*(3), 812–815.

American Pain Society. (2005). *Guidelines for the management of cancer pain in adults and children.* Glenview, IL: Author.

American Pain Society. (2008). *Principles of analgesic use in the treatment of acute pain and cancer pain.* Glenview, IL: Author.

Anderson, B. J., & Palmer, G. M. (2006). Recent pharmacological advances in paediatric analgesics. *Biomedicine and Pharmacotherapy, 60*(7), 303–309.

Anghelescu, D., Oakes, L., & Popenhagan, M. (2006). Management of pain due to cancer in neonates, children, and adolescents. In O. A. de Leon-Casasola (Ed.), *Cancer pain: Pharmacologic, interventional, and palliative care approaches* (pp. 509–521). Philadelphia, PA: Elsevier.

Banning, M. (2008). Topical diclofenac: Clinical effectiveness and current uses in osteoarthritis of the knee and soft tissue injuries. *Expert Opinion on Pharmacotherapy, 9*(16), 2921–2929.

Berde, C. B., Jaksic, T., Lynn, A. M., Maxwell, L. G., Soriano, S. G., & Tibboel, D. (2005). Anesthesia and analgesia during and after surgery in neonates. *Clinical Therapeutics, 27*(6), 900–921.

Berde, C. B., & Sethna, N. F. (2002). Analgesics for the treatment of pain in children. *The New England Journal of Medicine, 347*(14), 1094–1103.

Brislin, R. P., & Rose, J. B. (2005). Pediatric acute pain management. *Anesthesiology Clinics of North America, 23*(4), 789–814.

Dowden, S. J. (2009). Palliative care in children. In A. Twycross, S. J. Dowden, & E. Bruce (Eds.), *Managing pain in children: A clinical guide* (pp. 171–200). Oxford, United Kingdom: Wiley-Blackwell.

Endo-Pharmaceutical. (2009). Voltaren gel [Package insert]. Retrieved from http://www.voltarengel.com/

Greco, C., & Berde, C. (2005). Pain management for the hospitalized pediatric patient. *Pediatric Clinics of North America, 52*(4), 995–1027.

Kearns, G. L., Abdel-Rahman, S. M., Alander, S. W., Blowey, D. L., Leeder, J. S., & Kauffman, R. E. (2003). Developmental pharmacology—drug disposition, action, and therapy in infants and children. *The New England Journal of Medicine, 349*(12), 1157–1167.

Kienzler, J. L., Gold, M., & Nollevaux, F. (2010). Systemic bioavailability of topical diclofenac sodium gel 1% versus oral diclofenac sodium in healthy volunteers. *The Journal of Clinical Pharmacology, 50*(1), 50–61.

King Pharmaceuticals. (2009). Flector Patch [Package insert]. Retrieved from www.flectorpatch.com/references.cfm

Kraemer, F. W., & Rose, J. B. (2009). Pharmacologic management of acute pediatric pain. *Anesthesiology Clinics, 27*(2), 241–268.

Litalien, C., & Jacqz-Aigrain, E. (2001). Risks and benefits of nonsteroidal anti-inflammatory drugs in children: A comparison with paracetamol. *Paediatric Drugs, 3*(11), 817–858.

Lynn, A. M., Bradford, H., Kantor, E. D., Seng, K. Y., Salinger, D. H., Chen, J., . . . Anderson, G. D. (2007). Postoperative ketorolac tromethamine use in infants aged 6–18 months: The effect on morphine usage, safety assessment, and stereo-specific pharmacokinetics. *Anesthesia and Analgesia, 104*(5), 1040–1051.

Maunuksela, E. L., & Olkkola, K. T. (2003). Nonsteroidal anti-inflammatory drugs in pediatric pain management. In N. L. Schechter, C. B. Berde, & M. Yaster (Eds.), *Pain in infants, children, and adolescents* (2nd ed., pp. 171–180). Philadelphia, PA: Lippincott Williams & Wilkins.

McCarver, D. G., & Hines, R. N. (2002). The ontogeny of human drug-metabolizing enzymes: Phase II conjugation enzymes and regulatory mechanisms. *Journal of Pharmacology and Experimental Therapeutics, 300*(2), 361–366.

McNicol, E., Strassels, S., Goudas, L., Lau, J., & Carr, D. (2004). Nonsteroidal anti-inflammatory drugs, alone or combined with opioids, for cancer pain: A systematic review. *Journal of Clinical Oncology, 22*(10), 1975–1992.

Moffett, B. S., Wann, T. I., Carberry, K. E., & Mott, A. R. (2006). Safety of ketorolac in neonates and infants after cardiac surgery. *Paediatric Anaesthesia, 16*(4), 424–428.

Rainsford, K. D., Kean, W. F., & Ehrlich, G. E. (2008). Review of the pharmaceutical properties and clinical effects of the topical NSAID formulation, diclofenac epolamine. *Current Medical Research and Opinion, 24*(10), 2967–2992.

Remy, C., Marret, E., & Bonnet, F. (2006). State of the art of paracetamol in acute pain therapy. *Current Opinion in Anaesthesiology, 19*(5), 562–565.

World Health Organization. (1998). *Cancer pain relief and palliative care in children.* Geneva, Switzerland: Elsevier.

Yaster, M., Tobin, J. R., & Kost-Byerly, S. (2003). Local anesthetics. In N. L. Schechter, C. B. Berde, & M. Yaster (Eds.), *Pain in infants, children, and adolescents* (2nd ed., pp. 241–264). Philadelphia, PA: Lippincott Williams & Wilkins.

Zempsky, W. T., & Cravero, J. P. (2004). Relief of pain and anxiety in pediatric patients in emergency medical systems. *Pediatrics, 114*(5), 1348–1356.

Zernikow, B., Smale, H., Michel, E., Hasan, C., Jorch, N., & Andler, W. (2006). Paediatric cancer pain management using the WHO analgesic ladder—results of a prospective analysis from 2,265 treatment days during a quality improvement study. *European Journal of Pain, 10*(7), 587–595.

4

Opioids

Opioids remain the single most important group of medications for the relief of moderate to severe pain caused by serious illnesses and injuries. Opioid receptors are present throughout the body but are concentrated in the dorsal horn of the central nervous system (CNS). When the mu-opioid receptors are blocked by the administration of opioids or somewhat by the naturally produced endorphins, the transmission of the pain signal is lessened or inhibited along the ascending pain pathways, thus reducing the sensation of pain in the brain. Opioids are converted into metabolites (active and inactive) in the liver and then excreted via the renal system. These metabolites may accumulate in patients with renal impairment.

RECOMMENDED OPIOIDS

Because there is little proven difference between opioids in efficacy or adverse effects, the choice depends on availability, the prescribing health care provider's experience, and the child's experience of the effectiveness or adverse effects (American Pain Society [APS], 2008). The clinical effects are virtually identical among opioids at equal analgesic doses. However, research in genetic polymorphisms in opioid receptors (APS, 2008) is attempting to elucidate significant interindividual variations in response.

▓ *Morphine Sulfate*

Indications: Morphine is considered as the gold standard for opioid analgesia (McNicol et al., 2003; Yaster, Kost-Byerly, & Maxwell, 2003; Zernikow, Michel, Craig, & Anderson, 2009; Zernikow et al., 2006).

Dosage: Recommended initial doses are available in Table 4.1.

Forms: Intravenous (IV) and oral immediate-release formulations in both tablet and elixir are available, as well as several controlled-release formulations (Oramorph, MS-Contin, Kadian, and Avinza) that must be swallowed as intact tablets. One form of controlled-release morphine (Kadian) is approved for administration by emptying the contents of the capsule into soft food that can be swallowed without chewing. This is particularly useful for young children who are unable to swallow whole tablets (APS, 2008; Collins & Weisman, 2003).

Table 4.1 ▓ *Opioid Dosing Guidelines for Children Older Than 6 Months*

Recommended starting dose for children older than 6 months; for children younger than 6 months consider 50% of the following doses.

Opioid	Initial Pediatric Dose (<50 kg)		Initial Adult Dose (>50 kg)	
	Oral	IV	Oral	IV
Codeine	0.5–1 mg/kg q 4 h up to 10 mg/kg/day caused by ceiling effect	NA	Up to 60 mg/dose q 4 h	NA
Morphine	0.15–0.3 mg/kg q 2–4 h	0.05–0.1 mg/kg q 1–4 h	15–30 mg q 2–4 h	5–10 mg q 2 h
Oxycodone	0.1–0.2 mg/kg q 2–4 h	NA	5–10 mg q 2–4 h	NA
Hydro-morphone	0.02–0.1 mg/kg q 2–4 h	0.015–0.02 mg/kg q 2–4 h	2–4 mg q 2–4 h	0.5–1 mg q 2–4 h
Fentanyl	NA	0.5–2 mcg/kg q 30–60 min	NA	50 mcg

Abbreviations: h, hour; IV, intravenous; NA, not applicable; q, every.
Source: From APS, 2005, 2008; Anghelescu et al., 2006b; Berde & Sethna, 2002; Brislin & Rose, 2005; Greco & Berde, 2005; Williams, Hatch, & Howard, 2001; Yaster et al., 2003; Zernikow et al., 2009.

Warnings. For children with renal or hepatic dysfunction, morphine should be used with caution because of the potential accumulation of its active metabolites, which can increase the risk of adverse effects (Anghelescu, Oakes, & Popenhagan, 2006; Johnson, 2006).

▓ *Codeine*

Indications: Often prescribed for mild to moderate pain, codeine is actually inactive by itself and requires conversion via the cytochrome P450 enzyme CYP2D6 to the active form, which is morphine. However, 10% to 15% of Caucasians lack the enzyme needed for this conversion, so codeine will not provide analgesia for them (Brislin & Rose, 2005; Greco & Berde, 2005; Kraemer & Rose, 2009; Zernikow et al., 2006). In at least one study, up to 47% of children in the United Kingdom younger than 12 years were found to lack the enzyme to convert codeine to morphine (Williams, Patel, & Howard, 2002). Conversely, 40% of North African descents are "ultrarapid metabolizers," resulting in plasma levels of morphine higher than expected, with excellent analgesia, but also adverse opioid effects (Kraemer & Rose, 2009). Because many mothers who breastfeed are also prescribed codeine products for postpartum pain, the U.S. Food and Drug Administration (FDA) has issued a warning to health care providers regarding the possibility of overdose in infants whose mothers are ultrarapid metabolizers of codeine (FDA, 2007).

Codeine has a ceiling dose of 10 mg/kg/day (Zernikow et al., 2009) and is more strongly associated with nausea and constipation than other opioids (APS, 2008). These findings have led pain experts to question its continued use (Greco & Berde, 2005; Harrison, Loughnan, Manias, & Johnston, 2009; Williams, Hatch, & Howard, 2001; Zernikow et al., 2009).

Dosage: Recommended initial doses are available in Table 4.1.

▓ *Oxycodone*

Indications: Oxycodone is useful for moderate to severe pain with a relative potency between 1.5 and 2 times that of oral morphine (Friedrichsdorf & Kang, 2007).

Dosage: Recommended initial doses are available in Table 4.1.

Forms: Oxycodone is available only in oral formulations, both tablets and elixir. Health care providers should be specific as to elixir dosing, as 1 mg per 1 ml and 20 mg per 1 ml preparations are available. For continuous pain, the total daily dose of oxycodone can be converted to the controlled-release preparation of oxycodone hydrochloride (Oxycontin), which must be swallowed as a whole tablet.

Warnings: Oxycodone's active metabolite, oxymorphone, can accumulate in patients with renal failure (Johnson, 2007; Kraemer & Rose, 2009). It is often compounded with other agents, such as acetaminophen (Tylenol). Although there is no ceiling dose of oxycodone, there is a maximum daily dose of acetaminophen to avoid the risk of hepatic toxicity (see Chapter 3). Therefore, noncompounded oxycodone may be preferable.

▓ *Hydromorphone Hydrochloride (Dilaudid)*

Indications: Hydromorphone hydrochloride is used for moderate to severe pain, with the oral preparation having a relative potency between 5 and 8 times that of oral morphine (Zernikow et al., 2009).

Dosage: Recommended initial doses are available in Table 4.1.

Forms: Hydromorphone is available in oral preparations, including a controlled-release tablet called hydromorphone hydrochloride (Exalgo) and IV preparations.

Warnings: Hydromorphone is reportedly safe in patients with modest kidney failure, but increased adverse effects may occur in those with severe renal failure (Estfan, LeGrand, Walsh, Lagman, & Davis, 2005). It produces one main metabolite, hydromorphone-3-glucuronide, which can cause neurotoxic effects, including confusion, tremor, and agitation (Dowden, 2009b).

▓ *Fentanyl (Sublimaze)*

Indications: Fentanyl is used for moderate to severe pain, with a relative potency 50 to 100 times that of morphine and a rapid onset of action after IV administration. Because of its high lipid solubility and rapid entry into the brain, as well as a much shorter duration of action than other opioids, fentanyl is especially useful for brief painful procedures when systemic analgesia is indicated. However, for relief of ongoing pain, its short duration of action necessitates frequent doses, intravenous infusion, or transdermal patches.

Warnings: Fentanyl has no known toxic metabolites, although prolonged infusions may result in drug accumulation and a potential increase in adverse effects (Dowden, 2009b). The clearance of fentanyl is faster in infants and young children than in adults (Collins & Weisman, 2003). Fentanyl clearance is dependent on hepatic blood flow; consequently, dose reduction may be needed for children with cardiac failure and hepatic failure (Johnson, 2007). Although no dose adjustment is usually necessary in renal failure because its metabolites are inactive, caution should be used in profound renal failure because fentanyl is poorly dialyzable (Johnson, 2007). Tolerance and physical dependence may occur within 5 to 10 days of continuous infusions, leading to frequent dose escalation.

Adverse Effects: One specific adverse effect of IV fentanyl that does not occur with other opioids is chest wall rigidity caused by the opioid's action on dopaminergic transmission. Typically, this occurs only when fentanyl is administered rapidly and in high doses (>5 mcg/kg) (Friedrichsdorf & Kang, 2007). If this occurs, the adverse effect is best managed by administering a neuromuscular-blocking agent with ongoing ventilator support, naloxone, or both (Anghelescu et al., 2006).

Dosage: Recommended initial doses are available in Table 4.1.

Forms: The IV route is the usual method of administration. No oral preparation is available. However, because of the high lipid solubility of fentanyl, other novel routes of administration are possible: transdermal and oral transmucosal. The intranasal route is also used for acute procedural pain for patients who do not have immediate IV access (Borland, Bergesio, Pascoe, Turner, & Woodger, 2005; Borland, Jacobs, King, & O'Brien, 2007).

Transmucosal Route

Several formulations of fentanyl are available for oral transmucosal delivery with distinctly different pharmacokinetic properties: an oral lozenge, fentanyl citrate (Actiq), a buccal tablet, fentanyl citrate

(Fentora), and a buccal film, fentanyl (Onsolis). None of these formulations are indicated for acute or postoperative pain because of the difficulty in quickly and safely titrating an effective dose (APS, 2008; Kraemer & Rose, 2009). These formulations are indicated for the treatment of breakthrough pain in adult patients with cancer who are opioid tolerant, taking at least 60 mg of morphine equivalent dose every day for 1 week (APS, 2008). However, the dose of the transmucosal formulations cannot be calculated based on previous doses of opioids, and no pharmacokinetic studies have been done for breakthrough pain in children (Zernikow et al., 2009). The 200 mcg lozenge is equivalent to 2 mg of morphine given IV or 6 mg morphine given orally (Zernikow et al., 2009).

Use has been reported in children for preoperative sedation and procedure-related pain (Anghelescu et al., 2006; Kraemer & Rose, 2006) and for incident-related pain (e.g., pain related to movement) in patients with cancer (Gardner-Nix, 2001) at doses of 10 to 15 mcg/kg (Brislin & Rose, 2005), with an onset of analgesia in 5 to 15 minutes and a duration of about 2 hours (APS, 2008). Adult pharmacokinetic data indicate only 25% of a fentanyl dose is transmucosally absorbed, with two thirds of the remaining swallowed fentanyl degraded as a result of the hepatic first-pass effect. However, the bioavailability in children is presumed to be higher because of a greater proportion of fentanyl being swallowed by children than by adults (Zernikow et al., 2009). Safety and efficacy concerns, such as the need to supervise children to prevent chewing instead of sucking, the large time variability for complete consumption of the lozenge, and the frequency of vomiting as a side effect, may limit its usefulness for children (Brown, Taddio, & McGrath, 2010; Kraemer & Rose, 2009; Zernikow et al., 2009).

Transdermal Fentanyl

Because of its lipophilic properties, fentanyl can be absorbed through the skin. After applying a patch for 12 to 16 hours, a depot of fentanyl will form in subcutaneous tissues and will be released into the systemic circulation, with each patch providing 72 hours of fairly stable drug delivery. Oral doses of opioids may still be required for breakthrough pain. Transdermal administration via a fentanyl patch permits a sustained analgesic effect for select patients who are unable to tolerate oral opioids and for whom IV access is limited. Patches should never be prescribed for opioid-naïve patients because of the likelihood of overdosing and respiratory arrest and should not be used in patients with rapidly changing pain intensity (Friedrichsdorf & Kang, 2007; Zernikow et al., 2009). Before application of the patch, the pain should be managed with other forms of opioids to determine the equianalgesic dose of transdermal fentanyl.

Health care providers should be reminded that the patch with the lowest dose (12 mcg/hr) provides the equivalent of a morphine IV of 1.2 mg/hr (or 30 mg/day IV or 90 mg/day PO [by mouth]). Therefore, this method needs to be reserved for children who have used such opioid doses for an extended time and are likely to need significant doses for at least the next 72 hours (Finkel, Finley, Greco, Weisman, & Zeltzer, 2005). Titration to optimal effect takes patience, because the time to peak effect is delayed and normally requires close monitoring. The use of additional immediate release opioids may be necessary to reach adequate pain relief over the first 48 to 72 hours. Likewise, when the dose needs to be decreased to less than 12 mcg/hr, careful downward titration using fentanyl IV or an oral opioid needs to be provided to prevent withdrawal. When the patch is not replaced and doses are discontinued, fentanyl will remain in the subcutaneous reservoir, diminishing over the next 12 to 16 hours. The practice of cutting fentanyl patches with the intention of reducing the dose is not recommended because delivery characteristics may be altered. Safety considerations that need to be shared with patients and their caretakers are the following:

- Absorption is increased with fever. Never use a heating pad over the patch.
- Dispose of used patches safely in a tamper-proof container because residual fentanyl could affect a small child or pet if applied or ingested.

▨ *Methadone (Dolophine)*

Indications: Methadone has unique pharmacokinetic properties that may offer advantages over other opioids in treating neuropathic pain (Anghelescu et al., 2006; Esphani & Bruera, 2006; Jacob, 2006; Nicholson, 2006) and as an alternative to very high doses of other opioids for analgesia in adults (Manfredi & Houde, 2003; Ripamonti & Bianchi, 2002) and children (Davies, DeVlaming, & Haines, 2008). Opioid receptors mediate effective analgesics, whereas the N-methyl-D-aspartate (NMDA) receptors have a role in maintaining chronic pain states and modulating responses to analgesics. Methadone has both mu-opioid receptor agonist activity as well as NMDA receptor antagonist activity, which prevent opioid tolerance and hyperalgesia (the loss of mu receptors and an increase in activity in the NMDA receptors). The mu receptor is the main mediator of analgesia, whereas NMDA receptor activation can lead to pain. Morphine, unlike methadone, has little antagonism for NMDA receptors. Methadone has similar potency to morphine for mu receptors; however, its efficacy with chronic dosing is greater. Blockade of NMDA receptors reduces pain and hyperalgesia in many forms of inflammatory and neuropathic pain (Moulin et al., 2007) and partially prevents or reverses tolerance to mu opioids.

Warnings: Methadone has a long and unpredictable half-life of 12 to 200 hours (APS, 2005; Friedrichsdorf & Kang, 2007) with an associated risk of accumulation, leading to overdose and delayed sedation. Methadone appears to be safe for patients with renal failure (Estfan et al., 2005; Johnson, 2007). Because of multiple potential drug interactions (Bryson, Tamber, Seccareccia, & Zimmermann, 2006), consultation with a pain specialist experienced in methadone dosing is advised (Nicholson, 2007).

Dosage: The conversion between methadone and other opioids is based on the potency of methadone compared with other opioids, which varies according to a patient's current exposure to other opioids. Conversion from other opioids to methadone is one of the most challenging aspects of methadone use, with no consensus on how to safely determine the methadone dose. The potency ratio of methadone to other opioids is related to the magnitude of the opioid dose; in other words, the higher the preexisting opioid dose, the more potent the methadone becomes in this conversion calculation.

Several methods for rotating from morphine to methadone based on dose-dependent ratios have been recommended for adults (see Table 4.2), but similar data specific for children have not been published (Zernikow et al., 2009). Methadone should be started at lower than anticipated doses and slowly titrated upward while providing adequate short-acting doses of opioid pain medications during the titration period. Safe rotation to methadone is best practiced when there is close monitoring with initial doses and with each dose escalation to ensure adequate analgesia and minimal adverse effects. Limited information has been published for reverse rotation from methadone to alternative opioids, making it necessary to monitor for adverse effects and possible severe pain exacerbations (Manfredi & Houde, 2003; Moryl et al., 2002).

Forms: Methadone is available in oral tablets and elixir, as well as a parenteral form. The conversion from IV to PO doses is 1:1 because of high oral bioavailability (Manfredi & Houde, 2003). However, the one-to-one conversion does not apply to a continuous infusion, and experts advise a more conservative ratio with assistance from experienced health care providers (Shaiova et al., 2008).

Adverse Effects: Methadone can prolong the QTc and in high doses may cause ventricular tachycardia. Further studies are needed to determine predisposing factors. Although evidence is not clear regarding the overall implications, an electrocardiogram is recommended when

Table 4.2 ▨ *Suggested Safe and Effective Starting Doses for Methadone When Rotating From Oral Morphine Equivalent*

Usually divide the total dose into 3 equal doses every 8 hours.

Morphine Dose (PO total dose/day)	Conversion Ratio to Determine PO Methadone Dose	Example
30–90 mg	4:1	60 mg morphine ~ 15 mg methadone
90–300 mg	6:1 to 8:1	300 mg morphine ~ 35 mg methadone
>300 mg	8:1 to 12:1	400 mg morphine ~ 35 mg methadone

Abbreviation: PO, by mouth.
Source: From APS, 2008; Manfredi & Houde, 2003.

methadone is initiated (Cruciani et al., 2005; Shaiova et al., 2008). Use of other medications that can prolong the QTc, such as antiviral agents, antifungals, and selective serotonin reuptake inhibitors (SSRIs), as well as electrolyte imbalances and underlying cardiac disease, may increase the risk of cardiac toxicity. The potential advantages of methadone must be weighed against relative risk of QTc prolongation and goals of care, especially if indicated for pain in patients who have advanced diseases (Reddy et al., 2009).

▨ *Tramadol (Ultram)*

Indications: Tramadol is a unique analgesic agent that has weak mu-opioid receptor activity and inhibits reuptake of norepinephrine and serotonin, making it useful for both nociceptive and neuropathic pain with a lower risk of respiratory depression and constipation (Brown et al., 2010; Dowden, 2009a; Moulin et al., 2007; Zernikow et al., 2009). The reported experience in using it in children is very limited (Zernikow et al., 2009), and it should not to be used in infants because of immaturity in metabolism, with delayed clearance leading to a risk of respiratory depression (Anderson & Palmer, 2006). Some health care providers report tramadol may be as effective as morphine for postoperative pain, especially for children with risk factors for opioid-induced respiratory depression, such as sleep apnea or neuro-muscular disorders (Anderson & Palmer, 2006; Engelhardt, Steel, Johnston, & Veitch, 2003).

Dosage: The oral dose is 1 to 2 mg/kg every 8 to 12 hours, with a maximum of 8 to 10 mg/kg/day (Brown et al., 2010; Dowden, 2009b; Zernikow et al., 2009). Because its structure is similar to that of codeine with associated CYP2D6 polymorphisms, effective analgesia is uncertain (Zernikow et al., 2009).

Adverse Effects: Health care providers should be aware of the risk of nausea, vomiting, dizziness, and especially seizures, making it contraindicated in patients who have a history of seizures (Kraemer & Rose, 2009), especially with rapid escalation of doses (Dowden, 2009b; Zernikow et al., 2009). Recent information has been released warning health care providers of tramadol-related deaths from suicide for patients who have a history of drug addiction and misuse (FDA, 2010).

▩ *Tapentadol Hydrochloride (Nucynta)*

Indications: Tapentadol is a newer analgesic agent, similar to tramadol, and has weak mu-opioid receptor activity and inhibits reuptake of norepineprhine, making it useful for moderate to severe acute pain with a lower risk of respiratory depression and constipation compared with opioids.

Dosage: Current dosage recommendations apply only to patients 18 years or older as 50 to 100 mg every 4 to 6 hours (Wade & Spruill, 2009).

Adverse Effects: CNS adverse effects associated with other opioids have been reported with tapentadol, and it should be prescribed with caution in patients with a history of seizure (Wade & Spruill, 2009). Less gastrointestinal adverse effects (e.g., constipation and nausea) have been reported with tapentadol, presumably because of less reliance on the mu-opioid receptor activity compared with other opioids (Candiotti & Gitlin, 2010).

OPIOIDS NOT RECOMMENDED FOR PAIN MANAGEMENT

Meperidine (Demerol) has no advantage over other opioids and is not recommended as an analgesic because of the accumulation of its metabolite, normeperidine, which causes CNS toxicity (e.g., dysphoria, agitation, and seizures) especially in children with renal or hepatic dysfunction (APS, 1999, 2005, 2008; Greco & Berde, 2005; Johnson, 2007; Zernikow et al., 2006).

Pentazocine (Talwin), butorphanol tartrate (Stadol), and nalbuphine hydrochloride (Nubain), as mixed agonist–antagonists, were thought to reduce the risk of respiratory depression; however, these agents are not recommended to manage continuing pain states such as cancer. Their use in severe pain is limited by their ceiling effects, dysphoric reactions reported in adults, and the risk of evoking withdrawal symptoms in patients who have been receiving other opioids (APS, 2006; Anghelescu, Oakes, & Popenhagan, 2006; Kraemer & Rose, 2006).

PRINCIPLES OF OPIOID ADMINISTRATION

Determination of Opioid Dose

The recommended dosage ranges for children with no prior exposure to opioids, known as being *opioid naïve*, are outlined in Table 4.1. Even though weight, generally, is used to predict analgesic effect, the starting doses of opioids are merely estimates. No opioids, except codeine and tramadol, have a standard, optimal, or maximum dose (*ceiling dose*). Therapeutic plasma concentrations of opioids are affected by age, hepatic function, renal function, and clinical condition.

Dosages of opioids should be individualized based on age and disease status, including comorbidities and pain intensity, and previous or current opioid exposure. In other words, the absolute opioid dose is unimportant as long as the balance between pain relief and adverse effects is favorable. Further determination of the optimal dose should be done by titration, with a goal of using the lowest dose that provides satisfactory pain relief with the fewest adverse effects. Wide variability in response to opioid doses reinforces the need for prompt and individualized attention to unrelieved pain. Across all age groups, enormous variability exists in the dose of any opioid needed to provide pain relief, even for patients with identical sources of pain (APS, 2008).

Infants show a marked degree of individual variability in the rate of elimination and adverse effects of opioids (Bouwmeester, van den Anker, Hop, Anand, & Tibboel, 2003). For infants younger than 6 months of age, their immature livers and associated immature metabolic capacity cause drug accumulation and subsequent adverse effects (Dowden, 2009b; Greco & Berde, 2005; Kraemer & Rose, 2009; Zernikow et al., 2009). Starting doses should be reduced to approximately 50% to 75% of the dosing recommendations for older children of equal weight (APS, 2006; Anghelescu et al., 2006; Taddio, 2006), with increased vigilance for potential adverse effects, especially respiratory depression.

Equianalgesia

The term *equianalgesia* refers to the fact that different opioids require different doses to provide approximately the same pain relief. The equianalgesic doses in Table 4.3 are necessary to conduct an opioid rotation or change from one opioid to another because the current opioid causes (Zernikow et al., 2009) the following:

- Side effects other than constipation, which are unacceptable even when pain is controlled
- Uncontrolled pain even with rapid escalation of dose
- An inconvenience of route (e.g., the patient no longer has IV access)

Often during opioid rotation, the patient has improved pain control because of an *incomplete cross-tolerance* with the new opioid (APS, 2008); thus, the dose should be reduced by 25% to 50% of the calculated equianalgesic dose to avoid unacceptable adverse effects (Fine & Portenoy, 2009). Further adjustments of the dose of the new opioid should be based on clinical response (Zernikow et al., 2009). Methadone is not included in Table 4.3 because the conversion requires a dose-dependent calculation rather than a fixed ratio.

Methods of Administration

Oral Route

The oral route for pain medicines is generally preferred because it is less expensive, easier for parents to administer, and avoids the need for vascular access with the related risks of infection. The type of oral opioid preparation used is based on its available dosage forms, the pattern, and the expected duration of the source of the pain. Immediate-release

Table 4.3 ■ *Opioid Equianalgesic Doses*

	Equianalgesic Dose (mg/kg)	
Drug	IV/IM	PO
Morphine	10	30
Hydromorphone	1.5	7.5
Fentanyl	0.1–0.2	NA
Oxycodone	NA	15–30

Abbreviations: IM, intramuscular; IV, intravenous; NA, not applicable; PO, by mouth.
Source: From APS, 2008; Yaster et al., 2003.

opioid tablets or elixir have a short duration of action (1–4 hours) and are useful for intermittent or breakthrough pain.

For patients with pain requiring several days to resolve, and for whom pain is likely to persist throughout the day or require analgesic doses during the night, controlled-release opioid preparations provide a more consistent plasma level and convenient method of analgesia. The dose of the controlled-release forms of opioids is usually determined after first relieving pain with immediate-release opioids or using the IV route with the patient-controlled analgesia method for 24 hours. Additional immediate-release doses should be available for any unexpected exacerbations of moderate to severe pain (Dunlop & Bennett, 2006; Friedrichsdorf, Finney, Bergin, Stevens, & Collins, 2007). Patients, particularly those with communication limitations, need to be closely monitored for accumulation of drug leading to adverse effects during the initial hours of adding controlled-release doses.

With all controlled-release opioid preparations, as well as transdermal fentanyl, there is a possibility of "end-of-dose failure," or unacceptable pain levels during the last few hours of the recommended dosing interval, presumably because the opioid level has fallen below the therapeutic level. A shortened dosing interval of the controlled-release opioid preparation may be necessary to provide a more steady therapeutic plasma concentration.

Intramuscular Route

The intramuscular route is not recommended because of children's fear of needles and wide fluctuations of opioid level caused by erratic absorption patterns (APS, 2008). Children cannot understand why a "shot," which is painful, would help relieve pain.

Intravenous Route

When the oral route is not possible, IV boluses of opioids provide prompt relief for the following:

- Rapid control of pain for a dressing change or reduction of a bone fracture in the emergency department (ED)

- Postoperative pain when the patient cannot tolerate oral opioid doses
- Breakthrough pain when the patient cannot tolerate oral doses

---

| *Clinical Pearl* | To treat severe pain, consider prompt treatment by providing opioid doses until relief of pain is achieved (APS, 2008). |

- One method is to administer morphine in 0.05 mg/kg IV boluses every 5 to 10 minutes with a health care provider at the bedside until the pain intensity score is reduced by 50%.
- If rapid pain control is not achieved, the bolus dose may be increased by 50% to 100%.
- Once pain is controlled, readjustments of the continuous IV dose, including the use of a patient-controlled analgesia pump or controlled-release opioid doses, will be necessary to lessen the likelihood of recurrence of severe pain.
- If pain is not controlled without unacceptable side effects, consider regional interventions (see Chapters 6 and Chapter 7).

Continuous Intravenous Infusions

To avoid large variations in plasma concentrations of opioids associated with IV bolus regimens, which increase the risk of side effects during peak levels and increased pain during trough levels, continuous infusions are often optimal for continuing pain when the patient cannot swallow oral medications.

Continuous Subcutaneous Infusions

For children with poor IV access, subcutaneous infusions of opioids via a small butterfly needle or catheter may be an effective option. The dose of the opioid is equivalent to the IV dose with the volume limited to a rate of 1 to 3 ml per hour (APS, 2008).

Patient-Controlled Analgesia

Patient-controlled analgesia (PCA) methods deliver analgesics via a programmable infusion pump, allowing children to self-administer small amounts of opioids (boluses) based on their pain intensity and desire for pain relief. Although usually referring to IV routes, PCA drug delivery also may include medications given subcutaneously or neuroaxially via epidural or peripheral nerve block infusions. Indications for PCA include moderate to severe pain, such as pain experienced after major surgery (abdominal, thoracic, or orthopedic; Dowden, 2009a), sickle-cell crises (APS, 1999; Jacob et al., 2003; Melzer-Lange, Walsh-Kelly, Lea, Hillery, & Scott, 2004), burns (Dowden, 2009a), and cancer treatment (mucositis or bone marrow transplantation; APS, 2005; Zernikow et al., 2009). A particular advantage of PCA therapy is that it gives patients some sense of control in their own care.

Clinical Pearl	When is a patient-controlled analgesia the optimal choice (APS, 2005; Anghelescu, Burgoyne, Oakes, & Wallace, 2005; Brislin & Rose, 2005; Oakes, 2008)?

- The medical condition is associated with moderate to severe pain, requiring frequent administration of opioids.
- The child is able to comprehend the appropriate use of the bolus button and is motivated to use it when anticipating or experiencing pain.
- The child has the physical ability to activate the bolus dose.
- The child has no preexisting conditions associated with risks using a PCA, such as a history of sleep apnea, obesity, asthma, or upper airway obstruction.
- The nurse can assess the child's level of sedation every 1 to 2 hours to be aware of the earliest signs of opioid-induced sedation.

The initial doses for opioid-naïve children are listed in Table 4.4. For children who already take opioids, higher starting doses are needed. Considerations in providing PCA analgesia include the following:

- Boluses prescribed to cover intermittent or breakthrough pain.
- A lockout time usually set for 5 to 15 minutes. This allows each bolus to reach peak effect before the patient has another bolus, thus reducing the risk of overdose.

Table 4.4 ▓ *Initial PCA Settings for Opioid-Naïve Children*

Opioid	Continuous Infusion Dose	Bolus Dose/Frequency
Morphine	0–0.02 mg/kg/hr	0.02 mg/kg q 15–30 min
Hydromorphone	0–0.004 mg/kg/hr	0.004 mg/kg q 15–30 min
Fentanyl	0–0.5 to 1 mcg/kg/hr	0.5–1 mcg/kg q 10–15 min

Abbreviations: PCA, patient-controlled analgesia; q, every.
Source: From APS, 2008; Brislin & Rose, 2005; Dowden, 2009b; Greco & Berde, 2005; Kraemer & Rose, 2009; Zernikow et al., 2009.

▓ Adding a continuous infusion (also called *background* or *basal*) to the bolus if appropriate for pain relief, usually only for non-opioid-naïve (tolerant) patients who have continuous pain. It is especially useful in providing a more restful sleep by preventing the child from awakening in pain (Yaster et al., 2003). Continuous infusions will increase the risk of adverse effects, thus requiring more frequent reassessment for opioid-induced sedation and respiratory effects (Berde & Solodiuk, 2003; Brislin & Rose, 2005; Verghese & Hannallah, 2005).

▓ Addressing inadequate pain relief with gradual escalation of the opioid dose by calculating the total dose given in the previous hour and then adjusting the PCA bolus or the continuous infusion, or both, until adequate analgesia is achieved or intolerable adverse effects occur. Health care providers are to be reminded to evaluate coexisting medical conditions, as well as the use of concurrent sedatives, which could put the patient at risk for sedation and possible respiratory depression (Monitto et al., 2000; Voepel-Lewis, Marinkovic, Kostrzewa, Tait, & Malviya, 2008).

▓ The optional use of setting the pump with a limited amount of the opioid the patient may receive in a 4-hour period. However, there is no good evidence that this practice provides any increased safety in using PCA, and using this limit may prevent adequate pain relief in rapidly escalating pain.

The physical and cognitive ability to understand how to use a PCA effectively does not usually develop until at least 5 years of age (APS, 2008; Brislin & Rose, 2005; Verghese & Hannallah, 2005). Because the safety of PCA relies on the idea that patients who become sedated will stop pushing the bolus button, the use of parent- or nurse-controlled analgesia has been controversial, with limited recommendations (Berde & Solodiuk, 2003) and research to support control by selected family members for patients who are too young or too ill or who have developmental delays that make them unable to self-bolus (Anghelescu et al., 2005; Czarnecki et al., 2008; Monitto et al., 2000; Voepel-Lewis et al., 2008). Recent guidelines have been issued regarding "authorized" family members and nurses providing bolus doses with specific education, monitoring, and quality assurance activities to maximize patient safety (Wuhrman et al., 2007). Health care providers need to carefully evaluate parents in terms of their ability to provide parent-controlled analgesia. Parents of children with chronic illnesses such as cancer may wish to retain some control over their children's care during a hospital stay and often are familiar with technology. Institutions must establish mechanisms to ensure unauthorized use of PCA does not occur.

Clinical Pearl	If parents are authorized to press the bolus button for their child, they should be taught the following:

- To push the bolus button if their child is awake and his words or behavior indicate pain and he cannot push the button.
- To not press the bolus button for their sleeping child.
- To notify the nurse immediately and not press the bolus button if they are not able to wake their child easily or if the child is breathing abnormally.

When the PCA is no longer needed, the infusion should be stopped or its rate should be reduced while the patient is allowed to continue to self-administer boluses of opioids. Most children self-wean from the PCA by reducing the bolus attempts over time. For those who have had major surgery, leaving the bolus doses available even after discontinuing the basal may be reassuring for 24 hours after oral analgesia is initiated.

Tolerance, Physical Dependence, and Addiction

All opioids have the same potential risk for tolerance, physical dependence, and addiction.

Tolerance is an expected result of prolonged use of opioids and refers to the progressive decline in the analgesic effect of a drug over time so it is necessary to increase the dose, add appropriate coanalgesics, or change to another opioid to achieve the same pain control. Concerns about tolerance should not lead to reluctance in using opioids when necessary to achieve pain relief.

Physical dependence occurs when a person adapts to the continuous presence of certain medications, such as opioids, sedatives, antihypertensive agents, or steroids in the body. Similar to tolerance, physical dependence is an expected outcome of opioid use, especially when they are taken for more than 5 days (Franck, Harris, Soetenga, Amling, & Curley, 2008). The hallmark of physical dependence is the withdrawal syndrome, which occurs when the opioid dose is significantly reduced or abruptly discontinued (Savage et al., 2003; see Table 4.5). The onset of withdrawal symptoms is related to the half-life of the opioid. Renal or hepatic dysfunction will delay the onset of withdrawal because of prolonged clearance of any active metabolites of the opioid.

Preventing these distressing symptoms when opioids are no longer needed is best achieved by gradually reducing doses, commonly called *weaning*. The longer children receive opioids, the longer it will take to discontinue the opioid without withdrawal symptoms. Health care providers are to consider the following:

- For children who have used opioids for fewer than 5 days, it is advisable to decrease the opioid dose by 20% to 30% every 1 to 2 days.
- If opioids have been used for more than 5 to 7 days; however, a slower wean by a 20% reduction the first day with subsequent reductions of 5% to 10% each day as tolerated is recommended until a total daily dose of morphine (or its equivalent) of 30 mg for an adolescent or 0.6 mg/kg/day is reached (APS, 2006; Anghelescu et al., 2006; Zernikow et al., 2006). This process may take several weeks.

Table 4.5 ■ *Symptoms of Opioid Withdrawal*

System	Symptoms (Children and Adults)	Symptoms (Infants)
Central nervous hyperirritability	Agitation Irritability Insomnia, increased wakefulness Tremors Hyperactive reflexes Ataxia Inability to concentrate Anxiety Increased muscle tone Increased motor activity/myoclonus Abnormal movements	Neonates: high-pitched cry, exaggerated Moro reflex (normal for newborns up to 3 months of age)
Gastrointestinal (not seen with benzodiazepine withdrawal) dysfunction	Vomiting Diarrhea	Feeding intolerance Uncoordinated sucking/swallowing
Sympathetic nervous (autonomic system dysregulation)	Tachycardia Hypertension Tachypnea Sweating Fever Frequent yawning Nasal stuffiness	Mottling

Source: From Dowden, 2009b; Ista, van Dijk, Gamel, Tibboel, & de Hoog, 2007.

■ Observing children carefully for signs and symptoms of withdrawal and increase the opioid dose if these signs occur. The health care provider should reassure the child and parents that the need to carefully decrease the dosages does not mean the child is addicted to the opioid.

■ Use of oral methadone regimens, which are more often provided for children who are being weaned from opioids recovering from a critical illness or injury (See Chapter 14).

In conjunction with guidelines on methods to best discontinue opioids, objectively validated methods of assessing signs of withdrawal would be useful. However, a gold standard in assessing withdrawal does not exist at this time. Many tools are in development to assess withdrawal for patients in pediatric intensive care and to determine a scale with a threshold to alert the health care provider to potential opioid and benzodiazepine withdrawal syndrome (see Chapter 14).

Addiction

Addiction is a primary, chronic, neurobiological disease with genetic, psychosocial, and environmental factors characterized by a continuous craving for a drug and the need to use it for effects other than its medical indications (Savage et al., 2003). Behaviors associated with addiction include craving and impaired control over drug use with compulsive and continued abuse despite harm (APS, 2008). People who are addicted to opioids use drugs for their mind-altering properties, not for the medical purpose of pain relief, leading to a pattern of antisocial and criminal behavior to obtain the drug.

Health care providers also care for patients who have experienced repetitive episodes of untreated severe pain, such as from sickle-cell crises. These patients learn that they have to "appear" to be in pain to be believed and offered effective treatment. Health care providers may misidentify their requests for specific analgesia, and even aggressive behavior, as "drug seeking," labeling them as "clock watchers" (Jacob, 2001; McCaffery, Grimm, Pasero, Ferrell, & Uman, 2005).

Many health care providers and parents fear drug addiction and may withhold opioids from their children after a certain dose has been reached. For parents, an explanation of the difference in using opioids for their euphoric effects as opposed to using them to help recover from illness and injury may lessen these fears. Because opioids are a necessary part of the armamentarium of pain management, a growing trend toward prescription drug abuse and diversion in our society exists. Meeting the goal of treating pain while not contributing to drug abuse and diversion requires vigilance and education.

What Is Known About Substance Abuse in Children and Adolescents?

Any review of the literature on substance abuse needs to be done with the caveat that no standardized definitions exist for *misuse, abuse, dependence,* and *addiction,* with authors applying these terms in idiosyncratic ways. The exact prevalence of substance abuse for adults and children is not known (APS, 2008; Ballantyne & LaForge, 2007), but significant increases in prescription drug abuse over the past decade are worrisome with recognition of a growing public health concern (Twombly & Holtz, 2008). Limited research in middle- and high-school age children indicates approximately 10% have misused prescription drugs, including opioids, such as oxycodone and hydrocodone products, along with stimulants and sedatives (McCabe, Boyd, Cranford, & Teter, 2009; Passik, Heit, & Kirsh, 2006; Twombly & Holtz, 2008). The reason for misuse was reported to be for the relief of physical pain (McCabe et al., 2009) or anxiety, as well as for sleeping or "getting high" (Boyd, McCabe, Cranford, & Young, 2006).

Health care providers should seek educational resources to learn how to prescribe controlled substances, minimizing the opportunity for either the patient or a family member to misuse the prescribed medication. With the aging population suffering from pain related to arthritis, diabetes, and other chronic debilitating conditions, health care providers offer pain relief with opioids using appropriate rationale; however, other family members, including adolescents, are reported to be using them with or without the prescribed family member's knowledge. Use of prescribed medications is seen by adolescents as "safer" than "street drugs." Therefore, at the very least, health care providers should discuss the proper use of prescription medications with all patients and advise them about safekeeping and sharing them with others (see Appendix for more information).

Health care providers need to conduct appropriate risk assessments of patients and their caregivers when prescribing chronic opioid therapy. Considerable interest in identifying patients at risk for abuse has generated several screening tools for health care providers who prescribe to adults: the Screener and Opioid Assessment for

Patients with Pain (Akbik et al., 2006), the Opioid Risk Tool (Webster & Webster, 2005), and the Pain Assessment and Documentation Tool (Passik et al., 2004). One tool has been used in adolescents, the Drug Abuse Screening Test (Boyd et al., 2006). At this time, no reliable evidence exists on the accuracy of urine drug screening, pill counts, or prescription drug monitoring programs (Chou et al., 2009).

Although the increase in the abuse of opioids is a growing public health problem, interfering with legitimate use of opioids is to be avoided. Treatment of adolescents who have a history of opioid abuse but need opioids for the treatment of a serious illness or injury is best provided by a multidisciplinary team, including a pain management specialist, social worker, and psychologist. The team must work together to develop a plan to prescribe appropriate medicines while minimizing the risk of illicit use. Setting boundaries within an agreed-upon treatment plan based on mutual trust and honesty is recommended (see Chapter 11).

Opioid-Induced Hyperalgesia

Opioid-induced hyperalgesia is a state of nociceptive sensitization caused by prolonged exposure to opioids characterized by a paradoxical response in which a patient receiving opioids for the treatment of pain may actually become more sensitive to certain painful stimuli (Chu, Angst, & Clark, 2008). Animal and adult human studies suggest opioids may increase rather than decrease sensitivity to noxious stimuli (Zernikow et al., 2009). Although the precise molecular mechanism is not yet understood, it is generally thought to result from changes in the peripheral nervous system and CNS, which lead to sensitization of nerve pathways attributed to several mechanisms, including activation of the NMDA-receptor system (Zernikow et al., 2009). Health care providers should suspect opioid-induced hyperalgesia when pain relief is not achieved despite increased opioid doses in the absence of disease progression. A reduction in the opioid dose or opioid rotation typically results in reestablishing pain control.

OPTIMIZING SAFETY

Concerns about the safety of administration of opioids to infants and children should not prevent health care providers from using these when necessary (American Academy of Pediatrics and Canadian Paediatric Society, 2000). When appropriately prescribed and administered, opioids are no more dangerous for children than they are for adults. Successful opioid therapy requires that the benefits of analgesia outweigh the risk of adverse effects, most of which are dose related and disappear within the first week of opioid administration. However, the risk of constipation does not diminish over time. Because children and adolescents do not necessarily report all side effects, health care providers should ask about their occurrence. Many patients report an "allergy" to opioids when the reality is they experience adverse effects such as pruritus. Health care providers need to ask patients to describe what happened to confirm the rare true allergy.

Clinical Pearl	Opioid adverse effects are to be treated by (Zernikow et al., 2009) the following:

- Symptomatic treatment of the adverse effect itself
- Changing to another opioid with less association of the symptom
- Providing multimodal therapy with NSAIDs, coanalgesics, or a nonpharmacologic strategy to decrease the dose of the opioid
- Changing the dosing regimen or route of the same drug with the goal of a constant blood level rather than a pattern of high peak serum levels

Adverse Effects of Opioids
Opioid-Induced Sedation

Characterized by drowsiness and impaired mental and physical performance, opioid-induced sedation is usually transient, resolving after a few days of opioid use. All patients are at risk for excessive sedation when they take their first opioid dose, even when the doses are appropriate. Sedation is more likely if too large a dose of opioid is given or if their metabolites accumulate (McNicol et al., 2003; Pasero & McCaffery, 2002). If an opioid-naïve child is experiencing unintended advancing sedation, it is possible that stimulation can be sufficient to arouse him or her to answer questions. However, the child may then fall back into an oversedated state immediately afterward. Therefore, frequent direct nurse reassessment of children during the initial titration of any opioid is needed.

A child who has been in severe pain may have had problems sleeping, and then after the pain is controlled, the child is more likely to fall asleep because of the previous sleep deprivation. Therefore, sleep is not always a sign of overdosage as long as the patient can be easily aroused. Also, because pain stimulates respiration, patients in whom pain is controlled after a period of poor control can be at risk for respiratory depression and should be observed closely until a steady state of analgesia is achieved. If reducing the dose or rotating to another opioid does not resolve the sedation, a mild stimulant such as methylphenidate (Ritalin, 0.05 mg/kg to 0.2 mg/kg) may be added early in the day with the only other dose no later than early afternoon so that it will not interfere with sleep (APS, 2008; Greco & Berde, 2005). Such stimulants may reduce opioid-related cognitive dysfunction and allow dose escalation in patients who have somnolence as a limiting side effect (Esphani & Bruera, 2006).

Assessing the level of sedation is the key to early identification and treatment of opioid-induced respiratory depression. Sedation scales developed for *intentional sedation,* such as the Ramsay Scale (Ramsay, Savage, Simpson, Goodwin, 1974) or Richmond Agitation Sedation Scale (RASS) (Sessler et al., 2002), may be less useful for assessment of sedation associated with the use of opioids, in which sedation is considered an adverse effect. One sedation scale developed to recognize distinct changes in level of alertness and arousability of patients as early signs of advancing unintended sedation from opioids is the Pasero Opioid-Induced Sedation Scale (POSS) (Pasero & McCaffery, 2002). This tool has been found to be the

Table 4.6 ▦ *Pasero Opioid-Induced Sedation Scale*

Level	Description of Patient	Action to be Considered
S	Sleep, easy to arouse	Acceptable, no action necessary
1	Awake and alert	
2	Slightly drowsy, easily aroused	
3	Frequently drowsy, but arousable, drifts off to sleep during conversation	Unacceptable ▦ Decrease opioid dose by 25%–50% ▦ Add an opioid-sparing analgesic such as an NSAID ▦ Monitor the patient's level of sedation and respiratory status closely ▦ Consider stimulant
4	Somnolent, minimal or no response to physical stimulation	Unacceptable ▦ Stop opioid ▦ Consider administering naloxone ▦ Consider need for oxygen or bag-mask ventilation

Abbreviation: NSAID, nonsteroidal anti-inflammatory drug.
Source: From "Monitoring Sedation" by C. Pasero & M. McCaffery, 2002, *American Journal of Nursing, 102*, pp. 67–69. Copyright 1994 by Chris Pasero. Used with permission.

most applicable and easy to use for optimizing safety in patients who are receiving opioids (Nisbet & Mooney-Cotter, 2009). (See Table 4.6 for the POSS scale and recommended actions for the health care provider to follow.) If there is any concern about a child who is sleeping regarding any effect of the opioid causing excessive sedation, health care providers are to awaken the patient to determine arousability (Pasero, 2009). However, prior to awakening the patient, careful assessment of the respiratory status (e.g., depth, regularity, rate, and noisiness) needs to be noted as stimulation will change what the child's usual respiratory status is during sleep.

Opioid-Induced Respiratory Depression

Unintended advancing sedation has been identified as a precedent to clinically significant respiratory depression (Pasero & McCaffery,

2002). Opioids, binding to opioid receptors in the pontine and ventral medulla of the brain stem, suppress the respiratory center in the brain stem, leading to a decrease in tidal volume and respiratory rate, with an accumulation of carbon dioxide that causes further sedation and further respiratory depression. A decrease in blood oxygen saturation level has been recognized as a late indicator of opioid overdose (APS, 2008). The risk of respiratory depression is not more probable with any particular opioid when equipotent doses are administered. Respiratory depression is rare for patients who have been taking opioids for longer than a week (APS, 2008; McNicol et al., 2003). A risk assessment tool to identify children who would benefit from increased vigilance and technological monitoring has not yet been developed. However, individual and iatrogenic risk factors for opioid-induced sedation and respiratory depression are largely extrapolated from adult literature and include the following:

- A history of obstructive or central sleep apnea, upper airway obstruction, mediastinal masses, sleep disordered breathing, or other causes of respiratory insufficiency (APS, 2008).
- Renal insufficiency or progressive liver function impairment leading to accumulation of active opioid metabolites (Zernikow et al., 2009)
- Metabolic encephalopathy
- Marked obesity
- Infants younger than 6 months caused by decreased metabolic rates and less restrictive blood-brain barriers (Greco & Berde, 2005)
- Concurrent use of medications with known risks of sedative effects (e.g., antihistamines, antiemetics, and anxiolytics)

These patients need more frequent observation to detect any increase in sedation that could signal impending respiratory depression.

Electronic monitoring, such as pulse oximetry or apnea monitoring with alarms that sound in a centralized nursing area, can be useful for high-risk patients but cannot substitute for frequent clinical assessments by nurses skilled in noting early signs of opioid toxicity. Pulse oximetry is not as effective for patients receiving supplemental oxygen because peripheral oxygenation levels can be maintained during hypoventilation for a prolonged period even as carbon dioxide is rising (Fu, Downs, Schweiger, Miguel, & Smith, 2004; Keidan et al., 2008). End-tidal carbon dioxide ($EtCO_2$) monitoring is an early indicator of respiratory compromise for children undergoing sedation during procedures (Lightdale et al., 2006) but is technologically challenging to use in children who are not mechanically ventilated. At this time, no consensus or conclusive evidence exists regarding which forms of electronic monitoring are most useful for patients who are at high risk for respiratory depression.

Mild respiratory depression can be managed by reducing the opioid dose, whereas with moderate to severe depression, stimulation, airway support, and bag-mask ventilation are to be considered. After the patient's respiration and level of consciousness return to baseline, the health care provider is to consider the appropriate actions:

- Resuming the PCA, restarting at a lower dose, or providing only bolus doses
- Withholding controlled-release opioid doses
- Optimizing doses of nonopioids and coanalgesics
- Reviewing all medications to determine whether concurrent medicines are contributing to the patient's compromised status

---

Clinical Pearl

If significant opioid-induced respiratory depression occurs, the health care provider must do the following:

- Interrupt the opioid administration
- Stimulate the patient (e.g., shake, call by name, ask to breathe)
- Administer oxygen
- Administer naloxone (Narcan), if indicated
  - For patients less than 40 kg, administer 2 mcg/kg every 30 seconds or dilute the naloxone to make a 10 mcg/ml solution and administer at a rate of 0.5 mcg/kg every 2 minutes (APS, 2008).
  - For patients more than 40 kg, dilute 0.4 mg of naloxone in 10 ml of saline and administer 0.5 ml every 2 minutes until the child becomes responsive and the respiratory rate and depth increase (APS, 2008).

Because of the risk of opioid withdrawal, an opioid antagonist should be used only for children with impending respiratory arrest or symptomatic respiratory depression, and then only with small, carefully titrated doses to improve respiratory function without reversing analgesia (McNicol et al., 2003). Naloxone (Narcan) is a pure opioid antagonist that occupies and displaces opioids from all opioid receptors (Dowden, 2009b). Many patients achieve rapid reversal of adverse opioid effects after very small doses of naloxone; thus, doses should be titrated to effect if possible, to avoid inducing severe pain. It is important to recognize that rapid administration of a large dose of naloxone can precipitate withdrawal, with the dramatic onset of severe pain, seizure, and sympathetic instability (APS, 2008). Because the duration of action for naloxone is 45 minutes, it is advisable to prepare to repeat doses of naloxone because the half-life of some opioids is longer than the half-life of naloxone (Dowden, 2009b).

Constipation

The most frequently reported side effect of opioids is constipation, which will not diminish over time. Because opioids slow bowel motility, constipation should be anticipated and prophylactically treated unless diarrhea is already present (Greco & Berde, 2005; Zernikow et al., 2009). Ileus rarely occurs, but hard, dry stools and incomplete evacuation can lead to pseudo-obstruction of the bowel, causing anorexia, nausea, and vomiting. Health care providers should be alert for other related conditions and comorbidities, such as inactivity or dehydration, and recommend increasing the child's fiber and oral fluids, if possible. A stool softener alone will not be sufficient and must be combined with a mild peristaltic stimulant (Thomas, 2008). (See Table 4.7 for various agents and dosage recommendations.) Less constipation has been reported with the fentanyl patch (Zernikow et al., 2009).

Naloxone given by the oral route may be efficacious and well tolerated (Meissner, Schmidt, Hartmann, Kath, & Reinhart, 2000). A more recent and similar agent, not yet approved for children, methylnaltrexone (Relistor), may be given to older adolescents as a subcutaneous injection, effective without reversing opioid analgesia

Table 4.7 ■ *Prevention and Treatment of Constipation (Oral Doses)*

Drug	Preparation	Age in Years	Recommended Maximum Dose/ Day

Docusate/senna (Senna-S)	Tablets 50 mg/ 8.6 mg	2–5: 1/2 tab daily
		6–12: 1 tab daily
		  10–40 mg
		  PO daily
		≥12: 2 tabs daily
			1 tab bid
			2 tabs bid
			
			4 tabs bid

Bisacodyl (Dulcolax)	Tablets: repeat doses q 12 hours until desired effect	3–12: 5–10 mg PO ≥12: 5–15 mg/hr PO	
	Suppository (give per rectum)	<2: 5 mg (1/2 supp) ≥2: 10 mg (1 supp)	5 mg 10 mg

Type of Drug	Name	Age in Years	Recommended Dose/Day
Saline	Magnesium citrate (Citroma)	<6 6–12 ≥12	2–4 ml/kg PO* 100–150 ml PO 150–300 ml PO
	Magnesium hydroxide (Phillips' Milk of Magnesia)	<2 2–5 6–12 ≥12	0.5 ml PO 5–15 ml PO* 15–30 ml PO* 30–60 ml PO *
	Sodium phosphate/ biphosphate enema (Fleet enema)	2–12 ≥12	2.25 oz pediatric enema 4.5 oz enema
Lubricant: Mineral oil (avoid PO at bedtime due to risk of aspiration)		5–11 ≥12 2–11 ≥12	5–15 ml PO* 15–45 ml PO* 30–60 ml rectally 60–150 ml retention enema

(Continued)

Table 4.7 ▪ *Prevention and Treatment of Constipation (Oral Doses)*
(Continued)

Type of Drug	Name	Age in Years	Recommended Dose/Day
Surfactant/stool softener	Docusate (Colace; give in 1–4 divided doses)	<3 3–5	10–40 mg PO 20–60 mg PO
	capsules or oral liquid of various mg per unit	6–12 ≥12	40–150 mg PO 50–400 mg PO
Miscellaneous	Glycerin	<6	1 infant suppository, 1–2 times or 2–5 ml as an enema
		≥6	1 adult suppository 1–2 times or 5–15 ml as an enema
	Lactulose (Lactugal; can be diluted in water, juices, milk)	Children	7.5 ml PO after breakfast 15–30 ml PO increased up to maximum of 60 ml
	Polyethylene glycol (Miralax; mix in 4–8 oz of fluid)	Adults	1/2 to 1 packet (17 g) PO every day up to tid dosing

Note. *May be given in single or divided doses.
Abbreviations: bid, two times a day; PO, by mouth; tid, three times a day.
Source: From Avila, 2004; Santucci & Mack, 2007.

with minimal abdominal cramping (APS, 2008; Kraemer & Rose, 2009; Thomas, 2008).

Pruritus

Itching is usually limited to the face, neck, and upper chest and is a fairly common side effect of opioids that results from the release of histamine from mast cells, occurring more often with morphine (Zernikow et al., 2006) and less with fentanyl. It usually resolves within a few days, and health care providers can consider adding an antihistamine or changing to an alternative opioid.

Nausea/Vomiting

Stimulation of the chemoreceptor trigger zone in the medulla with the associated feeling of nausea usually resolves soon after opioids are started (APS, 2005; Dowden, 2009a; Zernikow et al., 2009). Antiemetics, preferably those with minimal sedative effects, or changing to another opioid that causes less nausea may be appropriate.

Urinary Retention

Increased bladder smooth muscle tone and sphincter spasm can develop, resulting in urinary retention. This adverse effect occurs when opioids are delivered by any route but more often when delivered epidurally or intrathecally (Wheeler, Oderda, Ashburn, & Lipman, 2002). Other possible etiologies, including disease progression (e.g., bladder obstruction by tumor or impending cord compression associated with neurogenic bladder), precipitating drugs (e.g., tricyclic antidepressants), or other conditions, such as hypovolemia or renal failure, should be excluded before decreasing the opioid dose. Children will need reassurance that this symptom will resolve, along with calming measures, local application of a warm wet towel, and the sound of running water to induce voiding. Short-term bladder catheterization may be needed, as urinary retention usually resolves within a few days of initiating an opioid. All opioids can cause urinary retention. Therefore, as with all side effects, rotating to another opioid may provide relief of this symptom for specific patients.

Myoclonus

A less common opioid-related adverse effect, ranging from mild twitching to generalized spasms, myoclonus often occurs when entering the sleep state and is usually seen with high-dose opioids or rapid escalation, especially with morphine and hydromorphone (Zernikow et al., 2009). If myoclonus is infrequent or not distressing to the child, no treatment is warranted. If myoclonus is problematic, health care providers can consider an opioid dose reduction or rotation. Another option is to add clonazepam (Klonopin) 0.01 mg/kg orally every 12 hours to a maximum dose of 20 mg/day (Brown & McGrath, 2006) or parenteral benzodiazepine if the oral route is not possible (McNicol et al., 2003).

Central Nervous System Effects

Euphoria, dysphoria, confusion, dizziness, and hallucinations can occur initially but usually disappear within a few days (Dowden, 2009a). Patients also report disturbances in sleep that usually are described as vivid dreams that may or may not be frightening.

PREVENTING OPIOID GAPS

When transitioning opioids among routes, the need to avoid an "analgesic gap" is critical, with a need for careful planning for discharge from the inpatient setting (APS, 2008). If the source of the pain is resolving and the patient's medical stability is increasing, the oral route is often optimal for outpatient care, including a plan for managing pain related to rehabilitation plans. Ensuring a safety net for children to have adequate doses of opioids as needed is comforting for children and their parents at the time of discharge (Dowden, 2009a). Clear and precise written instructions for the opioids as well as contact information for any concerns, including what actions to take if side effects or inadequate pain control occurs, needs to be carefully reviewed with the parents (see Appendix).

Clinical Pearl

In evaluating the current pain management plan, ask:

▓ Is the current dose and frequency sufficient for normal function?

▓ Does the child wake during night or limit activities because of pain?

▓ Does the controlled-release dose wear off before the next dose is due?

▓ Does the child frequently have breakthrough pain between doses?

▓ Is the breakthrough rescue dose sufficient?

▓ How many rescue doses are needed in 24 hours?

REFERENCES

Akbik, H., Butler, S. F., Budman, S. H., Fernandez, K., Katz, N. P., & Jamison, R. N. (2006). Validation and clinical application of the Screener and Opioid Assessment for Patients with Pain (SOAPP). *Journal of Pain and Symptom Management, 32*(3), 287–293.

American Academy of Pediatrics and Canadian Paediatric Society. (2000). Prevention and management of pain and stress in the neonate. American Academy of Pediatrics. Committee on Fetus and Newborn. Committee on Drugs. Section on Anesthesiology. Section on Surgery. Canadian Paediatric Society. Fetus and Newborn Committee. *Pediatrics, 105*(2), 454–461.

American Pain Society. (1999). *Guidelines for management of acute and chronic pain in sickle cell disease.* Glenview, IL: Author.

American Pain Society. (2005). *Guidelines for the management of cancer pain in adults and children.* Glenview, IL: Author.

American Pain Society. (2008). *Principles of analgesic use in the treatment of acute pain and cancer pain.* Glenview, IL: Author.

Anderson, B. J., & Palmer, G. M. (2006). Recent developments in the pharmacological management of pain in children. *Current Opinion in Anaesthesiology, 19*(3), 285–292.

Anghelescu, D. L., Burgoyne, L. L., Oakes, L. L., & Wallace, D. A. (2005). The safety of patient-controlled analgesia by proxy in pediatric oncology patients. *Anesthesia and Analgesia, 101*(6), 1623–1627.

Anghelescu, D., Oakes, L., & Popenhagan, M. (2006). Management of pain due to cancer in neonates, children, and adolescents. In O. A. de Leon-Casasola (Ed.), *Cancer pain: Pharmacologic, interventional, and palliative care approaches* (pp. 509–521). Philadelphia, PA: Elsevier.

Avila, J. G. (2004). Pharmacologic treatment of constipation in cancer patients. *Cancer Control, 11*(3 Suppl.), 10–18.

Ballantyne, J. C., & LaForge, K. S. (2007). Opioid dependence and addiction during opioid treatment of chronic pain. *Pain, 129*(3), 235–255.

Barkin, R. L., Barkin, S. J., & Barkin, D. S. (2006). Propoxyphene (dextropropoxyphene): A critical review of a weak opioid analgesic that should remain in antiquity. *American Journal of Therapeutics, 13*(6), 534–542.

Berde, C. B., & Sethna, N. F. (2002). Analgesics for the treatment of pain in children. *The New England Journal of Medicine, 347*(14), 1094–1103.

Berde, C. B., & Solodiuk, J. (2003). Multidisciplinary programs for management of acute and chronic pain in children. In N. L. Schechter, C. B. Berde, & M. Yaster (Eds.), *Pain in infants, children, and adolescents* (2nd ed., pp. 471–486). Philadelphia, PA: Lippincott Williams & Wilkins.

Borland, M., Jacobs, I., King, B., & O'Brien, D. (2007). A randomized controlled trial comparing intranasal fentanyl to intravenous morphine for managing acute pain in children in the emergency department. *Annals of Emergency Medicine, 49*(3), 335–340.

Borland, M. L., Bergesio, R., Pascoe, E. M., Turner, S., & Woodger, S. (2005). Intranasal fentanyl is an equivalent analgesic to oral morphine in paediatric burns patients for dressing changes: A randomised double blind crossover study. *Burns, 31*(7), 831–837.

Bouwmeester, N. J., van den Anker, J. N., Hop, W. C., Anand, K. J., & Tibboel, D. (2003). Age- and therapy-related effects on morphine requirements and plasma concentrations of morphine and its metabolites in postoperative infants. *British Journal of Anaesthesia, 90*(5), 642–652.

Boyd, C. J., McCabe, S. E., Cranford, J. A., & Young, A. (2006). Adolescents' motivations to abuse prescription medications. *Pediatrics, 118*(6), 2472–2480.

Brislin, R. P., & Rose, J. B. (2005). Pediatric acute pain management. *Anesthesiology Clinics of North America, 23*(4), 789–814.

Brown, S. C., & McGrath, P. A. (2006). Evaluation and control of cancer pain in the pediatric patient. In O. A. de Leon-Casasola (Ed.), *Cancer pain: Pharmacologic, interventional, and palliative care approaches* (pp. 33–52). Philadelphia, PA: Elsevier.

Brown, S. C., Taddio, A., & McGrath, P. A. (2010). Pharmacological considerations in infants and children. In P. Beaulieu, D. Lussier, F. Porreca, & A. H. Dickenson (Eds.), *Pharmacology of pain* (pp. 529–545). Seattle: IASP Press.

Bryson, J., Tamber, A., Seccareccia, D., & Zimmermann, C. (2006). Methadone for treatment of cancer pain. *Current Oncology Reports*, *8*(4), 282–288.

Candiotti, K. A., & Gitlin, M. C. (2010). Review of the effect of opioid-related side effects on the undertreatment of moderate to severe chronic non-cancer pain: Tapentadol, a step toward a solution? *Current Medical Research and Opinion*, *26*(7), 1677–1684.

Chou, R., Fanciullo, G. J., Fine, P. G., Miaskowski, C., Passik, S. D., & Portenoy, R. K. (2009). Opioids for chronic noncancer pain: Prediction and identification of aberrant drug-related behaviors: A review of the evidence for an American Pain Society and American Academy of Pain Medicine clinical practice guideline. *Journal of Pain*, *10*(2), 131–146.

Chu, L. F., Angst, M. S., & Clark, D. (2008). Opioid-induced hyperalgesia in humans: Molecular mechanisms and clinical considerations. *Clinical Journal of Pain*, *24*(6), 479–496.

Collins, J., & Weisman, S. (2003). Management of pain in childhood cancer. In N. L. Schechter, C. B. Berde, & M. Yaster (Eds.), *Pain in infants, children, and adolescents* (2nd ed., pp. 517–538). Philadelphia, PA: Lippincott Williams & Wilkins.

Cruciani, R. A., Sekine, R., Homel, P., Lussier, D., Yap, Y., Suzuki, Y., . . . Portenoy, R. K. (2005). Measurement of QTc in patients receiving chronic methadone therapy. *Journal of Pain and Symptom Management*, *29*(4), 385–391.

Czarnecki, M. L., Ferrise, A. S., Jastrowski Mano, K. E., Garwood, M. M., Sharp, M., Davies, H., & Weisman S. J. (2008). Parent/nurse-controlled analgesia for children with developmental delay. *Clinical Journal of Pain*, *24*(9), 817–824.

Davies, D., DeVlaming, D., & Haines, C. (2008). Methadone analgesia for children with advanced cancer. *Pediatric Blood & Cancer*, *51*(3), 393–397.

Dowden, S. J. (2009a). Managing acute pain in children. In A. Twycross, S. J. Dowden, & E. Bruce (Eds.), *Managing pain in children: A clinical guide* (pp. 109–144). Oxford, United Kingdom: Wiley-Blackwell.

Dowden, S. J. (2009b). Palliative care in children. In A. Twycross, S. J. Dowden, & E. Bruce (Eds.), *Managing pain in children: A clinical guide* (pp. 171–200). Oxford, United Kingdom: Wiley-Blackwell.

Dunlop, R. J., & Bennett, K. C. (2006). Pain management for sickle cell disease. *Cochrane Database of Systematic Reviews*, (2), CD003350.

Engelhardt, T., Steel, E., Johnston, G., & Veitch, D. Y. (2003). Tramadol for pain relief in children undergoing tonsillectomy: A comparison with morphine. *Paediatric Anaesthesia*, *13*(3), 249–252.

Esphani, N., & Bruera, E. (2006). Current trends in cancer pain management. In O. A. de Leon-Casasola (Ed.), *Cancer pain: Pharmacologic, interventional, and palliative care approaches* (pp. 13–23). Philadelphia, PA: Elsevier.

Estfan, B., LeGrand, S. B., Walsh, D., Lagman, R. L., & Davis, M. P. (2005). Opioid rotation in cancer patients: Pros and cons. *Oncology*, *19*(4), 511–516.

Fine, P. G., & Portenoy, R. K. (2009). Establishing "best practices" for opioid rotation: Conclusions of an expert panel. *Journal of Pain and Symptom Management*, *38*(3), 418–425.

Finkel, J. C., Finley, A., Greco, C., Weisman, S. J., & Zeltzer, L. (2005). Transdermal fentanyl in the management of children with chronic severe pain: Results from an international study. *Cancer*, *104*(12), 2847–2857.

Franck, L. S., Harris, S. K., Soetenga, D. J., Amling, J. K., & Curley, M. A. (2008). The withdrawal assessment tool-1 (WAT-1): An assessment instrument for monitoring opioid and benzodiazepine withdrawal symptoms in pediatric patients. *Pediatric Critical Care Medicine*, *9*(6), 573–580.

Friedrichsdorf, S. J., Finney, D., Bergin, M., Stevens, M., & Collins, J. J. (2007). Breakthrough pain in children with cancer. *Journal of Pain and Symptom Management*, *34*(2), 209–216.

Friedrichsdorf, S. J., & Kang, T. I. (2007). The management of pain in children with life-limiting illnesses. *Pediatric Clinics of North America*, *54*(5), 645–672.

Fu, E. S., Downs, J. B., Schweiger, J. W., Miguel, R. V., & Smith, R. A. (2004). Supplemental oxygen impairs detection of hypoventilation by pulse oximetry. *Chest, 126*(5), 1552–1558.

Gardner-Nix, J. (2001). Oral transmucosal fentanyl and sufentanil for incident pain. *Journal of Pain and Symptom Management, 22*(2), 627–630.

Greco, C., & Berde, C. (2005). Pain management for the hospitalized pediatric patient. *Pediatric Clinics of North America, 52*(4), 995–1027.

Harrison, D., Loughnan, P., Manias, E., & Johnston, L. (2009). Utilization of analgesics, sedatives, and pain scores in infants with a prolonged hospitalization: A prospective descriptive cohort study. *International Journal of Nursing Studies, 46*(5), 624–632.

Ista, E., van Dijk, M., Gamel, C., Tibboel, D., & de Hoog, M. (2007). Withdrawal symptoms in children after long-term administration of sedatives and/or analgesics: A literature review. "Assessment remains troublesome." *Intensive Care Medicine, 33*(8), 1396–1406.

Jacob, E. (2001). Pain management in sickle cell disease. *Pain Management Nursing, 2*(4), 121–131.

Jacob, E. (2004). Neuropathic pain in children with cancer. *Journal of Pediatric Oncology Nursing, 21*(6), 350–357.

Jacob, E., Miaskowski, C., Savedra, M., Beyer, J. E., Treadwell, M., & Styles, L. (2003). Changes in intensity, location, and quality of vaso-occlusive pain in children with sickle cell disease. *Pain, 102*(1–2), 187–193.

Johnson, S. J. (2007). Opioid safety in patients with renal or hepatic dysfunction (Electronic Version). *Pain Topics.* Retrieved from www.Pain-Topics.org

Keidan, I., Gravenstein, D., Berkenstadt, H., Ziv, A., Shavit, I., & Sidi, A. (2008). Supplemental oxygen compromises the use of pulse oximetry for detection of apnea and hypoventilation during sedation in simulated pediatric patients. *Pediatrics, 122*(2), 293–298.

Kraemer, F. W., & Rose, J. B. (2009). Pharmacologic management of acute pediatric pain. *Anesthesiology Clinics, 27*(2), 241–268.

Lightdale, J. R., Goldmann, D. A., Feldman, H. A., Newburg, A. R., DiNardo, J. A., & Fox, V. L. (2006). Microstream capnography improves patient monitoring during moderate sedation: A randomized, controlled trial. *Pediatrics, 117*(6), e1170–e1178.

Manfredi, P. L., & Houde, R. W. (2003). Prescribing methadone, a unique analgesic. *The Journal of Supportive Oncology, 1*(3), 216–220.

McCabe, S. E., Boyd, C. J., Cranford, J. A., & Teter, C. J. (2009). Motives for nonmedical use of prescription opioids among high school seniors in the United States: Self-treatment and beyond. *Archives of Pediatrics and Adolescent Medicine*, *163*(8), 739–744.

McCaffery, M., Grimm, M. A., Pasero, C., Ferrell, B., & Uman, G. C. (2005). On the meaning of "drug seeking." *Pain Management Nursing*, *6*(4), 122–136.

McNicol, E., Horowicz-Mehler, N., Fisk, R. A., Bennett, K., Gialeli-Goudas, M., Chew, P. W., . . . American Pain Society. (2003). Management of opioid side effects in cancer-related and chronic noncancer pain: A systematic review. *Journal of Pain*, *4*(5), 231–256.

Meissner, W., Schmidt, U., Hartmann, M., Kath, R., & Reinhart, K. (2000). Oral naloxone reverses opioid-associated constipation. *Pain*, *84*(1), 105–109.

Melzer-Lange, M. D., Walsh-Kelly, C. M., Lea, G., Hillery, C. A., & Scott, J. P. (2004). Patient-controlled analgesia for sickle cell pain crisis in a pediatric emergency department. *Pediatric Emergency Care*, *20*(1), 2–4.

Monitto, C. L., Greenberg, R. S., Kost-Byerly, S., Wetzel, R., Billett, C., Lebet, R. M., & Yaster M. (2000). The safety and efficacy of parent-/nurse-controlled analgesia in patients less than six years of age. *Anesthesia & Analgesia*, *91*(3), 573–579.

Moryl, N., Santiago-Palma, J., Kornick, C., Derby, S., Fischberg, D., Payne, R., & Manfredi, P. L. (2002). Pitfalls of opioid rotation: Substituting another opioid for methadone in patients with cancer pain. *Pain*, *96*(3), 325–328.

Moulin, D. E., Clark, A. J., Gilron, I., Ware, M. A., Watson, C. P., Sessle, B. J., & Canadian Pain Society. (2007). Pharmacological management of chronic neuropathic pain—consensus statement and guidelines from the Canadian Pain Society. *Pain Research & Management*, *12*(1), 13–21.

Nicholson, A. B. (2007). Methadone for cancer pain. *Cochrane Database of Systematic Reviews*, (4), CD003971.

Nisbet, A. T., & Mooney-Cotter, F. (2009). Comparison of selected sedation scales for reporting opioid-induced sedation assessment. *Pain Management Nursing*, *10*(3), 154–164.

Oakes, L. (2008). Patient controlled analgesia. In J. Verger & R. Lebet (Eds.), *American Association of Critical-Care Nurses procedure manual for pediatric acute and critical care* (pp. 1269–1279). St. Louis, MO: Saunders Elsevier.

Pasero, C. (2009). Assessment of sedation during opioid administration for pain management. *Journal of Perianesthesia Nursing, 24*(3), 186–190.

Pasero, C., & McCaffery, M. (2002). Monitoring sedation. *American Journal of Nursing, 102*(2), 67–69.

Passik, S. D., Heit, H., & Kirsh, K. L. (2006). Reality and responsibility: A commentary on the treatment of pain and suffering in a drug-using society. *Journal of Opioid Management, 2*(3), 123–127.

Passik, S. D., Kirsh, K. L., Whitcomb, L., Portenoy, R. K., Katz, N. P., Kleinman, L., . . . Schein, J. R. (2004). A new tool to assess and document pain outcomes in chronic pain patients receiving opioid therapy. *Clinical Therapeutics, 26*(4), 552–561.

Ramsay, M., Savege, T., Simpson, B. R., & Goodwin, R. (1974). Controlled sedation with alphaxolone-alphadolone. *British Medical Journal, 2*, 656–659.

Reddy, S., Hui, D., El Osta, B., de la Cruz, M., Walker, P., Palmer, J. L., Bruera, E. (2009). The effect of oral methadone on the QTc interval in advanced cancer patients: A prospective pilot study. *Journal of Palliative Medicine, 13*(1), 33–38.

Ripamonti, C., & Bianchi, M. (2002). The use of methadone for cancer pain. *Hematology/Oncology Clinics of North America, 16*(3), 543–555.

Santucci, G., & Mack, J. W. (2007). Common gastrointestinal symptoms in pediatric palliative care: Nausea, vomiting, constipation, anorexia, cachexia. *Pediatric Clinics of North America, 54*(5), 673–689.

Savage, S. R., Joranson, D. E., Covington, E. C., Schnoll, S. H., Heit, H. A., & Gilson, A. M. (2003). Definitions related to the medical use of opioids: Evolution toward universal agreement. *Journal of Pain and Symptom Management, 26*(1), 655–667.

Sessler, C. N., Gosnell, M. S., Grap, M. J., Brophy, G. M., O'Neal, P. V., Keane, K. A., . . . Elswick, R. K. (2002). The Richmond Agitation-Sedation Scale: Validity and reliability in adult intensive care unit patients. *American Journal of Respiratory and Critical Care Medicine, 166*(10), 1338–1344.

Shaiova, L., Berger, A., Blinderman, C. D., Bruera, E., Davis, M. P., Derby, S., . . . Perlov, E. (2008). Consensus guideline on parenteral methadone use in pain and palliative care. *Palliative and Support Care, 6*(2), 165–176.

Taddio, A. (2002). Opioid analgesia for infants in the neonatal intensive care unit. *Clinics in Perinatology, 29*(3), 493–509.

Thomas, J. (2008). Opioid-induced bowel dysfunction. *Journal of Pain and Symptom Management, 35*(1), 103–113.

Twombly, E. C., & Holtz, K. D. (2008). Teens and the misuse of prescription drugs: Evidence-based recommendations to curb a growing societal problem. *Journal of Primary Prevention, 29*(6), 503–516.

U.S. Food and Drug Administration. (2007). *Use of codeine products in nursing mothers.* Retrieved from http://www.fda.gov/Drugs/DrugSafety/PostmarketDrugSafetyInformationforPatientsandProviders/ucm118108.htm

U.S. Food and Drug Administration. (2010). *Ultram (tramadol hydrochloride), Ultracet (tramadol hydrochloride/acetaminophen): Label change.* Retrieved from http://www.fda.gov/Safety/MedWatch/SafetyInformation/Safety-AlertsforHumanMedicalProducts/ucm213264.htm

Verghese, S. T., & Hannallah, R. S. (2005). Postoperative pain management in children. *Anesthesiology Clinics of North America, 23*(1), 163–184.

Voepel-Lewis, T., Marinkovic, A., Kostrzewa, A., Tait, A. R., & Malviya, S. (2008). The prevalence of and risk factors for adverse events in children receiving patient-controlled analgesia by proxy or patient-controlled analgesia after surgery. *Anesthesia and Analgesia, 107*(1), 70–75.

Wade, W. E., & Spruill, W. J. (2009). Tapentadol hydrochloride: A centrally acting oral analgesic. *Clinical Therapeutics, 31*(12), 2804–2818.

Webster, L. R., & Webster, R. M. (2005). Predicting aberrant behaviors in opioid-treated patients: Preliminary validation of the Opioid Risk Tool. *Pain Medicine, 6*(6), 432–442.

Wheeler, M., Oderda, G. M., Ashburn, M. A., & Lipman, A. G. (2002). Adverse events associated with postoperative opioid analgesia: A systematic review. *Journal of Pain, 3*(3), 159–180.

Williams, D. G., Hatch, D. J., & Howard, R. F. (2001). Codeine phosphate in paediatric medicine. *British Journal of Anaesthesia, 86*(3), 413–421.

Williams, D. G., Patel, A., & Howard, R. F. (2002). Pharmacogenetics of codeine metabolism in an urban population of children and its implications for analgesic reliability. *British Journal of Anaesthesia, 89*(6), 839–845.

Wuhrman, E., Cooney, M. F., Dunwoody, C. J., Eksterowicz, N., Merkel, S., & Oakes, L. L. (2007). Authorized and unauthorized ("PCA by Proxy") dosing of analgesic infusion pumps: Position statement with clinical practice recommendations. *Pain Management Nursing, 8*(1), 4–11.

Yaster, M., Kost-Byerly, S., & Maxwell, L. (2003). Opioid agonists and antagonists. In N. L. Schechter, C. B. Berde, & M. Yaster (Eds.), *Pain in infants, children, and adolescents* (2nd ed., pp. 181–224). Philadelphia, PA: Lippincott Williams & Wilkins.

Zernikow, B., Michel, E., Craig, F., & Anderson, B. J. (2009). Pediatric palliative care: Use of opioids for the management of pain. *Paediatric Drugs, 11*(2), 129–151.

Zernikow, B., Smale, H., Michel, E., Hasan, C., Jorch, N., & Andler, W. (2006). Paediatric cancer pain management using the WHO analgesic ladder—results of a prospective analysis from 2265 treatment days during a quality improvement study. *European Journal of Pain, 10*(7), 587–595.

5

Coanalgesics

Coanalgesic medications include a diverse group of drugs developed for the treatment of medical conditions other than pain but that have also been found to provide pain relief (American Pain Society [APS], 2008). Coanalgesics are usually prescribed along with nonsteroidal anti-inflammatory drugs (NSAIDs) or opioids but can be used alone for neuropathic pain. Because coanalgesics do not have an immediate onset of action and require slow titration to avoid toxicity, clinicians should explain to patients that an adequate trial of one drug should be attempted before changing to another. Although their efficacy and safety have not been evaluated in well-controlled studies in children, coanalgesics are often given *off-label*, drawing from anecdotal experience or extrapolated from adult studies, with the health care provider considering the child's comorbidities (APS, 2008).

ANTICONVULSANTS

Anticonvulsants are effective in treating neuropathic pain by a mechanism presumed to be related to their ability to control seizures by reducing neuronal excitability. Gabapentin (Neurontin) and pregabalin (Lyrica) have similar mechanisms of action, efficacies, and adverse effects. Older anticonvulsants, such as phenytoin (Dilantin) or carbamazepine (Tegretol), are less suitable because of their significant adverse effects, including bone marrow suppression (APS, 2005; Brown & McGrath, 2006). Newer anticonvulsants, such as topiramate (Topamax) and lamotrigine (Lamictal), have less evidence for efficacy in controlling neuropathic pain in adults (APS, 2008) but have recently been associated with a risk of suicide in patients who are 15 years and older (Patorno et al., 2010).

▨ *Gabapentin (Neurontin)*

Indications: Gabapentin has emerged as the first choice among coanalgesics for various neuropathic pain syndromes in children, including postherpectic neuralgia, spinal cord tumors or injuries, vincristine-induced neuropathy, phantom limb pain after amputation, postthoracotomy neuropathic pain, fibromyalgia, complex regional pain syndrome, and migraine headaches (APS, 2008; Golden, Haut, & Moshe, 2006; Stinson & Bruce, 2009). It has also provided beneficial effects on mood and anxiety disorders (Berde, Lebel, & Olsson, 2003). Perioperative administration of gabapentin (and pregabalin) for adults reduced postoperative pain, opioid consumption, and opioid-related adverse effects after surgery (Kong & Irwin, 2007; Tiippana, Hamunen, Kontinen, & Kalso, 2007). However, determination of the optimal dose and duration of treatment is not conclusive.

Dosage: Recommended initial and maximal doses are available in Table 5.1. Because of its short half-life, the optimal dosing frequency is three times a day (Dauri et al., 2009). Health care providers need to gradually increase the dosage every 2 to 3 days to minimize adverse effects. Patients should be informed that at least 3 days may be required to experience analgesic effects.

Forms: Gabapentin is available in various capsules or tablets of different strengths, as well as an oral solution. No intravenous (IV) formulation is available.

Drug Interactions: No drug interactions have been found with gabapentin.

Warnings: Because gabapentin is eliminated entirely by the kidneys, dosage reduction must be considered with renal insufficiency. When gabapentin is no longer indicated, clinicians should taper the dosages over a period of 1 to 3 weeks to prevent a withdrawal syndrome, which includes irritability, agitation, anxiety, headache, nausea, and diarrhea (Berde et al., 2003; Kong & Irwin, 2007).

Table 5.1 ▦ *Dosing Guidelines for Coanalgesics*

Medication	Pediatric Initial Dose	Maximum Dose	Adult Initial Dose	Maximum Dose
Gabapentin (Neurontin)	5–10 mg/kg/day up to 100 mg tid	70 mg/kg/day or 1200 mg tid	100–300 mg tid	3600 mg/day
Pregabalin (Lyrica)	Consider 1/6 of the gabapentin dose up to 75 mg bid*	Not known	150 mg bid	1200 mg/day
Amitriptyline (Elavil)	0.1 mg/kg/day up to 10 mg at bedtime**	1–2 mg/kg/day more than 2–3 weeks (max dose 150 mg at bedtime)	25 mg at bedtime	150 mg
Topical lidocaine (Lidoderm 5% patch)	1 patch cut to fit painful area	No more than 1 patch for 12 hours/day	1–3 patches cut to fit painful areas	No more than 3 patches for 12 hours/day
Ketamine (Ketalar)	0.05–0.2 mg/kg/hr IV infusion	0.2 mg/kg/hr	0.1–0.15 mg/kg/hr IV infusion	
	2–5 mg/kg PO	100 mg PO	0.5 mg/kg PO tid or qid, increasing by 0.5 mg/kg	
			100 mg/day PO up to 500 mg/day	
Baclofen (Lioresal)	5 mg/day PO	Increase by 5–15 mg/day up to 60 mg/day PO	5 mg/day tid PO up to 10–20 mg tid PO	200 mg/day
Cyclobenzaprine (Flexeril)	Not known*	Not known	5–10 mg tid	40 mg/day

(Continued)

Table 5.1 ▓ *Dosing Guidelines for Coanalgesics (Continued)*

Medication	Pediatric Initial Dose	Maximum Dose	Adult Initial Dose	Maximum Dose
Dexamethasone (Decadron)	0.02–0.3 mg/ kg/day in 3–4 divided doses	10 mg/day	4 mg bid	24 mg/day
Methylprednisolone (Solu-Medrol)	0.5 mg/kg up to initial adult dose		10 mg tid	40 mg tid

*Safety and efficacy have not been established for neonatal and pediatric patients.
**Safety and efficacy have not been established for use in infants.
Abbreviations: bid, two times a day; IV, intravenous; PO, by mouth; qid, four times a day; tid, three times a day.
Source: Compiled from American Pain Society, 2005, 2008; Blonk, Koder, Bemt, & Huygen, 2010; Brown, Taddio, & McGrath, 2010; Dauri et al., 2009; Dworkin et al., 2007; Friedrichsdorf & Kang, 2007; Krane, Leong, Golianu, & Leong, 2003.

Adverse Effects: These symptoms usually occur early in therapy and gradually disappear over the first week of therapy: mild sedation, dizziness, ataxia, fatigue, impaired concentration, hallucinations, headaches, weight gain, fluid retention, nausea, and myalgia (APS, 2008; Friedrichsdorf & Kang, 2007).

▓ *Pregabalin (Lyrica)*

Pregabalin, as a newer analogue of gabapentin, has demonstrated significant pain relief in adults; however, no data are currently available on its use in children (Friedrichsdorf & Kang, 2007). Therapeutic levels can be achieved earlier in therapy than with gabapentin; therefore, pain relief may be achieved more rapidly as well.

Indications: See the indications for gabapentin.

Forms: Pregabalin is available in oral capsules and solution. No IV preparation is available.

Dosage: Recommended initial and maximal doses are available in Table 5.1. Health care providers need to gradually increase the dosage every 2 to 3 days to minimize the side effects. Pregabalin dosing frequency has the advantage that only 2 doses are needed per day. Patients should be informed that at least 3 days may be required to experience analgesic effects.

Drug Interactions: No drug interactions have been found with pregabalin.

Warnings: Because pregabalin is eliminated entirely by the kidneys, dosage reduction must be considered with renal insufficiency. When pregabalin is no longer indicated, clinicians should taper the dosages over a period of 1 to 3 weeks to prevent a withdrawal syndrome.

Adverse Effects: Generally, pregabalin has the same adverse effects as gabapentin, but it is less associated with nausea and vomiting (Dauri et al., 2009).

ANTIDEPRESSANTS

Antidepressants relieve neuropathic pain because of their ability to increase levels of norepinephrine and serotonin, crucial neurotransmitters in pain modulation, as well as block sodium channels affecting the transmission of pain (APS, 2008; Dowden, 2009; Moulin et al., 2007). Their safety and efficacy in patients younger than 18 years have not been established (APS, 2008). Health care providers are to be vigilant in monitoring children and adolescents who are taking any type of antidepressant in regard to risk of suicide (Schneeweiss et al., 2010).

▒ *Tricyclic Antidepressants*

Indications: When given in lower doses than are needed for antidepressant effects, tricyclic antidepressants (TCAs) can be effective in treating neuropathic pain but are less preferred because of their more challenging adverse effect profile (APS, 2008; Moulin et al., 2007). If gabapentin is given at maximum doses without effectively relieving neuropathic pain, a TCA can be added. Various TCAs are available, such as amitriptyline (Elavil), nortriptyline (Pamelor), desipramine (Norpramin), imipramine (Tofranil), and doxepin (Siniquan), with no evidence that one is more effective than another for neuropathic pain (APS, 2008; Moulin et al., 2007).

Dosage: Recommended initial and maximal doses of amitriptyline are available in Table 5.1, usually initiated with a small single daily dose 1 hour before bedtime, which is advantageous to promote sleep and minimize daytime somnolence. The dose may be increased by 50% every 2 to 3 days (Brown & McGrath, 2006). Patients need to be informed that 5 to 7 days may be needed before the full analgesic effect is achieved at any particular dose.

Forms: Amitriptyline is available only in tablet form.

Warnings: Use TCAs with caution for patients with preexisting cardiac rhythm disturbances that can be worsened by TCAs (Berde et al., 2003) or if other cardiotoxic medications (i.e., doxorubicin) are being administered (APS, 2008). An electrocardiogram is recommended periodically during long-term use or if standard dosages are exceeded (Collins & Weisman, 2003). If TCAs are to be discontinued, tapering over 1 to 2 weeks is recommended to avoid withdrawal symptoms such as irritability and bothersome vivid dreaming at night owing to rapid eye movement sleep rebound (Berde et al., 2003).

Adverse Effects: Patients frequently complain of dry mouth and initial somnolence that subside after a few days. Less common complaints include orthostatic hypotension, disorientation, nightmares, weight gain, urinary retention, and constipation (Dworkin et al., 2007). These side effects can frequently be managed by a temporary reduction in dose followed by a gradual increase in the dose.

Drug Interactions: Many interactions have been reported between TCAs and other medications, making prescribing challenging for patients with complex medical problems, such as the need to avoid prescribing selective serotonin reuptake inhibitors (SSRIs) along with TCAs (APS, 2008; Dworkin et al., 2007).

Selective Serotonin Reuptake Inhibitors and Serotonin Noradrenaline Reuptake Inhibitors

Better tolerated than TCAs, SSRIs and serotonin noradrenaline reuptake inhibitors (SNRIs) have been used for adults with neuropathic pain, and limited success has been seen with paroxetine (Paxil), duloxetine (Cymbalta), and venlafaxine (Effexor) (APS, 2008; Moulin et al., 2007). Their safety and efficacy in children have not been established (APS, 2008). The preference of using SSRIs and SNRIs for older patients with neuropathic pain is for concurrent depression, anxiety, or insomnia and only after careful consideration that all drug interactions have been eliminated.

LOCAL ANESTHETICS

By blocking the sodium channels in the peripheral and central neurons, and therefore reducing spontaneous impulses, local anesthetics (LAs) reduce pain by preventing transmission of pain along peripheral and central nerve pathways. To be effective, LAs need to be physically injected, infused, or absorbed through the skin directly into the area of the nerves that are to be blocked from sending pain signals up the spinal pathways.

Indications: LAs are useful for the following:

- Providing pain relief for painful procedures involving the dermis or mucous membranes by using either LAs in the forms of creams or infiltrating LA solution (see Chapter 13).
- Providing relief of acute pain related to various surgical procedures or tumors (see Section III).
- Neuropathic pain states when other more conventional medications have not proved effective, specifically using lidocaine as an IV infusion (see later discussion for more information).
- Using lidocaine 5% patches is useful for localized areas of neuropathic pain, such as with postherpetic neuralgia (Lidoderm; Moulin et al., 2007)

Forms: Lidocaine (Xylocaine) is the most commonly administered LA, effective when administered by infiltration or topical preparations, and is the only LA that can be given as an IV infusion. The oral analogue to lidocaine is mexiletine (Mexitil), but is frequently associated with nausea, vomiting, and other unacceptable adverse effects. More detailed information about dosages of mexilitine is available (Krane, Leong, Golianu, & Leong, 2003). Lidocaine is also available as a 5% patch (Lidoderm) for topical application. Other LAs include bupivacaine (Marcaine), ropivacaine (Naropin), and chloroprocaine (Nesacaine), which are discussed further in Section III.

Dosage: Because lidocaine pharmacokinetics is similar in children and adults, dosing scheduled for children should correlate reasonably with published experience in adults. Lidocaine infusions of 150 mcg/kg/hr are recommended with plasma levels measured every 8 to 12 hours to maintain lidocaine plasma levels of 2–5 mcg/ml (Krane et al., 2003). Recommended doses for lidocaine patches are available in Table 5.1.

Adverse Effects: At recommended doses noted in Table 5.1, LA plasma levels usually remain well below the known toxic concentrations. Most of the adverse effects are caused by high plasma concentrations affecting the cardiac and central nervous systems (i.e., hypotension, vasodilation, and seizures). Specifically for the lidocaine patch, systemic side effects are rare because of minimal absorption but may have mild skin reactions (i.e., erythema or local rash). For patients with hepatic or renal insufficiency who receive a lidocaine infusion, dose adjustments are necessary to prevent toxicity.

KETAMINE *(KETALAR)*

A derivative of phenylcyclohexylpiperidine, ketamine is an anesthetic drug with analgesic properties, especially useful as a potent *N*-methyl-D-aspartate (NMDA) receptor antagonist (Blonk, Koder, Bemt, & Huygen, 2010). Clinical trials in humans have shown mixed results. It is best used in patients taking large doses of opioids and is best delivered as continuous infusion (Subramaniam, Subramaniam, & Steinbrook, 2004).

Clinical Pearl	The NMDA receptors in the dorsal horn of the spinal cord play a role in the development of central sensitization, specifically described as *hyperalgesia*, and the development of "wind up" phenomenon, which is observed during repetitive noxious stimulations resulting in progressively increasing pain intensity. Opioids when used alone in large doses for a prolonged period induce tolerance that may lead to increased pain in spite of escalating doses (opioid-induced hyperalgesia). Ketamine's reduction of opioid tolerance is attributed to its NMDA receptor-antagonist action.

Indications: Better known as an anesthetic, ketamine provides analgesia when given at very low doses and has increasing applications for managing complex acute and cancer pain in both adults and children (Anderson & Palmer, 2006; Blonk et al., 2010), specifically for the following:

- Treating neuropathic pain that has been unresponsive to other agents. However, the routine use of oral ketamine for chronic pain may have limited place in the armamentarium of health care providers because of limited data on efficacy and a poor safety profile.
- Severe pain refractory to high doses of opioids associated with advanced cancer. Adding ketamine has allowed opioid dose reductions of 25% to 50% (APS, 2008; Anghelescu & Oakes, 2005; Dowden, 2009). Limited literature is available for use in adults (Blonk et al., 2010; Mercadante, Arcuri, Tirelli, & Casuccio, 2000) or children (Klepstad, Borchgrevink, Hval, Flaat, & Kaasa, 2001).

However, ketamine does not interfere with spontaneous breathing, and laryngeal reflexes remain intact. Blood pressure and heart rate are maintained as well. When ketamine is no longer indicated, abrupt discontinuance of doses or infusion is not associated with any withdrawal syndrome.

Forms: Parenteral solutions are the only form available for ketamine. Because no oral preparation is commercially available, the parenteral form can be taken orally, mixed with fruit juice or soft drinks to mask the bitter taste.

Dosage: Recommended initial and maximal doses are available in Table 5.1.

Warnings: Caution is to be used with children who have increased intracranial pressure because ketamine increases cerebral blood flow (Kraemer & Rose, 2009).

Adverse Effects: Ketamine should only be prescribed by health care providers experienced in its use (APS, 2008) who are well aware of the associated adverse effects, which are less problematic in children younger than 5 years but can include central nervous system (effects of dysphoria, light-headedness, dizziness, diplopia, vivid dreams, hallucinations, disorientation, strange sensations, sleep difficulties, and confusion). These symptoms are dose related (i.e., low doses usually are not associated with hallucinations, excessive sedation, and dysphoria) (Anderson &

Palmer, 2006; Subramaniam et al., 2004). Because of the adverse effects of increased secretions and possible dysphoric/psychotropic effects, children are often given anticholinergic agents and a benzodiazepine (i.e., midazolam [Versed] infusion) to reduce the psychotropic effects (Kraemer & Rose, 2009). Ketamine is metabolized by the liver, with minimal drug remaining for renal excretion; thus, it is useful for children with renal dysfunction (Dowden, 2009). Health care providers need to assess liver function tests.

MUSCLE RELAXANTS AND ANTISPASMODIC AGENTS

▓ *Cyclobenzaprine (Flexeril)*

Cyclobenzaprine is the best studied of the muscle relaxants and has been found to be consistently effective with less sedative adverse effects than benzodiazepines. Cyclobenzaprine is available only in an oral tablet. Recommended initial and maximal doses are available in Table 5.1.

▓ *Baclofen (Lioresal)*

Baclofen (Lioresal) is a useful antispasmodic agent given to relieve intractable spasticity associated with cerebral palsy. Oral and intrathecal preparations are available. Recommended initial and maximal doses are available in Table 5.1. Adverse effects include weakness, sedation, confusion, and hypotension. A gradual reduction in doses before discontinuing baclofen is necessary to avoid adverse effects and possible seizures (APS, 2008).

ALPHA-2 AGONISTS

Alpha-2 receptors are located on primary afferent terminals (both peripheral and spinal endings) in the dorsal horn of the spinal cord and within the brain stem. Alpha-2 agonists work by reducing central sympathetic output and increasing firing inhibitory neurons within the descending pain pathways. Although these agents may cause sedation, they do provide some analgesia with the advantage of not suppressing spontaneous respiration (Dowden, 2009). These agents do not provide adequate analgesia when used alone and always serve as a coanalgesic along with opioids.

■ Clonidine (Catapres)

Clonidine is useful in reducing postoperative pain when administered in epidural or peripheral nerve block infusions (Anderson & Palmer, 2006). Transdermal clonidine is given for prevention of opioid withdrawal syndrome during rapid opioid weaning regimens.

■ Dexmedetomidine (Presedex)

A newer medication, dexmedetomidine, was originally developed as a sedative but has analgesic properties because of its alpha-2 agonist properties with minimal incidence of respiratory depression (Kraemer & Rose, 2009). It is also used to facilitate acute discontinuation of opioids after cardiac transplantation in children (Anderson & Palmer, 2006). Dexmedetomidine is available only as a continuous infusion.

CORTICOSTEROIDS

Indications: Corticosteroids inhibit prostaglandins and decrease inflammation and edema on the surrounding tissues and are especially useful in reducing pain associated with bone metastases and lymphedema. For neural tissues, they are particularly useful in ameliorating painful malignant lesions of the brachial or lumbosacral plexus or lesions compressing the spinal cord (Collins & Weisman, 2003).

Forms: Corticosteroids include prednisone (Deltasone), dexamethasone (Decadron), and methylprednisolone (Solu-Medrol).

Dosage: Recommended initial and maximal doses are available in Table 5.1. Rapid withdrawal of corticosteroids may exacerbate pain and is to be avoided.

Adverse Effects: Chronic use of corticosteroids can cause weight gain, hyperglycemia, osteoporosis, Cushing syndrome (less with dexamethasone), proximal myopathy, psychosis, and an increased risk of gastrointestinal bleeding, especially when used in combination with NSAIDs.

In summary, although acute pain is usually controlled with NSAIDs and opioids, coanalgesics are useful for chronic pain, especially for neuropathic pain syndromes. As understanding of multimodal strategies and molecular mechanisms of pain becomes more developed with more research in children, more coanalgesics may be found to be useful.

REFERENCES

American Pain Society. (2005). *Guidelines for the management of cancer pain in adults and children*. Glenview, IL: Author.

American Pain Society. (2008). *Principles of analgesic use in the treatment of acute pain and cancer pain*. Glenview, IL: Author.

Anderson, B. J., & Palmer, G. M. (2006). Recent pharmacological advances in paediatric analgesics. *Biomedicine and Pharmacotherapy, 60*(7), 303–309.

Anghelescu, D. L., & Oakes, L. L. (2005). Ketamine use for reduction of opioid tolerance in a 5-year-old girl with end-stage abdominal neuroblastoma. *Journal of Pain Symptom Management, 30*(1), 1–3.

Berde, C. B., Lebel, A. A., & Olsson, G. (2003). Neuropathic pain in children. In N. L. Schechter, C. B. Berde, & M. Yaster (Eds.), *Pain in infants, children, and adolescents* (2nd ed., pp. 620–638). Philadelphia, PA: Lippincott Williams & Wilkins.

Blonk, M. I., Koder, B. G., Bemt, P. M., & Huygen, F. J. (2010). Use of oral ketamine in chronic pain management: A review. *European Journal of Pain, 14*(5), 466–472.

Brown, S. C., & McGrath, P. A. (2006). Evaluation and control of cancer pain in the pediatric patient. In O. A. de Leon-Casasola (Ed.), *Cancer pain: Pharmacologic, interventional, and palliative care approaches* (pp. 33–52). Philadelphia, PA: Elsevier.

Brown, S. C., Taddio, A., & McGrath, P. A. (2010). Pharmacological considerations in infants and children. In P. Beaulieu, D. Lussier, F. Porreca, & A. H. Dickenson (Eds.), *Pharmacology of pain* (pp. 529–545). Seattle, WA: IASP Press.

Collins, J., & Weisman, S. (2003). Management of pain in childhood cancer. In N. L. Schechter, C. B. Berde, & M. Yaster (Eds.), *Pain in infants, children, and adolescents* (2nd ed., pp. 517–538). Philadelphia, PA: Lippincott Williams & Wilkins.

Dauri, M., Faria, S., Gatti, A., Celidonio, L., Carpenedo, R., & Sabato, A. F. (2009). Gabapentin and pregabalin for the acute post-operative pain management. A systematic-narrative review of the recent clinical evidences. *Current Drug Targets, 10*(8), 716–733.

Dowden, S. J. (2009). Pharmacology of analgesic drugs. In A. Twycross, S. J. Dowden, & E. Bruce (Eds.), *Managing pain in children: A clinical guide* (pp. 39–66). Oxford, United Kingdom: Wiley-Blackwell.

Dworkin, R. H., O'Connor, A. B., Backonja, M., Farrar, J. T., Finnerup, N. B., Jensen, T. S., . . . Wallace M. S. (2007). Pharmacologic management of neuropathic pain: Evidence-based recommendations. *Pain, 132*(3), 237–251.

Friedrichsdorf, S. J., & Kang, T. I. (2007). The management of pain in children with life-limiting illnesses. *Pediatric Clinics of North America, 54*(5), 645–672.

Golden, A. S., Haut, S. R., & Moshe, S. L. (2006). Nonepileptic uses of antiepileptic drugs in children and adolescents. *Pediatric Neurology, 34*(6), 421–432.

Klepstad, P., Borchgrevink, P., Hval, B., Flaat, S., & Kaasa, S. (2001). Long-term treatment with ketamine in a 12-year-old girl with severe neuropathic pain caused by a cervical spinal tumor. *Journal of Pediatric Hematology/Oncology, 23*(9), 616–619.

Kong, V. K., & Irwin, M. G. (2007). Gabapentin: A multimodal perioperative drug? *British Journal of Anaesthesia, 99*(6), 775–786.

Kraemer, F. W., & Rose, J. B. (2009). Pharmacologic management of acute pediatric pain. *Anesthesiology Clinic, 27*(2), 241–268.

Krane, E. J., Leong, M. S., Golianu, B., & Leong, Y. Y. (2003). Treatment of pediatric pain with nonconventional analgesics. In N. L. Schechter, C. B. Berde, & M. Yaster (Eds.), *Pain in infants, children, and adolescents* (2nd ed., pp. 225–240). Philadelphia, PA: Lippincott Williams & Wilkins.

Mercadante, S., Arcuri, E., Tirelli, W., & Casuccio, A. (2000). Analgesic effect of intravenous ketamine in cancer patients on morphine therapy: A randomized, controlled, double-blind, crossover, double-dose study. *Journal of Pain and Symptom Management, 20*(4), 246–252.

Moulin, D. E., Clark, A. J., Gilron, I., Ware, M. A., Watson, C. P., Sessle, B. J., . . . Canadian Pain Society. (2007). Pharmacological management of chronic neuropathic pain—consensus statement and guidelines from the Canadian Pain Society. *Pain Research & Management, 12*(1), 13–21.

Patorno, E., Bohn, R. L., Wahl, P. M., Avorn, J., Patrick, A. R., Liu, J., & Schneeweiss, S. (2010). Anticonvulsant medications and the risk of suicide, attempted suicide, or violent death. *Journal of the American Medical Association, 303*(14), 1401–1409.

Schneeweiss, S., Patrick, A. R., Solomon, D. H., Dormuth, C. R., Miller, M., Mehta, J., . . . Wang P. S. (2010). Comparative safety of antidepressant agents for children and adolescents regarding suicidal acts. *Pediatrics, 125*(5), 876–888.

Stinson, J., & Bruce, E. (2009). Chronic pain in children. In A. Twycross, S. J. Dowden, & E. Bruce (Eds.), *Managing pain in children: A clinical guide* (pp. 145–170). Oxford, United Kingdom: Wiley-Blackwell.

Subramaniam, K., Subramaniam, B., & Steinbrook, R. A. (2004). Ketamine as adjuvant analgesic to opioids: A quantitative and qualitative systematic review. *Anesthesia & Analgesia, 99*(2), 482–495.

Tiippana, E. M., Hamunen, K., Kontinen, V. K., & Kalso, E. (2007). Do surgical patients benefit from perioperative gabapentin/pregabalin? A systematic review of efficacy and safety. *Anesthesia & Analgesia, 104*(6), 1545–1556.

III

Regional Analgesia

6

Epidural Infusions

Neuraxial analgesia is the administration of medications into the epidural or intrathecal space to prevent the transmission of pain messages sent by the nerves to the brain. Providing a more targeted analgesia delivery, adverse effects of opioids associated with systemic delivery are reduced, potentially providing more effective analgesia compared with other routes (American Society of Anesthesiologists [ASA], 2004). However, these methods are not without risk and need to be managed by suitably trained and experienced staff to minimize complications.

This chapter will describe epidural analgesia. An extensive body of literature confirms that these approaches can be applied with excellent safety and efficacy for infants and children and can improve the course of postoperative recovery for many types of surgery (Berde et al., 2005; Greco & Berde, 2005; Jylli, Lundeberg, & Olsson, 2002). Discussion of providing analgesia to peripheral nerve plexus is found in Chapter 7. For the use of intrathecal catheters, refer to the available literature. The use of this method of neuraxial analgesia in pediatrics is limited.

The epidural space is between the dura mater and the vertebral canal, extending from the cranium to the sacrum and containing loose connective tissue, fat, lymph vessels, blood vessels, and nerves (see Figure 6.1). An epidural catheter has the (theoretical) advantage of having the dura as a natural barrier, preventing the spread of an infection to the spinal cord. Medications injected or infused into the epidural space diffuse across the dura and the subarachnoid space and bind to receptors in the dorsal horn of the spinal cord. Some degree of systemic absorption of medications, especially those that

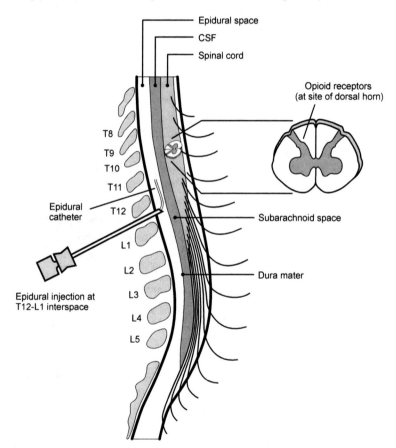

Figure 6.1 ■ Epidural needle and catheter placement. Delivery of analgesia by a catheter inserted into the epidural space.
From "Opioid Analgesics," by C. Pasero, R. K. Portenoy, and M. McCaffery, 1999. In M. McCaffery & C. Pasero (Eds.), *Pain: Clinical Manual*, 2nd ed., pp. 161–299. Used with permission from Elsevier.

are lipophilic, can occur via the epidural blood vessels. The catheter is inserted into the epidural space as close as possible to the dermatomes involved in the surgical procedure or painful area, usually between the lumbar (L3) and the thoracic (T3) area. In small infants, the catheter may be placed caudally via the sacrococcygeal membrane and threaded up the epidural space until the appropriate level has been reached (Sethna & Suresh, 2007).

Placement of the epidural catheter and ongoing medical direction of the epidural catheter are done by those trained in anesthesiology. Percutaneous catheters are usually placed for short-term use (several days), with tunneled catheters for long-term epidural analgesia.

INDICATIONS

Postoperative Pain

Epidural analgesia is provided for control of postoperative pain associated with thoracic, major abdominal, urologic, or lower extremity orthopedic surgical procedures for infants, children, and adolescents (Aram, Krane, Kozloski, & Yaster, 2001; Jylli et al., 2002).

Management of Pain Unresponsive to Parenteral and Enteral Opioids

Placement of an epidural catheter to control cancer-related pain below the T4 dermatome (nipple line) can be considered when systemic routes of analgesia no longer provide pain relief without intolerable adverse effects (e.g., opioid-induced sedation and respiratory depression) (Aram et al., 2001).

MEDICATIONS

Opioids and local anesthetics (LAs) are usually administered as epidural infusions, often as a combination to provide synergistic analgesic effects, minimizing the risk of opioid-related adverse effects as discussed later in this chapter (Desparmet, Hardart, & Yaster, 2003; Dowden, 2009; Verghese & Hannallah, 2005). When a continuous epidural infusion is not indicated, either the LA, preservative-free morphine (Duramorph), or a lipid-encapsulated morphine preparation (DepoDur) can be given as a single injection (commonly called a "one shot") into the epidural space. The resulting analgesia effect lasts for 12 to 24 hours and requires at least a 12-hour observation period for respiratory depression (American Pain Society [APS], 2008).

Local Anesthetics

▦ *Bupivacaine (Marcaine)*

The usual concentration for the infusion is 0.1% (1 mg/ml) to 0.125% (1.25 mg/ml). The maximum dose for patients 6 months or older is 0.4 mg/kg/hr (Berde et al., 2005). Higher doses can be given with careful consideration of risk versus benefits and monitoring for adverse effects. However, because of delayed clearance in infants less than 6 months old, infusions should be no greater than 0.2 mg/kg/hr, and the infusion should be limited to less than 72 hours (Berde et al., 2005).

Opioids

One major consideration in the choice of opioid in the epidural infusion is determining the need or avoidance of having the opioid spread away from the catheter tip. Hydrophilic opioids, such as morphine and hydromorphone hydrochloride (Dilaudid), remain longer in the cerebrospinal fluid (CSF) than lipophilic opioids, such as fentanyl (Sublimaze), with more opportunity for rostral spread increasing the risk of suppression in the respiratory center of the brain. Lipophilic opioids are readily absorbed by the epidural blood vessels with some risk of systemic adverse effects and shorter duration of action but offer the advantage of less rostral spread with less risk of respiratory depression. When the catheter tip is at the dermatome level covering the surgical incision, fentanyl is usually the opioid of choice. However, when the incision is above the catheter tip, hydromorphone may be chosen with the expectation of some beneficial rostal spread to the painful area.

▓ *Fentanyl*

The maximum initial dose is 0.05 mg/kg. The usual concentration in the infusion is 2 to 5 mcg/ml and infused with a maximum recommended hourly rate of 1 mcg/kg/hr (Desparmet et al., 2003).

▓ *Hydromorphone*

The maximum initial dose is 1 mcg/kg/bolus. The usual concentration in the infusion is 5 to 10 mcg/ml at a maximum recommended rate of 4 mcg/kg/hr (Desparmet et al., 2003).

▓ *Morphine*

The usual concentration in the infusion is 10 to 50 mcg/ml infused initially at 4 mcg/kg/hr with a maximum recommended rate of 12 mcg/kg/hr (Desparmet et al., 2003).

Clonidine (Catapres)

Opioids and clonidine act on receptors involved in pain transmission in the spinal dorsal horn providing markedly synergistic analgesia when combined with dilute LA infusions. By using the combination of LA with opioid *and* clonidine, the amount of opioid in the infusion can be reduced with minimal loss of efficacy, along with potentially less incidence of adverse effects of epidural opioids (e.g., respiratory depression, pruritus, and nausea) (Cucchiaro, Adzick, Rose, Maxwell, & Watcha, 2006; De Negri, Ivani, Visconti, & De Vivo, 2001) or LAs (i.e., motor block) (Berde et al., 2005; Cucchiaro et al., 2006). However, epidural administration of clonidine does carry some risk of hypotension and excessive sedation. Because of limited safety data available, epidural clonidine is not advisable in infants younger than 1 year (Sethna & Suresh, 2007).

Dosage. For children 1 year or older, the usual concentration of clonidine is 0.4 mcg/ml at a maximum rate of 0.5 mcg/kg/hr (Berde et al., 2005; Sethna & Suresh, 2007) while observing for undesired hemodynamic effects or sedation.

ONGOING MONITORING AND CARE

Clinically significant central nervous system (CNS) or respiratory depression can be avoided by slow titration, careful monitoring of sedation levels and respiratory status, and dose modifications when increased sedation is detected (Ingelmo et al., 2007; Oakes, 2008; Pasero, Eksterowicz, Primeau, & Cowley, 2007).

Recommended assessments for the duration of the epidural infusion (Dowden, 2009; Ingelmo et al., 2007; Kraemer & Rose, 2009) include the following:

- Pain intensity score every 4 hours while awake using an age-appropriate, validated pediatric scale
- Sedation score every 1 to 2 hours
- Respiratory rate and heart rate every 1 to 2 hours
- Continuous oxygen saturation
- Blood pressure every 4 hours
- Motor function (i.e., hip or knee flexion every 4 hours while awake)
- Tubing and dressing as intact every 4 hours while awake
- Insertion site for redness, tenderness, or leakage as well as for possible catheter migration by comparing the number of exposed catheter marks to the previous assessment once a shift

---

Clinical Pearl

Vigilance is required to identify signs and provide immediate management for rare but serious complications, such as epidural hematoma or abscess (Dowden, 2009; Oakes, 2008; Pasero et al., 2007):

- Severe back pain
- Significant changes in motor function
- Reduced motor function of hands and digits with a thoracic catheter
- High sensory block (above dermatome T3)
- Fever >38.5°C
- Signs of local infection at the epidural entry site (erythema or discharge)

Assessing Sensory Block

The goal is to provide optimal sensory block with minimal effect on the motor nerves, conserving the children's ability to ambulate and perform all routine recovery activities to the extent of their medical or surgical condition. Because sensory nerve fibers respond similarly to pain and temperature changes, the level of sensory block is assessed with a cold stimulus to determine the highest dermatome to ensure that the coverage is not so extensive as to increase the risk of respiratory depression as follows (Dowden, 2009):

- Explain to the child and parent, when the cold object (i.e., ice or alcohol swab) touches his skin, he will be asked, "Do you feel something cold, warm, or the same on your skin?"
- The first touch needs to be on an area well away from the possible dermatome level (e.g., face or forearm) to determine that the child understands the process.
- Next, apply the touch to an area well below the possible dermatome level and ask the same question again, expecting the response to be that he does not feel the cold object.
- Repeat the process on the opposite side of the body (blocks may be uneven or unilateral).
- Document the blocked dermatomes (upper and lower margins) using a dermatome chart (see Figure 6.2). Example: "T8-L2, L = R"; or for uneven blocks: L: T9-L3, R: T7-L4.
- For nonverbal children, using the same process and observing for flinching or facial expression changes when the cold object is felt may be useful.

Consider increasing the infusion if the sensory block is lower than T3 and the pain is unrelieved.

Skin breakdown in pressure-exposed areas is possible because children have decreased sensation, prompting them to voluntarily reposition themselves. Consider use of a pressure-relieving mattress for children at significant risk for skin breakdown.

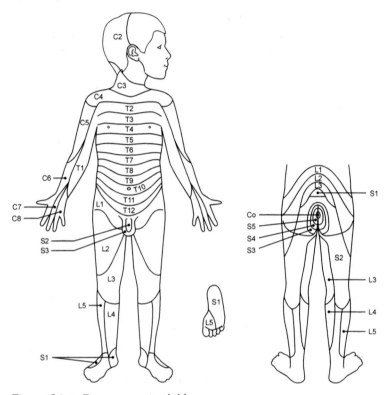

Figure 6.2 ▨ Dermatomes in children.
From "Managing Acute Pain in Children," by S. J. Dowden, 2009. In A.
Twycross, S. J. Dowden, & E. Bruce (Eds.), *Managing Pain in Children: A
Clinical Guide*, pp. 109–144. Used with permission from Wiley-Blackwell.

Assessing Motor Block

Because motor nerves as well as sensory nerves may be affected by
local anesthetics, patients are to be assessed for the following:

▨ Weakness of the lower limbs. If present, assistance will be required during ambulation. Assess for orthostatic hypotension before ambulation.
▨ Ability to flex the knees and hips every 4 hours. For young children,
ask them to move their feet (Oakes, 2008). Document the assessment indicating differences in the right versus the left, if not equal.

Numbness, "heaviness," and motor weakness may be quite distressing and frightening to children and may indicate the need to reduce the dose of the LA. Reduction in the concentration of the LA or removing all LAs from the infusion may be required to improve motor function.

Inadequate Analgesia

Unrelieved pain may occur from incorrect placement of the catheter relative to the site of pain, disruption of the infusion system (e.g., kinking or obstruction), or catheter migration or dislodgement from the original placement location, requiring the need to:

- Check the catheter site to determine placement of the catheter is consistent with previous markings, indicating migration has not occurred since the last assessment.
- Check the infusion system to rule out that any kinks or clamps could be preventing the infusion and to be certain that the pump is functioning properly. If no source is found, contact the anesthesia staff for further direction, including the need for an alternative dose of systemic analgesia.
- Consider increasing the infusion rate or providing an epidural bolus if the maximum dose has not been achieved.
- Provide systemic analgesics (e.g., opioids or nonsteroidal anti-inflammatory drugs [NSAIDs]), if safely appropriate.

> *Clinical Pearl*
>
> The use of systemic opioids along with epidural infusions, especially if the epidural infusion also includes an opioid, significantly increases the risk of opioid-induced sedation and respiratory depression and is controversial (Sethna & Suresh, 2007). However, it may be appropriate for patients who require opioid therapy prior to surgery, have significant pain within the surgical site in which multimodal therapy using NSAIDs is contraindicated, or have pain outside the coverage of the epidural infusion (Anghelescu, Ross, Oakes, & Burgoyne, 2008).

Leaking at the Epidural Site

A small amount of serosanguineous drainage is expected because of back pressure out of the exit tract around the catheter. If pain control is adequate, indicating the catheter is still in position and infusing into the epidural space, the health care provider is to reinforce the dressing and reassess the leakage every 4 hours. However, if the patient is complaining of increased pain, the health care provider is to contact the anesthesia staff for further direction.

Disconnection of the Catheter at the Junction of the Catheter Adapter

Wrap the free end of the catheter and maintain the infusion system with as much sterility as possible. Contact the anesthesia staff for further direction, which will require consideration of the risks versus benefits for reconnecting and restarting the epidural infusion. Reconnecting the catheter to a sterile infusion system will require cleaning the catheter, cutting with sterile scissors and reapplying a new catheter adapter (see Figure 6.3).

Urinary Retention

The delivery of LAs and opioids close to the micturition center of the spinal cord relaxes the detrusor muscle, interfering with sphincter tone. The central effects of opioids and sensory blockade of the anesthetics can interfere with perception of bladder fullness and the child's attention to bladder distension. Patients with lumbar epidural infusions are at increased risk, especially if opioids are included in the infusion. Therefore, most patients will require an indwelling Foley catheter during the epidural infusion.

PATIENT-CONTROLLED EPIDURAL ANALGESIA

Patient-controlled epidural analgesia (PCEA) allows older children to effectively provide additional boluses needed to supplement a

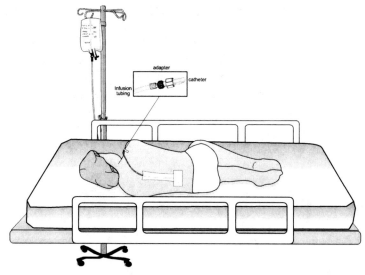

Figure 6.3 ■ Epidural catheter and infusion system.
From "Epidural Catheter: Care and Management," by L. Oakes, 2008. In J.
Verger & R. Lebet (Eds.), *AACN Procedure Manual for Pediatric Acute and
Critical Care,* pp. 1243–1254. Used with permission from Elsevier.

superimposed continuous epidural maintenance infusion (Antok
et al., 2003; Birmingham et al., 2003; Gauger et al., 2009). PCEA,
particularly fentanyl, because of its rapid onset of analgesia, doses
may be of particular benefit for predictable episodes of incident
pain, such as getting out of bed, physical therapy, or dressing
changes. The child is to be the only one authorized to use the PCEA
button, except for home use in terminally ill children who are de-
bilitated and have a parent who can be taught appropriate use of
epidural boluses. PCEA boluses are usually available every 15 minutes with a maximum of only two boluses per hour. Prescribing the
infusion dose within the maximum limits for the local anesthetic
should be done with the assumption that the patient will use two
boluses per hour.

COMPLICATIONS

Drug-Related Problems

Only preservative-free solutions that have been approved for intraspinal use are to be infused to prevent local damage to the spinal cord. Catheters, IV tubing without rubber injection ports, and pumps that are distinctive for epidural infusions (i.e., color coded and boldly labeled) are recommended to prevent accidental introduction of unintended medications into the epidural space. Strict attention to drug concentrations and infusion rates to avoid toxic dose of medications is necessary. Health care providers are never to flush the catheter with saline or heparin.

Overdose/Toxicity of Local Anesthetics

Vascular uptake or injection of the LA directly into the systemic circulation can result in serious adverse reactions related to high blood levels of LAs. Injecting or infusing LAs into the intrathecal space will lead to progressive loss of sensory and motor function of the legs, trunk, and chest.

Symptoms. A continuum of toxic effects exists and depends on the rapidity of rise and the total plasma concentration achieved after the drug is administered, with CNS and cardiovascular symptoms. The occasional occurrence of minor temporary numbness or motor block of the affected extremities is usually resolved easily by decreasing the dose or removing the local anesthetic from the epidural analgesia solution. Other milder CNS effects may occur at lower plasma levels, such as tinnitus, light-headedness, dizziness, blurred vision, decreased ability to hear, restlessness, and tremors. More significant toxicity with higher plasma levels includes hypotension, bradycardia and other dysrhythmias, seizures, sudden loss of consciousness, and sympathetic blockade leading to cardiovascular collapse.

Interventions. Stop the epidural infusion, place the child in a supine position, notify the anesthesia service, and provide IV fluid bolus (10 ml/kg; Dowden, 2009).

Prevention. Before injecting a bolus or initiating the infusion, the nurse is to gently aspirate the catheter. If other than a scant (<1 ml) of clear liquid is aspirated, the nurse must collaborate with the anesthesia staff before administering the bolus or continuing the infusion. A return of free-flowing clear fluid (CSF) into the syringe indicates that the catheter may be in the subarachnoid space. Free-flowing blood aspirated into the syringe indicates that the catheter may be in a blood vessel.

Overdose/Toxicity of Opioids

Symptoms. Excessive sedation and respiratory depression will occur.

Interventions. Stop the epidural infusion, notify the anesthesia team, stimulate the patient and ask him to breathe, establish a patent airway, and provide 100% oxygen. Consider the need to administer naloxone (Narcan; see Chapter 4). Once vital signs and level of consciousness have returned to baseline, consider restarting the infusion at 50% of the previous rate (Ingelmo et al., 2007). Orders for any systemic medication that could add sedative effects (e.g., benzodiazepines or antihistamines) must include the input of the anesthesia or pain service staff.

Pruritus

Because of the opioid in the epidural infusion, itching is most frequently reported if fentanyl is at a rate of more than 1 mcg/kg/hr (Oakes, 2008). However, it may also be related to systemically administered opioids.

Interventions. Administering an antihistamine or removing the opioid from the epidural infusion may be necessary. (See Chapter 4 for the treatment of pruritus.)

Catheter-Related Problems

Epidural Hematoma

Puncture of epidural blood vessels during the placement of the epidural catheter leading to the formation of an epidural hematoma is a rare complication.

Symptoms. Patients report escalating, severe back pain with sensory deficits and dense motor block. Radicular pain, paraplegia, and urinary and fecal retention or incontinence prompt the need for urgent neurosurgical evaluation to avoid the risk of nerve compression, ischemia, and permanent neurological damage.

Interventions. Obtain complete blood counts and coagulation studies, radiological imaging (CT/MRI), and a neurosurgical consultation. Surgical removal of the hematoma may be required.

Prevention. Careful screening of candidates for epidural catheter use should include establishing a minimum platelet count for insertion (i.e., 100,000 mm^3) and ensuring that coagulation test results are in the normal range before placement. Coordination of the need for any anticoagulants is essential, usually avoiding administration during the placement or withdrawal of the epidural catheter (Horlocker et al., 2010).

Epidural Abscess

Infection of the epidural space is a very rare but serious complication, especially if it leads to formation of an epidural abscess. This complication is thought to be more common when epidural catheters are left in place for a prolonged time, such as to treat chronic pain, and associated with poor aseptic technique or migration of skin infections at the insertion site.

Symptoms. Early signs and symptoms can be difficult to detect because external signs of infection and fever may not be present.

Continued motor deficits along with moderate to severe back pain with localized tenderness, radicular pain, malaise, and paraplegia, and urinary and fecal retention or incontinence prompt the need for urgent neurosurgical evaluation to avoid the risk of nerve compression, ischemia, and permanent neurological damage.

Interventions. Laboratory and diagnostic work-up includes a complete blood count, blood cultures, radiological imaging (CT/MRI), and a neurosurgical consultation. Treatment ranges from antibiotics to surgical removal of the abscess.

Prevention. Limiting the duration of the catheter to 72 hours as well as meticulous aseptic technique minimizes the risk of this complication (Aram et al., 2001).

Catheter Shearage or Breakage

Prevention. At the time of catheter removal, apply gentle traction and avoid excessive force. The catheter should come out easily and painlessly with the tip of the catheter intact. If the catheter breaks during removal and a small piece remains in the patient, observation is required to determine the need for surgical removal which is necessary only in the rare complication such as infection.

Postdural Puncture Headache

Patients may complain of headaches, which may be caused by the insertion needle puncturing the dura and subsequent leakage of CSF (Dowden, 2009).

Symptoms. The child may not complain of the headache until he becomes upright.

Intervention. Relief of the headache is best achieved by analgesics, bed rest, fluids, and caffeine. An epidural autologous blood patch may be considered for prolonged headaches.

LONG-TERM USE OF EPIDURAL INFUSIONS

Even for skilled health care providers in pain management taking care of children with challenging sources of pain, some patients, such as those with progressive cancer causing painful nerve compression, will not have their pain satisfactorily relieved without systemic side effects from conventional analgesics described in previous chapters. Therefore, neuraxial techniques may be required, including epidural infusions for weeks to months. The maximum length of time to avoid serious systemic infections is not known. Using a catheter normally for percutaneous use but tunneling a segment in the subcutaneous tissue may decrease unintended dislodgement and at least theoretically provide additional protection against colonization, much like it does for central lines. One retrospective series of pediatric experience of the use of tunneled epidural catheters indicated significant benefit with a substantial reduction in pain and minimizing the need for supplemental systemic opioids (Aram et al., 2001).

In summary, the short-term use of epidural analgesia has proved to be an attractive option in providing pain control for postoperative pain involving thoracic, abdominal, and lower extremity locations. For severe pain below the T4 dermatome and not responding to conventional analgesic regimens, the same principles for postoperative epidural analgesia can offer relief of suffering for hospitalized children, and when appropriate, may be continued in the home setting.

REFERENCES

American Pain Society. (2008). *Principles of analgesic use in the treatment of acute pain and cancer pain*. Glenview, IL: Author.

American Society of Anesthesiologists. (2004). Practice guidelines for acute pain management in the perioperative setting: An updated report by the American Society of Anesthesiologists Task Force on Acute Pain Management. *Anesthesiology, 100*(6), 1573–1581.

Anghelescu, D. L., Ross, C. E., Oakes, L. L., & Burgoyne, L. L. (2008). The safety of concurrent administration of opioids via epidural and intravenous routes for postoperative pain in pediatric oncology patients. *Journal of Pain and Symptom Management, 35*(4), 412–419.

Antok, E., Bordet, F., Duflo, F., Lansiaux, S., Combet, S., Taylor, P., . . . Chassard, D. (2003). Patient-controlled epidural analgesia versus continuous epidural infusion with ropivacaine for postoperative analgesia in children. *Anesthesia and Analgesia, 97*(6), 1608–1611.

Aram, L., Krane, E. J., Kozloski, L. J., & Yaster, M. (2001). Tunneled epidural catheters for prolonged analgesia in pediatric patients. *Anesthesia and Analgesia, 92*(6), 1432–1438.

Berde, C. B., Jaksic, T., Lynn, A. M., Maxwell, L. G., Soriano, S. G., & Tibboel, D. (2005). Anesthesia and analgesia during and after surgery in neonates. *Clinical Therapeutics, 27*(6), 900–921.

Birmingham, P. K., Wheeler, M., Suresh, S., Dsida, R. M., Rae, B. R., Obrecht, J., . . . Coté, C. J. (2003). Patient-controlled epidural analgesia in children: Can they do it? *Anesthesia and Analgesia, 96*(3), 686–691.

Cucchiaro, G., Adzick, S. N., Rose, J. B., Maxwell, L., & Watcha, M. (2006). A comparison of epidural bupivacaine-fentanyl and bupivacaine-clonidine in children undergoing the Nuss procedure. *Anesthesia and Analgesia, 103*(2), 322–327.

De Negri, P., Ivani, G., Visconti, C., & De Vivo, P. (2001). How to prolong postoperative analgesia after caudal anaesthesia with ropivacaine in children: S-ketamine versus clonidine. *Paediatric Anaesthesia, 11*(6), 679–683.

Desparmet, J. F., Hardart, R. A., & Yaster, M. (2003). Central blocks in children and adolescents. In N. L. Schechter, C. B. Berde, & M. Yaster (Eds.), *Pain in infants, children, and adolescents* (2nd ed., pp. 339–359). Philadelphia, PA: Lippincott Williams & Wilkins.

Dowden, S. J. (2009). Managing acute pain in children. In A. Twycross, S. J. Dowden, & E. Bruce (Eds.), *Managing pain in children: A clinical guide* (pp. 109–144). Oxford, United Kingdom: Wiley-Blackwell.

Gauger, V. T., Voepel-Lewis, T. D., Burke, C. N., Kostrzewa, A. J., Caird, M. S., Wagner, D. S., & Farley, F. A. (2009). Epidural analgesia compared with intravenous analgesia after pediatric posterior spinal fusion. *Journal of Pediatric Orthopaedics, 29*(6), 588–593.

Greco, C., & Berde, C. (2005). Pain management for the hospitalized pediatric patient. *Pediatric Clinics of North America, 52*(4), 995–1027.

Horlocker, T. T., Wedel, D. J., Rowlingson, J. C., Enneking, F. K., Kopp, S. L., Benzon, H. T., . . . Yuan, C. S. (2010). Regional anesthesia in the patient receiving antithrombotic or thrombolytic therapy: American Society of Regional Anesthesia and Pain Medicine Evidence-Based Guidelines (Third Edition). *Regional Anesthesia and Pain Medicine, 35*(1), 64–101.

Ingelmo, P. M., Gelsumino, C., Acosta, A. P., Lopez, V., Gimenez, C., Halac, A., . . . Fumagalli, R. (2007). Epidural analgesia in children: Planning, organization, and development of a new program. *Minerva Anestesiologica, 73*(11), 575–585.

Jylli, L., Lundeberg, S., & Olsson, G. L. (2002). Retrospective evaluation of continuous epidural infusion for postoperative pain in children. *Acta Anaesthesiologica Scandinavica, 46*(6), 654–659.

Kraemer, F. W., & Rose, J. B. (2009). Pharmacologic management of acute pediatric pain. *Anesthesiology Clinics, 27*(2), 241–268.

Oakes, L. (2008). Epidural catheter: Care and management. In J. Verger & R. Lebet (Eds.), *AACN procedure manual for pediatric acute and critical care* (pp. 1243–1254). St. Louis, MO: Saunders Elsevier.

Pasero, C., Eksterowicz, N., Primeau, M., & Cowley, C. (2007). Registered nurse management and monitoring of analgesia by catheter techniques: Position statement. *Pain Management Nursing, 8*(2), 48–54.

Pasero, C., Portenoy, R. K., & McCaffery, M. (1999). Opioid analgesics. In M. McCaffery & C. Pasero (Eds.), *Pain: Clinical manual* (2nd ed., pp. 161–299). St Louis, MO: Mosby.

Sethna, N. F., & Suresh, S. (2007). Central and peripheral regional analgesia and anaesthesia. In K. J. Anand, B. Stevens, & P. J. McGrath (Eds.), *Pain research and clinical management. Pain in neonates and infants* (3rd ed., pp. 155–176). Edinburgh, United Kingdom: Elsevier.

Verghese, S. T., & Hannallah, R. S. (2005). Postoperative pain management in children. *Anesthesiology Clinics of North America, 23*(1), 163–184.

7

Continuous Peripheral Nerve Block Infusions

By selectively blocking peripheral nerve plexuses, continuous peripheral nerve block infusions (CPNBIs) have emerged as a safe and effective technique useful for pain control in adult patients undergoing orthopedic surgery (Greco & Berde, 2005; Ilfeld, Morey, & Enneking, 2002; Ilfeld, Morey, Wright, Chidgey, & Enneking, 2003). More recently, anesthesiologists have provided CPNBIs for children as well (Brislin & Rose, 2005; Dadure et al., 2009; Ludot et al., 2008). Administration of local anesthetics (LAs) can be done as a "single shot" or continuous infusion via percutaneously placed catheters as part of a balanced pain management strategy aimed at reducing the need for opioid therapy. Although opioids are not infused via CPNBI, clonidine (Catapres) can be added to the infusion to increase the level and duration of nerve blockade usually without perceptible hemodynamic effects in children (Dalen, 2003; Greco & Berde, 2005).

Placement and the management of the perineural catheter need to be provided by an anesthesiologist who has been trained in providing the appropriate block for each surgical procedure. For the upper extremities, specific blocks are usually provided as follows:

- Shoulder/arm/elbow: interscalene, infraclavicular, or supraclavicular block
- Elbow/forearm: infraclavicular block
- Forearm/hand: axillary block

For the lower extremities (see Figure 7.1), specific blocks are usually provided as follows:

- Anterior thigh/knee: femoral block
- Ankle/foot: ankle block
- Posterior thigh/ knee except saphenous area: sciatic block
- Hip/anterior thigh/knee: lumbar plexus block
- Complete unilateral lower extremity blockade: lumbar plexus and sciatic block

Placement of nerve block catheters usually requires the patient to be awake to assist in confirmation of the optimal site by confirming pain relief; however, children are usually anesthetized during placement of catheters, thus requiring another means of confirming placement, including the use of nerve stimulators, and ultrasound guidance of regional anesthetic blockade (Greco & Berde, 2005). These techniques have evolved as improvements in equipment, needle and catheter sets, pumps, and local anesthetic medications have occurred. Percutaneous catheters are usually placed for short-term use (several days). Infusions usually do not exceed 12 ml/hr for patients less than 50 kg or 20 ml/hr for patients more than 50 kg. Advantages of this neuraxial method of managing pain compared with epidural analgesia include the following:

- Less systemic effects of medications, including less cardiovascular effects (e.g., hypotension) and no opioid-associated adverse reactions, unless administered systemically
- No motor block of unaffected extremity
- Ability to provide analgesia for levels above dermatome T4 (e.g., shoulders and arms)
- Less significant potential complications (e.g., no risk of epidural hematoma)
- Less incidence of urinary retention (may be associated with femoral CPNBI)

Until recently, use of CPNBIs was restricted to inpatient care. However, use of the CPNBI in the outpatient setting for adults (Enneking & Ilfeld, 2002) and children (Brislin & Rose, 2005; Dadure et al., 2003) has revealed few complications, allowing early discharge

Lumbar Plexus Block = all areas except Sciatic (below the knee)

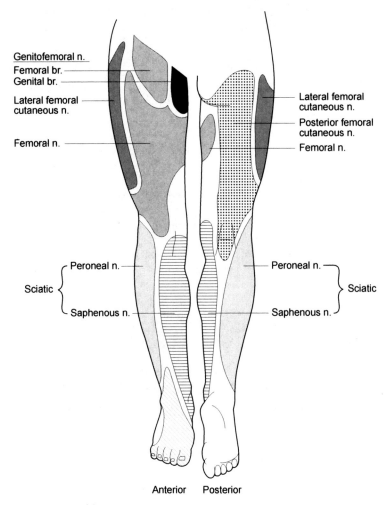

Figure 7.1 ▧ Nerve anatomy.
Adapted from *Atlas of Regional Anesthesia*, by D. L. Brown, 1992,
Philadelphia, PA: W. B. Saunders. Used with permission from Elsevier.

from the hospital (Ganesh et al., 2007). The development of disposable elastomeric balloon-type infusion devices has facilitated outpatient use of CPNBI (Dadure et al., 2003).

Clinical Pearl   Considerations regarding use of nerve block infusions for outpatient setting (Enneking & Ilfeld, 2002; Ganesh et al., 2007) include the following:

▪ Surgery is of such extent that pain is unlikely to be controlled by oral analgesics without unacceptable side effects.
▪ The patient and/or parent must be able to understand and follow instructions.
▪ Telephone communication must be available at all times to the prescriber.
▪ Communication with administering physician must occur at least every 24 hours.
▪ Patients with nerve block infusions must be able to demonstrate safe ambulation with or without an aid prior to discharge.

INDICATIONS

Postoperative Pain

CPNBI has successfully provided pain control for various orthopedic surgeries, including joint arthroplasty and replacements, amputation, and end-block resection of bone tumors.

Management of Pain Unresponsive to Parenteral and Enteral Opioids

Use of CPNBIs to control cancer-related pain can be considered when systemic routes of analgesia no longer provide pain relief without intolerable adverse effects (i.e., opioid-induced sedation and respiratory depression; Aram, Krane, Kozloski, & Yaster, 2001), such as for pathological fractures or tumor-related pain.

MEDICATIONS

Two preservative-free solutions are available for CPNBIs, both offering a similar degree of analgesia. Administrating LAs to reduce pain by blocking the sensory nerves with minimal motor nerve effects provides effective analgesia for the child to ambulate and begin any rehabilitation activities. No conclusive studies have been done to determine the exact dose of LAs needed to provide an adequate peripheral nerve block in infants and children. Dosage recommendations are based on what is currently known about the potential avoidance of adverse reactions to LA in infants and children.

Local Anesthetics

▦ *Ropivacaine (Naropin)*

The usual concentration for the infusion is from 0.1% (1 mg/ml) to 0.2% (2 mg/ml). The maximum dose for patients 6 months of age or older is from 0.4 to 0.5 mg/kg/hr to avoid toxicity (Dadure et al., 2003; Yaster, Tobin, & Kost-Byerly, 2003). Compared with bupivacaine, ropivacaine is associated with less motor block and hypotension (Enneking & Ilfeld, 2002; Ganesh et al., 2007; Kraemer & Rose, 2009).

▦ *Bupivacaine (Marcaine)*

The usual concentration for the infusion is from 0.125% (1.25 mg/ml) to 0.25% (2.5 mg/ml). The maximum dose for patients 6 months of age or older is 0.4 mg/kg/hr (Dalen, 2003). Larger doses can be given with careful consideration of risk versus benefits and monitoring for adverse effects.

Clonidine (Catapres)

The infusion is prepared with a concentration of 4 mcg/ml to infuse at a maximum dose usually not more than 1 mcg/kg/hr to improve analgesia but may also increase the incidence of motor block (Greco & Berde, 2005; Kraemer & Rose, 2009).

ONGOING MONITORING AND CARE

Recommended assessments for the duration of the CPNBI include the following:

- Pain intensity should be scored every 4 hours while awake (when inpatient) and with each clinic visit.
- Motor assessment of the affected limb should occur every 4 hours while awake (when inpatient) and with each clinic visit. Notify the anesthesia staff of any significant reduction in motor strength.
- The tubing and dressing should be intact with the pump infusing at the prescribed settings.
- The insertion site should be assessed for redness, tenderness, or leakage as well as for possible catheter migration by comparing the number of exposed catheter marks to the previous assessment once a shift.

Assessing Sensory Block

Mild paresthesias of the affected limb are to be expected.

Assessing Motor Block

Because motor nerves as well as sensory nerves may be affected by local anesthetics, patients are to be assessed for any reduced strength of unaffected limbs. If the CPNBI is provided in a lower limb, ambulation must be assisted. Patients with brachial or interscalene plexus block may have Horner's syndrome or unilateral vocal cord paralysis (hoarseness). Numbness, "heaviness," and motor weakness may be quite distressing and frightening to children and may indicate the need to reduce the dose of the LA. Reduction in the concentration or rate of the LA may be required to improve motor function.

Inadequate Analgesia

Assess and document the patient's pain level every 4 hours if inpatient and with each clinic visit if outpatient. Notify the anesthesia staff for unsatisfactory pain relief or any disturbing symptoms, such as paresthesia or profound motor block. Patients will likely need supplemental analgesics as well as the CPNBI.

Unrelieved pain may occur from incorrect placement of the catheter relative to the site of pain as well as disruption of the infusion system (i.e., kinking, obstruction), and catheter migration or dislodgement from the original placement location requiring the following:

- Check the catheter site to determine placement of the catheter is consistent with previous markings, indicating migration has not occurred since last assessment.
- Check the infusions system to rule out any kinks or clamps that could be preventing the infusion and the pump from functioning properly. If no source is found, contact the anesthesia staff for further direction, including the need for an alternate dose of systemic analgesia.
- Consider increasing the infusion rate and/or provide a bolus if the maximum dose has not been achieved.

Leaking at the Insertion Site

A small amount of serosanguineous drainage is expected because of back pressure out of the exit tract around the catheter. If pain control is adequate, indicating the catheter is still in position, the health care provider is to reinforce the dressing and reassess the leakage every 4 hours. However, if the patient is complaining of increased pain, the health care provider is to contact the anesthesia staff for further direction.

Disconnection of the Catheter at the Junction of the Catheter Adapter

Wrap the free end of the catheter and maintain the infusion system with as much sterility as possible. Contact the anesthesia staff for further direction that will require consideration of the risks versus benefits for reconnecting and restarting the CPNBI. Reconnecting the catheter to a sterile infusion system will require cleaning the catheter, cutting with sterile scissors, and reapplying a new catheter adapter.

COMPLICATIONS
Drug-Related Problems

Only preservative-free solutions that have been approved for intraspinal use are to be infused to prevent local damage to the nerve plexus. Catheters, IV tubing without rubber injection ports, and pumps that are distinctive for CPNBI (i.e., color coded and boldly labeled) are recommended to prevent accidental introduction of unintended medications into the nerve plexus. Strict attention to drug concentration and infusion rates to avoid toxic dose of medications is necessary. Health care providers are never to flush the catheter with saline or heparin.

Overdose/Toxicity of Local Anesthetics

Vascular uptake or injection of the LA directly into the systemic circulation can result in adverse reactions related to high blood levels of LAs.

Symptoms. Milder CNS effects may occur at lower plasma levels, such as tinnitus, metallic taste, light-headedness, dizziness, blurred vision, decreased ability to hear, restlessness, and tremors. More significant toxicity may occur with higher plasma levels, including hypotension, bradycardia and other dysrhythmias, seizures, sudden loss of consciousness, and sympathetic blockade leading to cardiovascular collapse.

Interventions. Stop the CPNBI, place the child in a supine position, notify the anesthesia service, and provide IV fluid bolus (10 ml/kg; Dowden, 2009).

Prevention. Before initiating the infusion, the nurse is to gently aspirate the catheter. If other than a scant (less than 1 ml) of clear liquid is aspirated, the nurse must collaborate with the anesthesia staff before administering the bolus or continuing the infusion. Free-flowing blood aspirated into the syringe indicates that the catheter may be in a blood vessel and the infusion of LA should be stopped immediately.

Catheter-Related Problems

Infection

Infection from CPNBIs are rare but more likely from femoral catheters (Ganesh et al., 2007).

Interventions. Notify the anesthesia staff if the child has fever or any signs of infection at the insertion site of the CPNBI.

Nerve Damage

Needle- or catheter-induced nerve injury is rare and usually transient (Ganesh et al., 2007).

Dislodgement

Prevention. Accidental catheter dislodgement can be minimized by tunneling the catheter and using an anchoring device to affix the catheter hub to the patient (Ilfeld et al., 2002).

Intervention. Notify the anesthesia staff for an alternate method of providing analgesia.

Skin Breakdown

Because children have decreased sensation prompting them to voluntarily reposition themselves, there is a need to assess the skin of the affected limb and assist the patients with repositioning every 2 hours while awake.

Intervention

Protect the affected areas and consider use of a pressure-relieving mattress for children at significant risk of skin breakdown.

PATIENT EDUCATION FOR CONTINUOUS PERIPHERAL NERVE BLOCK INFUSION

Patient selection is of utmost importance when considering the application of these techniques, especially for outpatients. Instructions, including cautions and limitations of continuous infusion, should be discussed with the patient and parents prior to discharge from the hospital. A written copy of these instructions should also be given to the patient and caregiver as a reference after discharge.

Before discharge, patients and parents need verbal and written instructions about the CPNBI, recognition of potential complications, what to do if catheter dislodgement or dislocation occurs, and actions to take for inadequate pain control, including (Ganesh et al., 2007) the following specific information:

- How to contact the anesthesia staff at any time
- Care in ambulation and how to protect numb areas from injury (e.g., heat, cold, or pressure)
- Common side effects of the medicines, including those that need to be reported immediately to the anesthesia staff
- How other pain medicines will be added if needed for pain not relieved by the nerve block infusion
- When to come to the outpatient clinic for troubleshooting infusion problems or bag or dose changes
- Optional: how to change the rate on a pump or remove the catheter when no longer needed under telephone direction from the anesthesia staff

In summary, the recent ability to provide CPNBI effectively and safely, both inpatient as well as on an outpatient basis, has been a major advance in ambulatory surgery (Enneking & Ilfeld, 2002).

REFERENCES

Aram, L., Krane, E. J., Kozloski, L. J., & Yaster, M. (2001). Tunneled epidural catheters for prolonged analgesia in pediatric patients. *Anesthesia & Analgesia*, *92*(6), 1432–1438.

Brislin, R. P., & Rose, J. B. (2005). Pediatric acute pain management. *Anesthesiology Clinics of North America, 23*(4), 789–814.

Brown, D. L. (1992). *Atlas of regional anesthesia.* Philadelphia, PA: W. B. Saunders.

Dadure, C., Bringuier, S., Raux, O., Rochette, A., Troncin, R., Canaud, N., . . . Capdevila, X. (2009). Continuous peripheral nerve blocks for postoperative analgesia in children: Feasibility and side effects in a cohort study of 339 catheters. *Canadian Journal of Anesthesia, 56*(11), 843–850.

Dadure, C., Pirat, P., Raux, O., Troncin, R., Rochette, A., Ricard, C., & Capdevila, X. (2003). Perioperative continuous peripheral nerve blocks with disposable infusion pumps in children: A prospective descriptive study. *Anesthesia & Analgesia, 97*(3), 687–690.

Dalen, B. (2003). Peripheral nerve blockade in the management of postoperative pain in children. In N. L. Schechter, C. B. Berde, & M. Yaster (Eds.), *Pain in infants, children, and adolescents* (2nd ed., pp. 363–394). Philadelphia, PA: Lippincott Williams & Wilkins.

Dowden, S. J. (2009). Managing acute pain in children. In A. Twycross, S. J. Dowden, & E. Bruce (Eds.), *Managing pain in children: A clinical guide* (pp. 109–144). Oxford, United Kingdom: Wiley-Blackwell.

Enneking, F. K., & Ilfeld, B. M. (2002). Major surgery in the ambulatory environment: Continuous catheters and home infusions. *Best Practice & Research Clinical Anaesthesiology, 16*(2), 285–294.

Ganesh, A., Rose, J. B., Wells, L., Ganley, T., Gurnaney, H., Maxwell, L. G., . . . Cucchiaro, G. (2007). Continuous peripheral nerve blockade for inpatient and outpatient postoperative analgesia in children. *Anesthesia & Analgesia, 105*(5), 1234–1242.

Greco, C., & Berde, C. (2005). Pain management for the hospitalized pediatric patient. *Pediatric Clinics of North America, 52*(4), 995–1027.

Ilfeld, B. M., Morey, T. E., & Enneking, F. K. (2002). Continuous infraclavicular brachial plexus block for postoperative pain control at home: A randomized, double-blinded, placebo-controlled study. *Anesthesiology, 96*(6), 1297–1304.

Ilfeld, B. M., Morey, T. E., Wright, T. W., Chidgey, L. K., & Enneking, F. K. (2003). Continuous interscalene brachial plexus block for postoperative pain control at home: A randomized, double-blinded, placebo-controlled study. *Anesthesia & Analgesia, 96*(4), 1089–1095.

Kraemer, F. W., & Rose, J. B. (2009). Pharmacologic management of acute pediatric pain. *Anesthesiology Clinics, 27*(2), 241–268.

Ludot, H., Berger, J., Pichenot, V., Belouadah, M., Madi, K., & Malinovsky, J. M. (2008). Continuous peripheral nerve block for postoperative pain control at home: A prospective feasibility study in children. *Regional Anesthesia and Pain Medicine, 33*(1), 52–56.

Yaster, M., Tobin, J. R., & Kost-Byerly, S. (2003). Local anesthetics. In N. L. Schechter, C. B. Berde, & M. Yaster (Eds.), *Pain in infants, children, and adolescents* (2nd ed., pp. 241–264). Philadelphia, PA: Lippincott Williams & Wilkins.

IV

Nonpharmacologic Methods

8

General Principles and Cognitive-Behavioral Techniques

Various nonpharmacologic techniques can be useful in reducing pain and its associated anxiety, either alone or as an adjunct to medications. Many of these methods fall within the independent scope of nursing practice and contribute to a holistic approach to pain management, building trusting relationships with children and their families. When discussing these techniques, it is important to reassure children that such strategies will "help the pain medicines work better." However, nonpharmacologic interventions cannot replace pharmacologic treatment in cases of severe pain.

The expectation is that older children and adolescents will learn to do these therapies on their own. Therefore, an educational component is needed for patients and parents to become active participants through practice and with feedback from the health care providers. Nonpharmacologic approaches to reducing pain are generally divided into three types of interventions:

1. Cognitive-behavioral techniques (CBTs), many of which can be provided by health care providers even with little additional training for toddler age through adolescence. Further details will be discussed in this chapter.
2. Cognitive techniques, which require specific additional training for health care providers, are found to be effective for school-age children through adolescence. See Chapter 9 for a further discussion about cognitive techniques.

3. Physical approaches, which are useful for patients of all ages, many of which can be provided by any health care provider in collaboration with a physical therapist. Some techniques require special training and qualifications. See Chapter 10 for a further discussion about physical approaches, including a specific section regarding methods for reducing pain in infants.

The mechanisms by which these methods reduce pain are still being studied but may include the promotion of natural self-regulatory processes, as well as sensory distraction and altering pain transmission and its perception in the brain. Across all of the nonpharmacologic interventions, research with adult patients is more prevalent, often with conflicting conclusions regarding the benefit (or lack thereof) of the intervention. Even when research studies are available, the sample sizes are small, with inadequate use of a control group and with understandable challenges in using blinded study designs because of the difficulty in providing a sham treatment. Most research with infants and children using these techniques has been for reducing pain during procedures (Bellieni et al., 2006; Franck, 2000; Klassen, Liang, Tjosvold, Klassen, & Hartling, 2008; Powers, 1999). More research is needed to determine their effectiveness for chronic pain and how to combine techniques to obtain maximum benefit without overstimulating the infant or child and how to match techniques to the specific needs of children (Palermo, Eccleston, Lewandowski, Williams, & Morley, 2010). The discussion in this chapter along with the next chapters will be centered on the most common techniques used in children and for which substantial research is available regarding their effectiveness.

GENERAL PRINCIPLES FOR NONPHARMACOLOGIC MANAGEMENT

Children have incredible inner resources that give them the ability to cope with distress. Specifically, children use their imaginations, along with their ability to focus to the extent of being unaware of their surroundings, to distract themselves through play, music, and other creative activities. Children have less negative bias about the efficacy of these techniques than adults and seem to be more adept at learning them. Health care providers may tap into these resources and teach children and their parents, which may reduce parental feelings of helplessness (Twycross, 2009).

Selection of a Nonpharmacologic Intervention

The choice of nonpharmacologic method is based on factors such as the child's age and cognitive abilities, culture, behavioral factors, coping ability, and type of pain. See Table 8.1 for age-appropriate recommendations. However, even among children at the same developmental stage, a wide variability in which specific technique is most useful in reducing pain has been found. In general:

- Preschoolers tend to do better with techniques that require less cognitive development.
- School-aged children and adolescents alike have fantastic imaginations and are often well able to tune out the environment around them, making them excellent candidates for cognitive techniques, while continuing to benefit from CBTs such as relaxation exercises.

Current practice continues to rely on the health care provider's clinical judgment to select the most effective strategies to help children cope with painful procedures. These interventions seem to work best when they are introduced early in the course of illness as part of a multidisciplinary effort. Recent interest on how to combine multiple nonpharmacologic techniques while caring for infants using a multisensory stimulation package has generated research (Bellieni et al., 2002; Stevens, Yamada, & Ohlsson, 2004; Tsao, Evans, Meldrum, Altman, & Zeltzer, 2008a).

Table 8.1 ■ *Cognitive-Behavioral Techniques for Pain Management*

Age	Activities	Method of Reinforcement by the Health Care Provider
Infants (birth to 1 year old)	Playing music or singing Rattles or mobiles Familiar items (e.g., blanket)	Recording lullabies featuring the parents' voices
Toddlers (1–3 years old)	Playing music, singing, reciting nursery rhymes Spinning pinwheels Puppet play Playing with a *familiar* toy	Reassure and praise Stickers provide visual reward
Preschoolers (3–5 years old)	Blowing bubbles Pretending to blow out candles Spinning pinwheels and kaleidoscopes Reading pop-up or sound books Playing music or singing Counting Talking about favorite things or places Tell stories Puppet play Playing with a *familiar* toy Medical play	Give simple choices (e.g., right arm or left arm for an injection) Stickers provide visual reward
School age (6–12 years old)	Playing music Squeezing a ball Kaleidoscopes Hand-held games Playing with a *novel* toy Medical play Art and art therapy Progressive muscle relaxation and controlled breathing Biofeedback	Give equally acceptable choices

(Continued)

Table 8.1 ▦ *Cognitive-Behavioral Techniques for Pain Management (Continued)*

Age	Activities	Method of Reinforcement by the Health Care Provider
Adolescents (12–18 years old)	Playing favorite music Handheld games Progressive muscle relaxation and controlled breathing Art and art therapy Biofeedback	Giving choices and more involvement in decision making

Source: From Anghelescu, Oakes, & Popenhagan, 2006; McGrath, Dick, & Unruh, 2003; Twycross, 2009; Uman, Chambers, McGrath, & Kisely, 2006; Windich-Biermeier, Sjoberg, Dale, Eshelman, & Guzzetta, 2007.

Clinical Pearl

In selecting effective techniques for children during painful procedures, consider the following:

▦ The child's age, cognitive level, and ability to follow directions
▦ The type of pain
▦ Asking the child (and parents) which techniques have been found more effective (and ineffective) with previously distressing procedures
▦ The skill level of the health care provider in providing the appropriate techniques

Optimizing Effectiveness

It is important to teach CBTs and cognitive techniques early in the illness experience before children have severe anxiety related to poorly controlled pain and coping during previous procedures (Anghelescu, Oakes, & Popenhagan, 2006; Poltorak & Benore, 2006). Introducing them as part of a multidisciplinary effort including children's input may give them more sense of control. Of note, despite what is known about the usefulness of nonpharmacologic methods as pain-relieving strategies, studies have found evidence that nurses do not use them in practice (Polkki, Vehvilainen-Julkunen, & Pietila, 2001; Twycross, 2007).

COGNITIVE-BEHAVIORAL TECHNIQUES

Children use their imaginative capacities to rehearse skills, cope with fears and challenges, and set goals for themselves. By achieving a sense of mastery over a situation such as a painful procedure, children learn to place the stressful and painful experiences at the periphery of awareness and focus elsewhere for a short period (Blount, Piira, Cohen, & Cheng, 2006; Uman, Chambers, McGrath, & Kisely, 2006). CBTs improve the child's ability to cope with the pain as well as actually decreasing the level of distress the child experiences in both acute and chronic pain. Positive reinforcement is a very important component of CBTs, encouraging future positive behaviors even if the child experiences difficulties or distress. Uncooperative behaviors should not be punished, and the child should never be threatened or made to feel ashamed for being unable to cooperate because of anxiety or distress.

Distraction

Distraction is actively focusing away from the pain and, instead, focusing on a more pleasant diversion activity. The underlying assumption is that when attention is occupied with another strong stimulus (e.g., hearing a story), the child undergoing the painful medical procedure will be less able to process painful stimuli.

Indications

For most children, distraction during medical procedures reduces the quantity of observed distress behaviors (e.g., pain and anxiety) with various procedures, including intramuscular injections, subcutaneous port access (Dahlquist, Pendley, Landthrip, Jones, & Steuber, 2002) and other needle procedures (Bellieni et al., 2006; Cassidy et al., 2002; Dahlquist, Busby, et al., 2002), and laceration repair (Sinha, Christopher, Fenn, & Reeves, 2006).

Contraindications

Distraction would be counterproductive for procedures in which the child must participate (e.g., to learn how to care for a wound or to learn how to give himself an injection).

Skills of Health Care Provider

This technique is considered natural and simple for health care providers to provide for children even with little formal training. Ideally, these strategies are introduced by a health care provider who teaches the parent how to be a future coach before another pain episode (Kleiber, Craft-Rosenberg, & Harper, 2001). See Chapter 12 for a further discussion about this technique.

Methods and Tools

To be effective, the distraction technique needs to be age-appropriate and must be appealing to the recipient. See Table 8.1 for suggested age-appropriate activities. Offering children choices provides them some control over this aspect of the experience. The activity needs to be consistent with their energy level and ability to concentrate (Twycross, 2009). After the procedure, reflecting on whether the distraction provided effective relief is helpful in reinforcing the child to become independent in such techniques. Some distraction techniques require specialized equipment.

Music and Music Therapy. Ranging from health care providers offering recorded music delivered via headphones to music therapy delivered by trained music therapists, music has long been used to enhance well-being and to assist in alleviation of pain and distress. Music is thought to exert its primary analgesic effect indirectly by the distraction of attention away from the pain related to the medical procedure (Klassen et al., 2008; Tsao, Evans, Meldrum, Altman, & Zeltzer, 2008b). Optimally, children need to be able to determine the type of music they want to hear (Clark et al., 2006). Music therapy in pediatric patients has been successful in decreasing pain intensity scores for children with chronic pain (Tsao, Meldrum, Kim, Jacob, & Zeltzer, 2007), cancer pain (Clark et al., 2006), and burn injuries (Miller, Rodger, Bucolo, Greer, & Kimble, 2009). Behavioral signs of distress associated with immunizations for preschool-age children were found reduced for those who were part of a music intervention group (Noguchi, 2006).

Virtual Reality. The ultimate distraction method is using virtual reality technologies with children becoming active participants in a virtual world, using visual and auditory stimuli that help "immerse" them into the computer-generated reality. The immersion process is commonly provided through a head-mounted display with a screen, stereo earphones, and a head tracking system reacting to the children's head movements. Virtual reality has been found to be more effective than general distraction methods for children with cancer undergoing invasive medical procedures, such as accessing a subcutaneous port (Gershon, Zimand, Pickering, Rothbaum, & Hodges, 2004). Others have found virtual reality to be an effective distraction method for peripheral intravenous insertion (Gold, Kim, Kant, Joseph, & Rizzo, 2006) and for wound care procedures for pediatric burn patients (Chan, Chung, Wong, Lien, & Yang, 2007).

Relaxation and Controlled Breathing

Relaxation, the state of relative freedom from anxiety and muscle tension, often includes controlled breathing techniques. Relaxation training is based on the belief that muscle tension can cause or exacerbate pain; therefore, muscle relaxation will reduce or alleviate pain. Progressive muscle relaxation involves focusing attention on each body part, starting with the toes, releasing the tension from each area of the body, and then gradually working toward the head. Controlled breathing is slow, deep, and rhythmic breaths to "blow away" the pain or to focus the attention away from the pain.

Indications

Relaxation and controlled breathing involve the relaxation of voluntary skeletal muscles, and thus, are effective only for older children and adolescents who can understand and follow the instructions of a health care provider. Medical conditions in which these techniques have been found to be most useful are procedure-related pain, acute or chronic pain associated with muscle tension, headache disorders, and myofascial pain.

Contraindications

Relaxation and controlled breathing are not useful for children who are too young or too ill to be able to understand and cooperate with the instructions.

Skills of a Health Care Provider

This technique is considered natural and simple for health care providers to provide for children even with little formal training. Ideally, these strategies are introduced by a health care provider who teaches the parent how to be a future coach before another pain episode (Kleiber et al., 2001). See Chapter 12 for a further discussion about this technique.

Methods and Tools

Health care providers can focus the attention of younger children on their movement of air in and out of their bodies during a medical procedure or "blowing away the pain." Often, asking children to breathe deeply five times followed by suggestions of calmness is effective. Older children and adolescents can learn progressive tension followed by relaxation of voluntary skeletal muscles for each of the eight muscle groups, specifically, lower arms, upper arms, legs, abdomen, chest, shoulders, eyes, and forehead. Combining these instructions with suggestions of heaviness and warmth and images of relaxing situations can improve the relaxation effort (e.g., the child saying to himself, "My arms are heavy and warm").

Clinical Pearl Guidelines for teaching controlled breathing (Poltorak & Benore, 2006) are as follows:

Instruct the child to sit or lie down in a comfortable position, modeling the following instructions before requiring his participation. Help the child locate his diaphragm muscle (i.e., the soft spot right underneath the middle of the ribcage and on top of the belly). Then instruct the child to do the following:

- Take a slow, easy breath in through the nose. Encourage the child to keep the upper body and shoulders relaxed. Using the metaphor of having a balloon in the belly, which the child will attempt to fill slowly as much as feels comfortable, will help the child to focus on the diaphragm muscle and keep the upper body relaxed.
- Hold his breath for a few seconds or as long as he feels comfortable and natural.
- Exhale slowly and gently through the mouth, slowly releasing the air from the balloon. The child can be encouraged to blow out in the same way as trying to blow a very large bubble with a wand.

The cycle can be repeated several times.

Medical Play

Through play, children gain more command and control over their hospital experience. By allowing children to play with and manipulate devices such as stethoscopes and needleless syringes, they gain a sense of mastery and become less sensitized with these objects at their bedside.

Indications

Medical play activities provide an outlet for emotions to help the child learn how to cope with acute, chronic, and procedural pain (McGrath, Dick, & Unruh, 2003).

Contraindications

Medical play is not useful for children who are too young or too ill to be able to actively participate.

Skills of a Health Care Provider

This technique is considered natural and simple for health care providers to provide for children even with little formal training. However, health care providers with specialized training (e.g., child life specialists and psychologists) offer additional expertise.

Methods and Tools

When verbal methods are unsuccessful, allowing children to express their feelings and concerns through the medium of play provides an opportunity to detect and correct misinformation. This technique is especially useful in the routine preparation of children for surgery or other painful and frightening procedures by prompting the child to act out a procedure with dolls or puppets while teaching him or her what will occur during the procedure.

Art and Art Therapy

The use of art with children can be the informal, playful, nondirected activity associated with childhood. The more formal directed use of art to allow children to use their creative processes to allow expression of what has happened to them is referred to as art therapy. Both forms are especially useful for children by providing a sense of normality through a familiar activity of childhood.

Indications

The informal provision of art as an activity serves as a normal outlet for children. Art therapy is used with children who have more serious psychosocial problems that may be related to chronic pain or the extreme fear of procedure-related pain (McGrath et al., 2003) and has been found useful to relieve cancer pain in adults (Nainis et al., 2006).

Contraindications

Art therapy is not useful for children who are too young or too ill to be able to actively participate.

Skills of a Health Care Provider

While prompting children to draw or otherwise express themselves through various media (e.g., markers and paints), various health care providers (e.g., nurses and physicians) provide a means for children to express themselves, often as a distraction technique. However, art therapy is usually coordinated by child life staff or art therapists who have knowledge of psychotherapeutic principles and the range of responses that the art therapy can elicit.

Methods and Tools

Various age-appropriate art supplies are required.

Biofeedback

Biofeedback consists of the measurement and self-control of physiological responses not usually considered to be under voluntary control, including blood pressure, heart rate, skin temperature, sweating, and muscle tension. The physiological responses are amplified or transformed in such a way that they can be monitored and understood by the children. Children quickly learn the significance of the auditory or visual feedback and can be taught how to modify their physiological responses (e.g., electromyography-feedback training for muscular-tension headaches) (McCarthy, Shea, & Sullivan, 2003; Twycross, 2009).

Indications

Biofeedback is used to reduce pain for children with migraine and tension headaches (Arndorfer & Allen, 2001; Scharff, Marcus, & Masek, 2002; Tsao & Zeltzer, 2005).

Contraindications

Biofeedback is not useful for children who are too young or too ill to be able to understand and cooperate with the instructions.

Skills of a Health Care Provider

Biofeedback requires health care providers specially trained in the technique.

Method and Tools

Biofeedback requires specialized equipment. The types of biofeedback include finger temperature, α-electroencephalography, muscle electromyography, and temporal pulse (McGrath et al., 2003). Each of these methods is used to alert children to muscle tension, which allows them to recognize the early signs of tension and implement relaxation techniques.

In summary, CBT is a pain-reducing strategy that diverts attention from pain by passively redirecting the child's attention or by actively involving the child in the performance of a more pleasant task. The legitimacy and effectiveness of CBT used adjunctively for relieving most types of pain in children and adolescents are widely reported but further research is needed (Velleman, Stallard, & Richardson, 2010).

REFERENCES

Anghelescu, D., Oakes, L., & Popenhagan, M. (2006). Management of pain due to cancer in neonates, children, and adolescents. In O. A. de Leon-Casasola (Ed.), *Cancer pain: Pharmacologic, interventional, and palliative care approaches* (pp. 509–521). Philadelphia, PA: Elsevier.

Arndorfer, R. E., & Allen, K. D. (2001). Extending the efficacy of a thermal biofeedback treatment package to the management of tension-type headaches in children. *Headache, 41*(2), 183–192.

Bellieni, C. V., Bagnoli, F., Perrone, S., Nenci, A., Cordelli, D. M., Fusi, M., . . . Buonocore, G. (2002). Effect of multisensory stimulation on analgesia in term neonates: A randomized controlled trial. *Pediatric Research, 51*(4), 460–463.

Bellieni, C. V., Cordelli, D. M., Raffaelli, M., Ricci, B., Morgese, G., & Buonocore, G. (2006). Analgesic effect of watching TV during venipuncture. *Archives of Diseases in Childhood, 91*(12), 1015–1017.

Blount, R. L., Piira, T., Cohen, L. L., & Cheng, P. S. (2006). Pediatric procedural pain. *Behavior Modification*, *30*(1), 24–49.

Cassidy, K. L., Reid, G. J., McGrath, P. J., Finley, G. A., Smith, D. J., Morley, C., . . . Morton, B. (2002). Watch needle, watch TV: Audiovisual distraction in preschool immunization. *Pain Medicine*, *3*(2), 108–118.

Chan, E. A., Chung, J. W., Wong, T. K., Lien, A. S., & Yang, J. Y. (2007). Application of a virtual reality prototype for pain relief of pediatric burn in Taiwan. *Journal of Clinical Nursing*, *16*(4), 786–793.

Clark, M., Isaacks-Downton, G., Wells, N., Redlin-Frazier, S., Eck, C., Hepworth, J. T., & Chakravarthy, B. (2006). Use of preferred music to reduce emotional distress and symptom activity during radiation therapy. *Journal of Music Therapy*, *43*(3), 247–265.

Dahlquist, L. M., Busby, S. M., Slifer, K. J., Tucker, C. L., Eischen, S., Hilley, L., & Sulc, W. (2002). Distraction for children of different ages who undergo repeated needle sticks. *Journal of Pediatric Oncology Nursing*, *19*(1), 22–34.

Dahlquist, L. M., Pendley, J. S., Landthrip, D. S., Jones, C. L., & Steuber, C. P. (2002). Distraction intervention for preschoolers undergoing intramuscular injections and subcutaneous port access. *Health Psychology*, *21*(1), 94–99.

Franck, L. (2000). Environmental and behavioral strategies to prevent and manage neonatal pain. In K. J. Anand, B. Stevens, & P. J. McGrath (Eds.), *Pain in infants* (2nd ed., Vol. 10, pp. 203–216). Amsterdam, The Netherlands: Elsevier.

Gershon, J., Zimand, E., Pickering, M., Rothbaum, B. O., & Hodges, L. (2004). A pilot and feasibility study of virtual reality as a distraction for children with cancer. *Journal of the American Academy of Child & Adolescent Psychiatry*, *43*(10), 1243–1249.

Gold, J. I., Kim, S. H., Kant, A. J., Joseph, M. H., & Rizzo, A. S. (2006). Effectiveness of virtual reality for pediatric pain distraction during IV placement. *Cyberpsychology & Behavior*, *9*(2), 207–212.

Klassen, J. A., Liang, Y., Tjosvold, L., Klassen, T. P., & Hartling, L. (2008). Music for pain and anxiety in children undergoing medical procedures: A systematic review of randomized controlled trials. *Ambulatory Pediatrics*, *8*(2), 117–128.

Kleiber, C., Craft-Rosenberg, M., & Harper, D. C. (2001). Parents as distraction coaches during IV insertion: A randomized study. *Journal of Pain and Symptom Management*, *22*(4), 851–861.

McCarthy, C. F., Shea, A. M., & Sullivan, P. (2003). Physical therapy management of pain in children. In N. L. Schechter, C. B. Berde, & M. Yaster (Eds.), *Pain in infants, children, and adolescents* (2nd ed., pp. 434–448). Philadelphia, PA: Lippincott Williams & Wilkins.

McGrath, P. J., Dick, B., & Unruh, A. M. (2003). Psychologic and behavioral treatment of pain in children and adolescents. In N. L. Schechter, C. B. Berde, & M. Yaster (Eds.), *Pain in infants, children, and adolescents* (2nd ed., pp. 303–316). Philadelphia, PA: Lippincott Williams & Wilkins.

Miller, K., Rodger, S., Bucolo, S., Greer, R., & Kimble, R. M. (2009). Multi-modal distraction. Using technology to combat pain in young children with burn injuries. *Burns, 36*(5), 647–658.

Nainis, N., Paice, J. A., Ratner, J., Wirth, J. H., Lai, J., & Shott, S. (2006). Relieving symptoms in cancer: Innovative use of art therapy. *Journal of Pain and Symptom Management, 31*(2), 162–169.

Noguchi, L. K. (2006). The effect of music versus nonmusic on behavioral signs of distress and self-report of pain in pediatric injection patients. *Journal of Music Therapy, 43*(1), 16–38.

Palermo, T. M., Eccleston, C., Lewandowski, A. S., Williams, A. C., & Morley, S. (2010). Randomized controlled trials of psychological therapies for management of chronic pain in children and adolescents: An updated meta-analytic review. *Pain, 148*(3), 387–397.

Polkki, T., Vehvilainen-Julkunen, K., & Pietila, A. M. (2001). Nonpharmacological methods in relieving children's postoperative pain: A survey on hospital nurses in Finland. *Journal of Advanced Nursing, 34*(4), 483–492.

Poltorak, D. Y., & Benore, E. (2006). Cognitive-behavioral interventions for physical symptom management in pediatric palliative medicine. *Child & Adolescent Psychiatric Clinics of North America, 15*(3), 683–691.

Powers, S. W. (1999). Empirically supported treatments in pediatric psychology: Procedure-related pain. *Journal of Pediatric Psychology, 24*(2), 131–145.

Scharff, L., Marcus, D. A., & Masek, B. J. (2002). A controlled study of minimal-contact thermal biofeedback treatment in children with migraine. *Journal of Pediatric Psychology, 27*(2), 109–119.

Sinha, M., Christopher, N. C., Fenn, R., & Reeves, L. (2006). Evaluation of nonpharmacologic methods of pain and anxiety management for laceration repair in the pediatric emergency department. *Pediatrics, 117*(4), 1162–1168.

Stevens, B., Yamada, J., & Ohlsson, A. (2004). Sucrose for analgesia in newborn infants undergoing painful procedures. *Cochrane Database of Systematic Reviews*, (3), CD001069.

Tsao, J. C., Evans, S., Meldrum, M., Altman, T., & Zeltzer, L. K. (2008a). A review of CAM for procedural pain in infancy: Part I. Sucrose and nonnutritive sucking. *Evidence-based Complementary and Alternative Medicine*, 5(4), 371–381.

Tsao, J. C., Evans, S., Meldrum, M., Altman, T., & Zeltzer, L. K. (2008b). A review of CAM for procedural pain in infancy: Part II. Other interventions. *Evidence-based Complementary and Alternative Medicine*, 5(4), 399–407.

Tsao, J. C., Meldrum, M., Kim, S. C., Jacob, M. C., & Zeltzer, L. K. (2007). Treatment preferences for CAM in children with chronic pain. *Evidence-based Complementary and Alternative Medicine*, 4(3), 367–374.

Tsao, J. C., & Zeltzer, L. K. (2005). Complementary and alternative medicine approaches for pediatric pain: A review of the state-of-the-science. *Evidence-based Complementary and Alternative Medicine*, 2(2), 149–159.

Twycross, A. (2007). Children's nurses' postoperative pain management practices: An observational study. *International Journal of Nursing Studies*, 44(6), 869–881.

Twycross, A. (2009). Non-drug methods of pain relief. In A. Twycross, S. J. Dowden, & E. Bruce (Eds.), *Managing pain in children: A clinical guide* (pp. 67–84). Oxford, United Kingdom: Wiley-Blackwell.

Uman, L. S., Chambers, C. T., McGrath, P. J., & Kisely, S. (2006). Psychological interventions for needle-related procedural pain and distress in children and adolescents. *Cochrane Database of Systematic Reviews*, (4), CD005179.

Velleman, S., Stallard, P., & Richardson, T. (2010). A review and meta-analysis of computerized cognitive-behaviour therapy for the treatment of pain in children and adolescents. *Child: Care and Health Development*, 36(4), 465–472.

Windich-Biermeier, A., Sjoberg, I., Dale, J. C., Eshelman, D., & Guzzetta, C. E. (2007). Effects of distraction on pain, fear, and distress during venous port access and venipuncture in children and adolescents with cancer. *Journal of Pediatric Oncology Nursing*, 24(1), 8–19.

9

Cognitive Techniques

Cognitive techniques useful in reducing pain include guided imagery and clinical hypnosis. Often, these techniques are referred to as self-regulation strategies, which are necessary life skills for the child or adolescent to use for pain, and also for other distressing symptoms, such as nausea and difficulties in sleeping. By redirecting the child's attention to something other than the pain, the assumption is that the brain is less aware of pain signals which reduces the pain intensity as the attention of the child is on something else more pleasant. As specific methods of distraction and attention, both guided imagery and clinical hypnosis are types of deliberate, directed daydreaming. Once taught to children, both techniques can be quicker and less expensive than pharmacologic interventions for mild pain and its related symptoms, and they have no side effects. What typically limit the use of these interventions are the lack of systematic training of health care providers and the misunderstanding by both health care providers and the public of what they provide.

| *Clinical Pearl* | Guided imagery and clinical hypnosis are very closely related, with common characteristics causing debate within the literature whether differentiating between the two interventions is worthwhile. Some distinctions between the two are the following: |

- For guided imagery, the health care provider plays a more active role, by *guiding* the child to an image that is more pleasant. For clinical hypnosis, the health care provider has a less active role unless asked to interject some direction by the child.
- For clinical hypnosis, during the deepest relaxation phase, the health care provider offers suggestions to promote the unconscious mind in such a way that pain or a related symptom is reduced in a similar future situation. For guided imagery, such suggestions are usually not offered with the intervention but focus only on the immediate situation requiring pain relief.

GUIDED IMAGERY

Engaging the child by focusing on a more pleasant activity, guided imagery provides distraction, changing the perception of the painful experience. The more vividly children imagine their positive experiences, the less pain they are likely to experience. Effective for children who are at least 3 years old, focusing on a pleasant mental picture or mentally traveling to a place of contentment can reduce pain and its associated anxiety as more of the senses are evoked (e.g., vision, hearing, smell, taste, and movement) (Huth, Broome, & Good, 2004).

Indications

Most work by health care providers has been done in using this technique for children undergoing medical procedures (Uman, Chambers, McGrath, & Kisely, 2006); however, it has also been used for recurrent abdominal pain (van Tilburg et al., 2009; Weydert et al., 2006) and postoperative pain (Huth et al., 2004; Pölkki, Pietilä, Vehviläinen-Julkunen, Laukkala, & Kiviluoma, 2008).

Contraindications

Guided imagery is contraindicated for those with severe emotional problems or a history of hallucinations.

Skills of a Health Care Provider

Guided imagery needs to be introduced by a trained health care provider who, prior to the pain experience, empowers the child to employ these skills, while encouraging the parents to act as coaches.

Methods and Tools

Effective use of imagery involves all of the child's senses and is more effective if outside stimuli are part of the "image." The health care provider is to prompt (guide) the child to imagine being in a more pleasant or otherwise positive situation (see Exhibit 9.1).

- The child can pretend to be or align with a powerful character in a book (e.g., a superhero). This diffuses feelings of powerlessness and promotes positive self-talk, such as "I'm as strong as Superman," "I have had this done before," and "I know what to do during an IV stick." This strategy can also be used to rehearse mentally or prepare for a stressful situation, such as being a soldier fighting a battle, to decrease feelings of powerlessness. Positive self-talk is part of imagery when a child is coached to say, "I will be okay" and "This procedure will help make me well."
- The incorporation of the sensory components of the medical procedure into the guided imagery exercise.
  - For younger children, during the povidone-iodine wash in preparation for a lumbar puncture, the health care provider can guide the child by using such words as "Feel the cool water the elephant has sprayed against your back."
  - For an adolescent who finds images of being at a beach pleasant, guiding him or her to feel the warmth of the water, see the colors, smell the scents, and hear the sounds during a wound care procedure may be effective.

Exhibit 9.1

An Example of an Exercise in Guided Imagery

- Make yourself as comfortable as possible.
- Take a few deep breaths through your nose, and breathe it out slowly.
- With each breath, notice that your body is becoming more comfortable.
- You may close your eyes if you wish.
- You may want to imagine your favorite place, a place that is special to you . . . .the _____ we talked about together.
- There may be other people with you, or you might want to be by yourself.
- You can enjoy this special place and know that your mind will remember it when you need to return.
- Your breathing is slow, deep, and easy.
- The muscles on your face are relaxed.
- Let yourself see, feel, smell, and hear the surroundings of that special place.
- It is yours.
- (*Pause, and let the child enjoy that special place for a few minutes.*)
- When you are ready to return from that special place, you will come back to your normal awareness.

Elements of relaxation and controlled breathing can be added for children who need to remain still during the procedure. Often health care providers skilled in this intervention offer individualized recordings for children to listen to on their own, with prompts to enhance guided imagery.

CLINICAL HYPNOSIS

Hypnosis is an altered state of consciousness, often but not always involving relaxation, in which an individual develops heightened concentration through which suggestions are accepted, allowing the use of natural mental and physical skills at optimal levels (Kuttner & Solomon, 2003). The goal of clinical hypnosis is a *therapeutic change in perception, emotion, behavior,* or *experience,* achieved by helping children to focus their attention away from the feared components of a procedure or persistent pain and to focus on an imaginative experience that is perceived as comforting, safe, fun, or intriguing (Kuttner & Catchpole, 2007).

Clinical Pearl

The Facts About Clinical Hypnosis

Hypnosis is used in a clinical setting supported by therapeutic rapport with the intention of reducing a symptom or changing maladaptive, conditioned response and is *not* for entertaining other people.

Clinical hypnosis is a state of intensified self-control in which children will be more focused. Clinical hypnosis is *not* sleep.

A trained professional can find helpful words to suggest ways to feel but *cannot* control children's minds in hypnosis.

Hypnotic suggestions can be tailored to an individual child, incorporating personal interests and using appropriate language for the child's age. Effective results come from flexibility in the intervention and *not* from a scripted conversation with the child.

Although the mechanisms of hypnotic analgesia are not completely understood, the use of neuroimaging studies has provided greater insight into the possible neural mechanisms underlying hypnotic states (Wood & Bioy, 2008). In hypnotic states, there is increased blood flow to occipital cortical areas, resulting in the acceptance of specific altered sensations, thereby mediating changes in perception of the painful experience (Casillas & Zeltzer, 2010).

Historically neglected, clinical hypnosis is now being increasingly recognized as an effective tool for children of all ages. Although possible for children as young as 3 years (Kuttner & Catchpole, 2007), the ability to benefit from hypnosis peaks between ages 7 and 14, after which there is a steady decline into adulthood (Wild & Espie, 2004).

It is a skill children can easily learn, providing a personal sense of mastery and control over their problems and reducing subsequent feelings of helplessness and powerlessness.

Clinical Hypnosis in Younger Children

Classic hypnosis does not occur with young children, who often prefer to follow the prompts of a health care provider with their eyes open and in motion more than older children and adolescents. For preschool children, hypnotic suggestions are integrated and externalized in play with relatively unstructured experiences, are more action oriented, and stay in the present time. This process is referred to as *imaginative involvement*, during which a child is intensely absorbed in a "here-and-now" fantasy experience in which present reality is suspended in the interests of the current imaginative experience (Kuttner & Catchpole, 2007). Children older than 6 years of age are more willing to close their eyes and "go inside," engaging their creative imagination in a structured hypnotic experience.

Clinical Hypnosis in Older Children and Adolescents

Older children and adolescents often prefer eye closure and physical relaxed states.

Adolescents may experience trance states when listening to music, "zoned out" with absorption on a pleasant experience. Effective clinical hypnosis is related to their ability and willingness to fantasize (Wild & Espie, 2004), such as "Let's pretend you are back in your room at home . . . ."

Indications

Clinical hypnosis can be used in various ways for children, including the following:

▪ Reduce anticipatory stress, develop coping strategies, and decrease the pain associated with various medical procedures (Gold, Kant, Belmont,

& Butler, 2007; Kuttner & Catchpole, 2007; Wood & Bioy, 2008), such as venipuncture (Liossi, White, & Hatira, 2009), lumbar punctures and bone marrow aspirations (Liossi, White, & Hatira, 2006; Richardson, Smith, McCall, & Pilkington, 2006), and voiding cystourethrography (Butler, Symons, Henderson, Shortliffe, & Spiegel, 2005).

- Block or manipulate the experience of pain related to cancer procedures and treatments (Gold et al., 2007; Liossi & Hatira, 2003; Richardson et al., 2006; Uman et al., 2006; Wild & Espie, 2004).
- Reduce chronic pain (Gold et al., 2007), such as chronic recurrent headaches (Kohen & Zajac, 2007), migraines (Hammond, 2007), and recurrent abdominal pain (Ball, Shapiro, Monheim, & Weydert, 2003).

To be effective, all of the following conditions need to be met:

- The child is responsive to hypnotic induction methods.
- The problem is treatable by clinical hypnosis.
- The child can relate positively to the health care provider.
- The child has at least minimal motivation to solve the problem.
- The parents agree to the use of clinical hypnosis.

Contraindications

Clinical hypnosis is contraindicated for those with severe emotional problems or a history of hallucinations. Absolute contraindications include (Sugarman & Wester, 2007) the following:

- The child is emotionally fragile.
- The child is asking to use the technique during an activity in which he would risk physical endangerment, such as while playing football.
- The adolescent is asking to use the technique for relief of certain problems for which hypnosis is not a solution (e.g., wants to have amnesia for breakup from a boyfriend or girlfriend).
- The child or parents want to "try it for fun."
- The medical or psychosocial conditions in which it is known that clinical hypnosis is not considered the most effective treatment.
- The request for clinical hypnosis is based on a misdiagnosis of the problem.

Skills of Health Care Provider

Clinical hypnosis is a tool, like medication, exercise, or diet, and should be used only as part of the treatment plan after a careful evaluation by a health care provider who has specialized training in clinical hypnosis. (See Appendix for suggested professional organizations that offer specialized training in clinical hypnosis.)

Methods and Tools

Two prerequisites that are necessary to provide effective clinical hypnosis include establishing a good rapport with the child and adapting the hypnotic technique to the child's cognitive developmental stage and preferences (Wood & Bioy, 2008). The confidence and expectations of the health care provider for the result to be a positive outcome are essential for success. Three types of suggestions can be made when dealing with pain (Wood & Bioy, 2008), adjusting for the developmental level of the child:

1. Suggestions of dissociations: Ask the child not to feel some parts of his or her body, or simply leave part of his or her body here and go elsewhere.
2. Suggestions of focused analgesia or sensory substitution: Replace the pain sensations by sensation of numbness or of complete analgesia. One technique useful for preschool and school-age children is the *magic glove*, which can be adapted to become a *magic hat* or *magic sock* (Kuttner & Solomon, 2003) and can be used in conjunction with lidocaine creams (Liossi et al., 2009).
3. Suggestions targeted at reinterpreting the sensations of pain as being less unpleasant: Ask the child to imagine a headache as an animal that gets smaller, or use a *pain switch* metaphor in which the child is told that he or she can switch off pain messages to various parts of his or her body (Kuttner & Solomon, 2003).

For the health care provider, guided imagery and clinical hypnosis present an opportunity to be inventive, spontaneous, and playful while building a stronger therapeutic relationship with a child and providing symptom relief (Liossi & Hatira, 2003). In spite of the need for more research using larger sample sizes and improved experimental designs, the literature to date should encourage consideration for clinical hypnosis to be incorporated into the clinical repertoire of efficacious and efficient procedures. The value of guided imagery and self-hypnosis goes well beyond the ability to help with these ailments by teaching the skills for self-regulation used to manage specific medical needs and other stressful events.

REFERENCES

Ball, T. M., Shapiro, D. E., Monheim, C. J., & Weydert, J. A. (2003). A pilot study of the use of guided imagery for the treatment of recurrent abdominal pain in children. *Clinical Pediatrics (Philadelphia)*, *42*(6), 527–532.

Butler, L. D., Symons, B. K., Henderson, S. L., Shortliffe, L. D., & Spiegel, D. (2005). Hypnosis reduces distress and duration of an invasive medical procedure for children. *Pediatrics*, *115*(1), e77–e85.

Casillas, J., & Zeltzer, L. K. (2010). Cancer pain in children. In S. M. Fishman, J. C. Ballantyne, & J. P. Rathmell (Eds.), *Bonica's management of pain* (4th ed., pp. 669–680). Philadelphia, PA: Wolters Kluwer/ Lippincott Williams & Wilkins.

Gold, J. I., Kant, A. J., Belmont, K. A., & Butler, L. D. (2007). Practitioner review: Clinical applications of pediatric hypnosis. *Journal of Child Psychology and Psychiatry*, *48*(8), 744–754.

Hammond, D. C. (2007). Review of the efficacy of clinical hypnosis with headaches and migraines. *The International Journal of Clinical and Experimental Hypnosis*, *55*(2), 207–219.

Huth, M. M., Broome, M. E., & Good, M. (2004). Imagery reduces children's postoperative pain. *Pain*, *110*(1–2), 439–448.

Kohen, D. P., & Zajac, R. (2007). Self-hypnosis training for headaches in children and adolescents. *The Journal of Pediatrics*, *150*(6), 635–639.

Kuttner, L., & Catchpole, R. E. (2007). Developmental considerations: Hypnosis with children. In L. Sugarman & W. C. Wester (Eds.), *Therapeutic hypnosis with children and adolescents* (pp. 25–44). Bethel, CT: Crown Publishing.

Kuttner, L., & Solomon, R. (2003). Hypnotherapy and imagery for managing children's pain. In N. L. Schechter, C. B. Berde, & M. Yaster (Eds.), *Pain in infants, children, and adolescents* (2nd ed., pp. 317–328). Philadelphia, PA: Lippincott Williams & Wilkins.

Liossi, C., & Hatira, P. (2003). Clinical hypnosis in the alleviation of procedure-related pain in pediatric oncology patients. *The International Journal of Clinical and Experimental Hypnosis, 51*(1), 4–28.

Liossi, C., White, P., & Hatira, P. (2006). Randomized clinical trial of local anesthetic versus a combination of local anesthetic with self-hypnosis in the management of pediatric procedure-related pain. *Health Psychology, 25*(3), 307–315.

Liossi, C., White, P., & Hatira, P. (2009). A randomized clinical trial of a brief hypnosis intervention to control venipuncture-related pain of pediatric cancer patients. *Pain, 142*(3), 255–263.

Pölkki, T., Pietilä, A. M., Vehviläinen-Julkunen, K., Laukkala, H., & Kiviluoma, K. (2008). Imagery-induced relaxation in children's postoperative pain relief: A randomized pilot study. *Journal of Pediatric Nursing, 23*(3), 217–224.

Richardson, J., Smith, J. E., McCall, G., & Pilkington, K. (2006). Hypnosis for procedure-related pain and distress in pediatric cancer patients: A systematic review of effectiveness and methodology related to hypnosis interventions. *Journal of Pain and Symptom Management, 31*(1), 70–84.

Sugarman, L., & Wester, W. C. (2007). Hypnosis with children and adolescents: A contextual framework. In L. Sugarman & W. C. Wester (Eds.), *Therapeutic hypnosis with children and adolescents* (pp. 3–24). Bethel, CT: Crown Publishing.

Uman, L. S., Chambers, C. T., McGrath, P. J., & Kisely, S. (2006). Psychological interventions for needle-related procedural pain and distress in children and adolescents. *Cochrane Database Systematic Review,* (4), CD005179.

van Tilburg, M. A., Chitkara, D. K., Palsson, O. S., Turner, M., Blois-Martin, N., Ulshen, M., & Whitehead, W. E. (2009). Audio-recorded guided imagery treatment reduces functional abdominal pain in children: A pilot study. *Pediatrics, 124*(5), e890–e897.

Weydert, J. A., Shapiro, D. E., Acra, S. A., Monheim, C. J., Chambers, A. S., & Ball, T. M. (2006). Evaluation of guided imagery as treatment for recurrent abdominal pain in children: A randomized controlled trial. *Boston Medical Center Pediatrics, 6,* 29.

Wild, M. R., & Espie, C. A. (2004). The efficacy of hypnosis in the reduction of procedural pain and distress in pediatric oncology: A systematic review. *Journal of Developmental and Behavioral Pediatrics, 25*(3), 207–213.

Wood, C., & Bioy, A. (2008). Hypnosis and pain in children. *Journal of Pain and Symptom Management, 35*(4), 437–446.

10

Physical Approaches

Physical approaches are primarily sensory, including touch, massage, stroking, and rocking, which health care providers and family members are innately prepared to use to comfort distressed children. It is not known whether the demonstrated efficacy of these techniques results from distraction of the painful stimulus or from stimulation of larger nerves, which then interferes with the transmission of pain. Studies on the efficacy of these approaches are difficult to design because of the inability to provide an adequate placebo.

COLD THERAPY

Superficial cooling decreases sensitivity to pain. Analgesic effects may be the result of muscle relaxation, cutaneous counterirritation, or effects on nerve conduction (Tanabe, Ferket, Thomas, Paice, & Marcantonio, 2002). Cold therapy will reduce the body temperature to depths of 1 to 2 cm, causing vasoconstriction, local hypoesthesia, and reduced inflammation and edema.

Indications

Cold therapy is often used for the treatment of acute injuries and trauma, recommended the first 24 to 48 hours to reduce swelling, followed by applying heat after 48 hours (McCarthy, Shea, & Sullivan, 2003). Typically, the application of cold by health care providers is done in conjunction with elevation, compression, and massage. Other uses of cold therapy include the acute management of first-degree skin burn, the reduction of muscle spasms, and decreasing swelling and inflammation from other conditions (e.g., arthritic flare-up or acute tendinitis).

Contraindications

Cold should not be applied to open wounds or areas with arterial insufficiency. It should not be used for an acute injury after 2 to 3 days because it may delay healing. Cold therapy should not be used for children with sickle-cell disease caused by likely exacerbation of the sickling process or for neonates because of the potential effect on thermoregulation.

Skills of a Health Care Provider

Because of the variable uses and contraindications to using cold in relation to a specific injury, collaboration with a physical therapist for specific uses is recommended.

Methods and Tools

Cold therapy methods include ice massage, cold or ice packs, and cold compression units. Health care providers should rotate ice packs to a new site at intervals of no longer than 10 minutes to allow the comfortable sensation of cold without damaging the skin. If the skin becomes blanched, discontinue the cold pack. The application of the ice compress allows children to participate in their own care and provides some distraction. Cold therapy may be less acceptable to children.

HEAT THERAPY

Superficial heating decreases pain by inducing vasodilation, improving circulation and the availability of nutrients and oxygen delivery to the injured site, reducing inflammatory edema, and promoting muscle relaxation. Depending on the type of heat therapy application and the duration of exposure, the involved depth is up to 1 cm.

Indications

Heat is useful for muscle and joint stiffness, subacute and chronic traumatic and inflammatory conditions, muscle spasms, tendonitis (McCarthy et al., 2003), and sickle-cell pain (Dampier & Shapiro, 2003). For traumatic injuries with intact skin (e.g., sprained joints), heat is used after 48 hours of cold therapy to reduce swelling.

Contraindications

Heat is not to be used over areas of circulatory compromise, on irradiated tissues, or on any area of impaired sensation, such that the child would not be able to communicate that the temperature is too hot leading to possible skin burns.

Skills of a Health Care Provider

Because of the variable uses and contraindications to using heat in relation to a specific condition, collaboration with a physical therapist for specific uses is recommended.

Methods and Tools

Various methods of applying heat can be used, including heat packs, heat lamps, hot showers, and baths. The heat is to be applied to the painful site, promoting relaxation and healing. Precautions should be taken to ensure the source of heat is wrapped, allowing a comfortable sensation of heat without damaging the skin. The application of heat allows children to participate in their own care and provides some distraction.

MASSAGE THERAPY

Massage is defined as the manual manipulation of soft tissue, increasing superficial circulation. In humans, touch is the first sense to develop. Proponents of massage explain that by receiving caring and purposeful touching of the skin, the stress response is reduced, inducing a release of endogenous opioids, and pain is reduced to a more tolerable level. Relaxation and drowsiness are promoted. The repetitive movements of the hands of the health care provider stimulate peripheral receptors in the skin. This stimulation also transmits impulses to the higher centers in the central nervous system, thereby resulting in feelings of well-being.

Indications

Massage is used to promote relaxation and to reduce pain associated with muscle spasms, achy or tense muscles, arthritis, and other chronic pain conditions (Beider, Mahrer, & Gold, 2007; Tsao, 2007).

Contraindications

Patients who are in the acute phase of musculoskeletal injury, serious head injuries, concussions, subdural hematomas, or meningitis should not have massage therapy (Beider et al., 2007). Clinicians are to avoid massaging areas of thrombophlebitis, acute inflammatory process, broken skin, burned skin, tissue necrosis, or infections such as herpes or chickenpox. Massage may be contraindicated in severe thrombocytopenia and sickle-cell disease. Although some research has been conducted in infants, more studies are needed in preterm and full-term infants to determine the safety and efficacy of this modality for daily care as an analgesic for procedural pain (Tsao, Evans, Meldrum, Altman, & Zeltzer, 2008b). Massage therapy should not be used as a substitute for active exercise.

Skills of a Health Care Provider

Massage therapy includes a wide range of variability in terms of pressure and pacing. A skilled massage therapist will know how to go from light touch to deeper massage (Beider et al., 2007), paying attention to the child's responses to tactile stimulation (e.g., amount of pressure and rate of movement).

Methods and Tools

Particular massage techniques and modalities have either stimulating or calming effects, including simple rhythmic rubbing, stroking, and kneading of the muscle and soft tissues (Beider et al., 2007). Favorite sites for massage are the back, hands, and feet. This technique can be taught to parents so they can provide it to their children.

EXERCISE THERAPY

Exercise therapy typically consists of the use of physical rehabilitation methods to regain lost motor strength, increase range of motion, regain balance, and prevent muscle deconditioning. Patients with persistent pain may withdraw from participation in normal physical activities, losing flexibility. The mechanism of action of exercise therapy in pain reduction is not fully understood but may be related to the production of endorphins and other endogenous pain-reducing mediators (McGrath, Dick, & Unruh, 2003).

Indications

General exercise regimens are an important component of pain management for children experiencing recurrent or persistent pain with the goal of improving functional ability and movement. Exercise is essential in the postoperative management of orthopedic surgeries, including amputation, in the rehabilitation plan following most injuries, and for the treatment of musculoskeletal conditions (i.e., fibromyalgia and complex regional pain syndrome).

Contraindications

Exercise is not recommended during the acute phase of most illnesses and injuries. Specific plans for exercise need to be individualized to the patient's condition by skilled health care providers (e.g., physical therapists).

Skills of a Health Care Provider

The skills of physical and occupational therapists are essential in determining and monitoring the treatment plan for children. Early guidance, including parent teaching, is useful in transitioning children to safe and effective home exercise programs.

Methods and Tools

Skilled therapists can prescribe appropriate exercises to strengthen weak muscles and mobilize stiff joints while focusing on activities that are most enjoyable to the child. The goal is for the child to return to his baseline functional activity level (McCarthy et al., 2003). Simple stretching exercises for 20 to 30 minutes, several times a week, can help patients to maintain their flexibility. Orthotics for muscle and nerve weakness are needed to prevent injury for many children with motor and sensory deficits.

TRANSCUTANEOUS ELECTRIC NERVE STIMULATION

Transcutaneous electric nerve stimulation (TENS) is a method for stimulating nerves via a portable battery-powered device that delivers a painless, low-voltage electrical current through electrodes placed on skin. The current competes with the transmission of pain messages (gate control theory) and promotes the release of pain inhibitors (e.g., endogenous opioids in the spinal cord) (Sluka & Walsh, 2003). The child will feel a buzzing, tingling, or vibrating sensation at the electrode site. TENS technologies are characterized by electrical pulse rate, pulse width, and pulse intensity.

Indications

TENS has been found to be effective as a safe and noninvasive method for relief of acute and chronic pain, including musculoskeletal discomfort, neuropathic pain, phantom limb pain, and postoperative pain (McCarthy et al., 2003; Smith & Madsen, 2003). Superficial pain appears more sensitive to the analgesic effects of TENS than deep, visceral pain. Adaptation to the stimulus, however, is common. Children need to be old enough (e.g., at least 8 years old) to understand the intention of the therapy and the explanation that the electrical current will not hurt them (McCarthy et al., 2003).

Contraindications

TENS should be used with caution for patients who have a seizure disorder and is contraindicated for those who have a pacemaker and should not be used over a pregnant uterus, carotid arteries, eyes, and malignant tumor, as well as while driving (McCarthy et al., 2003).

Skills of a Health Care Provider

A physical therapist is required to determine the appropriateness of TENS as well as the appropriate electrode placement and TENS settings, followed by ongoing monitoring to determine effectiveness.

Methods and Tools

The successful application of TENS involves a period of trial and error in the selection of several stimulation parameters, such as frequency and amplitude of the current, and the type, size, and location of the electrodes used to deliver the current. Standard self-adhesive electrodes are usually placed on the affected body part with the TENS unit turned on for an hour several times a day (McCarthy et al., 2003). A written patient and parent treatment plan and diary are beneficial, much like analgesic diaries (McCarthy et al., 2003; see Appendix). A glove electrode, which offers another option to provide a larger contact area to treat pain, has shown promising results for pain of the hand (Cowan et al., 2009).

ACUPUNCTURE

Acupuncture is a system of ancient medicine, healing, and Eastern philosophy originating in China, involving stimulation of specific anatomic locations on the skin by various techniques. Although the actual mechanism for acupuncture is not fully known, the theory is that energy (*chi*) flows through the body along channels known as meridians, which are connected by acupuncture points. Pain is theorized to be the result of the obstruction of the flow of energy (Kemper & Gardiner, 2003). By inserting very fine needles into the body at acupuncture points along the meridians involved, the energy flow is restored, eliminating or reducing the pain (Kemper & Gardiner, 2003). Several mechanisms for acupuncture have been postulated, such as endorphin activation by stimulating acupuncture points (Waterhouse, Tsao, & Zeltzer, 2009), with the needles stimulating A-delta fibers, leading to the release of the pain-reducing substances norepinephrine and serotonin (Kundu & Berman, 2007).

Additional psychological and physiological factors may mediate the response to acupuncture, including expectations, anxiety, patient motivation, placebo effects, and counter-irritation or distraction (Linde et al., 2007). The differences in efficacy of acupuncture among individual patients are probably influenced by some of these mechanisms. The efficacy, safety, and acceptance of acupuncture for pain management are well established for adults (Kundu & Berman, 2007). Because of children having an aversion to needles, acupuncture has been more accepted for use in adolescents, but there has been limited research in children (Kemper et al., 2000). Many children have accepted this method of treatment despite the insertion of needles. However, based on the limited research in children, the use of acupuncture is increasingly being included in pediatric pain management regimens (Kundu & Berman, 2007). When it has been combined with hypnotherapy for children with chronic pain, children and parents have reported significant improvement in pain and functioning with no adverse effects (Zeltzer et al., 2002).

Indications

Acupuncture is predominantly used for chronic pain associated with headaches, including migraine (Kundu & Berman, 2007; Pintov, Lahat, Alstein, Vogel, & Barg, 1997; Tsao & Zeltzer, 2005; Waterhouse et al., 2009), abdominal pain (Kundu & Berman, 2007), and musculoskeletal pain (Kemper et al., 2000; Kundu & Berman, 2007). Perioperative acupuncture may be a useful adjunct for acute postoperative pain management (Kundu & Berman, 2007; Sun, Gan, Dubose, & Habib, 2008; Wu et al., 2009). Limited research has been done in children with cancer and sickle-cell disease (Jindal, Ge, & Mansky, 2008; Kundu & Berman, 2007). Financial barriers frequently limit access to acupuncture treatment because of minimal third-party coverage of costs.

Contraindications

Acupuncture is contraindicated in the treatment of malignancy, mechanical obstruction, fulminant infection, hemorrhagic diseases, and conditions that require surgical repair.

Skills of a Health Care Provider

Acupuncture is described as a safe modality for pediatric patients but should be provided only by qualified health care providers (Jindal et al.,

2008; Kundu & Berman, 2007). The acceptance of acupuncture as a legitimate medical therapy for adults or children, however, is not a given (Ernst, 2009). More consistent licensing, certification, and accreditation are needed to assist patients in identifying qualified acupuncturists and ensure the quality of the treatments. Licensing for the practice of acupuncture is determined by the individual states, with requirements usually consisting of a formal training program and certification examination (Lin, 2003). Most pediatric acupuncture is given by physicians who meet these requirements (Lin, 2003).

Methods and Tools

Use of sterile technique and disposable needles is required. Each acupuncture point has a prescribed depth of insertion. After insertion, the acupuncture needle may be stimulated by manual manipulation (lifting or twisting the needle) or by electroacupuncture (attaching low-voltage electrodes to the needles) (Lin, 2003). During acupuncture, children should not feel pain from the therapy itself. Treatments last from 5 to 15 minutes, with 1 to 20 needles inserted. Although some patients experience immediate pain improvement, others require at least 3 treatments. Mild transient adverse effects, such as bleeding at needling sites, may occur, with the rare case reports of serious adverse effects, such as pneumothorax, cardiac tamponade, or infections.

NONPHARMACOLOGIC INTERVENTIONS SPECIFIC FOR INFANTS

Nonnutritive Sucking

Nonnutritive sucking refers to the placement of a pacifier in an infant's mouth to promote sucking behavior without breast milk or formula. The use of a pacifier can provide comfort during painful procedures, as measured by reduced crying, reduced heart rate, and lower behavioral distress (Gibbins et al., 2002; Tsao, Evans, Meldrum, Altman, & Zeltzer, 2008a). This intervention may elicit activation of the neuropeptide systems, which achieve an analgesic effect (Cignacco et al., 2007; Tsao et al., 2008a). See Chapter 13 for additional information about the additional benefits of sucrose with the pacifier.

Rocking

For infants, rhythmic movement in the form of rocking helps with relaxation and decreases pain (Twycross, 2009).

Positioning

Positioning to gently support infants in a naturally secure position may help to relieve procedural pain in neonates. Combining this action with facilitated tucking (wrapping a blanket snuggly around infants in such a way that their limbs are in proximity to their trunk) has been found to be effective in reducing procedural pain (e.g., heel sticks) (Cignacco et al., 2007; Prasopkittikun & Tilokskulchai, 2003; Tsao et al., 2008b; Twycross, 2009).

One specific positioning technique, called *kangaroo care*, involving parents holding their infants with skin-to-skin contact, has been shown to reduce the pain response (as measured by facial actions, maximum heart rate, and minimal oxygen saturation changes from baseline) in preterm infants (Johnston et al., 2003) and healthy newborns who undergo heel sticks and other painful procedures (Gray, Watt, & Blass, 2000; Tsao et al., 2008b). Others have proposed that the familiar odor of their mothers' milk would add a calming effect and diminish distress of infants during heel sticks (Rattaz, Goubet, & Bullinger, 2005). Generalizability and standardization of this intervention are complicated by variations in maternal attitudes and comforting styles.

In summary, physical approaches can be useful as a primary treatment modality or as an adjunct within the pain management plan (see Table 10.1 for age-appropriate techniques). Rigorous, carefully designed research studies are much needed to validate their usefulness for infants, children, and adolescents.

Table 10.1 ▪ *Physical Approaches for Pain Management*

Age	Techniques
Infants (from birth to 1 year old)	Stroking
	Touching
	Rocking
	Gentle massage
	Pacifier and nonnutritive sucking
	Positioning and kangaroo care
	Heat and cold therapies (excluding neonates)
Toddlers (1–3 years old) and Preschoolers (3–5 years old)	Heat and cold therapies
	Massage
	Exercise therapy
School age (6–12 years old) and Adolescents (12–18 years old)	Heat and cold therapies
	Massage
	Exercise therapy
	TENS
	Acupuncture

Abbreviation: TENS, transcutaneous electric nerve stimulation.
Source: From Lin, 2003; McCarthy, Shea, & Sullivan, 2003; Tsao & Zeltzer, 2005; Twycross, 2009.

REFERENCES

Beider, S., Mahrer, N. E., & Gold, J. I. (2007). Pediatric massage therapy: An overview for clinicians. *Pediatric Clinics of North America*, *54*(6), 1025–1041.

Cignacco, E., Hamers, J. P., Stoffel, L., van Lingen, R. A., Gessler, P., McDougall, J., & Nelle, M. (2007). The efficacy of nonpharmacological interventions in the management of procedural pain in preterm and term neonates. A systematic literature review. *European Journal of Pain*, *11*(2), 139–152.

Cowan, S., McKenna, J., McCrum-Gardner, E., Johnson, M. I., Sluka, K. A., & Walsh, D. M. (2009). An investigation of the hypoalgesic effects of TENS delivered by a glove electrode. *Journal of Pain*, *10*(7), 694–701.

Dampier, C., & Shapiro, B. (2003). Management of pain in sickle cell disease. In N. L. Schechter, C. B. Berde, & M. Yaster (Eds.), *Pain in infants, children, and adolescents* (2nd ed., pp. 489–515). Philadelphia, PA: Lippincott Williams & Wilkins.

Ernst, E. (2009). Acupuncture: What does the most reliable evidence tell us? *Journal of Pain and Symptom Management, 37*(4), 709–714.

Gibbins, S., Stevens, B., Hodnett, E., Pinelli, J., Ohlsson, A., & Darlington, G. (2002). Efficacy and safety of sucrose for procedural pain relief in preterm and term neonates. *Nursing Research, 51*(6), 375–382.

Gray, L., Watt, L., & Blass, E. M. (2000). Skin-to-skin contact is analgesic in healthy newborns. *Pediatrics, 105*(1), e14.

Jindal, V., Ge, A., & Mansky, P. J. (2008). Safety and efficacy of acupuncture in children: A review of the evidence. *Journal of Pediatric Hematology/Oncology, 30*(6), 431–442.

Johnston, C. C., Stevens, B., Pinelli, J., Gibbins, S., Filion, F., Jack, A., . . . Veilleux, A. (2003). Kangaroo care is effective in diminishing pain response in preterm neonates. *Archives of Pediatrics & Adolescent Medicine, 157*(11), 1084–1088.

Kemper, K. J., & Gardiner, P. (2003). Complementary and alternative medical therapies in pediatric pain. In N. L. Schechter, C. B. Berde, & M. Yaster (Eds.), *Pain in infants, children, and adolescents* (2nd ed., pp. 941–947). Philadelphia, PA: Lippincott Williams & Wilkins.

Kemper, K. J., Sarah, R., Silver-Highfield, E., Xiarhos, E., Barnes, L., & Berde, C. (2000). On pins and needles? Pediatric pain patients' experience with acupuncture. *Pediatrics, 105*(4), 941–947.

Kundu, A., & Berman, B. (2007). Acupuncture for pediatric pain and symptom management. *Pediatric Clinics of North America, 54*(6), 885–889.

Lin, Y. C. (2003). Acupuncture. In N. L. Schechter, C. B. Berde, & M. Yaster (Eds.), *Pain in infants, children, and adolescents* (2nd ed., pp. 462–469). Philadelphia, PA: Lippincott Williams & Wilkins.

Linde, K., Witt, C. M., Streng, A., Weidenhammer, W., Wagenpfeil, S., Brinkhaus, B., & Melchart, D. (2007). The impact of patient expectations on outcomes in four randomized controlled trials of acupuncture in patients with chronic pain. *Pain, 128*(3), 264–271.

McCarthy, C. F., Shea, A. M., & Sullivan, P. (2003). Physical therapy management of pain in children. In N. L. Schechter, C. B. Berde, & M. Yaster (Eds.), *Pain in infants, children, and adolescents* (2nd ed., pp. 434–448). Philadelphia, PA: Lippincott Williams & Wilkins.

McGrath, P. J., Dick, B., & Unruh, A. M. (2003). Psychologic and behavioral treatment of pain in children and adolescents. In N. L. Schechter, C. B. Berde, & M. Yaster (Eds.), *Pain in infants, children, and adolescents* (2nd ed., pp. 303–316). Philadelphia, PA: Lippincott Williams & Wilkins.

Pintov, S., Lahat, E., Alstein, M., Vogel, Z., & Barg, J. (1997). Acupuncture and the opioid system: Implications in management of migraine. *Pediatric Neurology, 17*(2), 129–133.

Prasopkittikun, T., & Tilokskulchai, F. (2003). Management of pain from heel stick in neonates: An analysis of research conducted in Thailand. *Journal of Perinatal & Neonatal Nursing, 17*(4), 304–312.

Rattaz, C., Goubet, N., & Bullinger, A. (2005). The calming effect of a familiar odor on full-term newborns. *Journal of Developmental & Behavioral Pediatrics, 26*(2), 86–92.

Sluka, K. A., & Walsh, D. (2003). Transcutaneous electrical nerve stimulation: Basic science mechanisms and clinical effectiveness. *Journal of Pain, 4*(3), 109–121.

Smith, J. L., & Madsen, J. R. (2003). Neurosurgical procedures for the treatment of pediatric pain. In N. L. Schechter, C. B. Berde, & M. Yaster (Eds.), *Pain in infants, children, and adolescents* (2nd ed., pp. 329–362). Philadelphia, PA: Lippincott Williams & Wilkins.

Sun, Y., Gan, T. J., Dubose, J. W., & Habib, A. S. (2008). Acupuncture and related techniques for postoperative pain: A systematic review of randomized controlled trials. *British Journal of Anaesthesia, 101*(2), 151–160.

Tanabe, P., Ferket, K., Thomas, R., Paice, J., & Marcantonio, R. (2002). The effect of standard care, ibuprofen, and distraction on pain relief and patient satisfaction in children with musculoskeletal trauma. *Journal of Emergency Nursing, 28*(2), 118–125.

Tsao, J. C. (2007). Effectiveness of massage therapy for chronic, nonmalignant pain: A review. *Evidence-based Complementary and Alternative Medicine, 4*(2), 165–179.

Tsao, J. C., & Zeltzer, L. K. (2005). Complementary and alternative medicine approaches for pediatric pain: A review of the state-of-the-science. *Evidence-based Complementary and Alternative Medicine, 2*(2), 149–159.

Tsao, J. C., Evans, S., Meldrum, M., Altman, T., & Zeltzer, L. K. (2008a). A review of CAM for procedural pain in infancy: Part I. Sucrose and non-nutritive sucking. *Evidence-based Complementary and Alternative Medicine, 5*(4), 371–381.

Tsao, J. C., Evans, S., Meldrum, M., Altman, T., & Zeltzer, L. K. (2008b). A review of CAM for procedural pain in infancy: Part II. Other interventions. *Evidence-based Complementary and Alternative Medicine, 5*(4), 399–407.

Twycross, A. (2009). Nondrug methods of pain relief. In A. Twycross, S. J. Dowden, & E. Bruce (Eds.), *Managing pain in children: A clinical guide* (pp. 67–84). Oxford, United Kingdom: Wiley-Blackwell.

Waterhouse, M., Tsao, J. C., & Zeltzer, L. K. (2009). Commentary on the use of acupuncture in chronic pediatric pain. *Journal of Developmental & Behavioral Pediatrics, 30*(1), 69–71.

Wu, S., Sapru, A., Stewart, M. A., Milet, M. J., Hudes, M., Livermore, L. F., & Flori, H. R. (2009). Using acupuncture for acute pain in hospitalized children. *Pediatric Critical Care Medicine, 10*(3), 291–296.

Zeltzer, L. K., Tsao, J. C., Stelling, C., Powers, M., Levy, S., & Waterhouse, M. (2002). A phase I study on the feasibility and acceptability of an acupuncture/hypnosis intervention for chronic pediatric pain. *Journal of Pain and Symptom Management, 24*(4), 437–446.

V

Integration of Methods of Treatment

11

Multidisciplinary Approaches

Caring for children with pain is optimal when various disciplines, including nurses, anesthesiologists, pediatricians, oncologists, pharmacists, psychologists, child life specialists, and physical and occupational therapists contribute their expertise through a comprehensive pain assessment and treatment plan (Connelly & Schanberg, 2006). Different forms of multidisciplinary approaches exist across health care systems based on institutional resources and the needs of their patients, ranging from informal communication among colleagues to clearly defined pain teams. Each institution needs to determine the best multidisciplinary approach suited for its patient population and organizational culture. The critical factor is identifying a core group of health care providers from various disciplines who are committed to improve pain management for patient referrals if a pain service is available, and, even more importantly, to indirectly improve pain management for all patients served by the institution with the development of the following (Berde & Solodiuk, 2003):

- Institutional standardized protocols that are useful in providing consistency in analgesic regimens; for example, multidisciplinary teams can develop analgesic drug cards or online resources, including information such as equianalgesic doses and how to minimize adverse effects (e.g., opioid-induced constipation or pruritus)
- Mechanisms to include timely nonpharmacologic approaches to reduce needle-related pain, and augment medications by offering other

209

approaches "to make the pain medicines work better" through collaboration with child life specialists and psychologists
- Quality improvement monitoring processes to identify and develop plans to minimize analgesic dosing errors
- Quality improvement initiatives to improve compliance with pain assessment documentation and effective treatment of significant pain (Oakes, Anghelescu, Windsor, & Barnhill, 2008)
- Educational programs for all levels of staff regarding appropriate pain assessment, updating the latest in new medications or other treatment approaches with an emphasis on the need to consider multimodal approaches to pain management

Clinical Pearl	Multidisciplinary care is defined as follows:

- Is an integrated approach of pharmacologic and psychological therapies using a pharmacologic multimodal regimen to reduce or block ascending and/or descending pain pathways as well as modifying situational factors (Stinson & Bruce, 2009)
- Emphasizes the acceptance of the need to function with a commitment to follow the rehabilitation plan with an acceptable level of chronic pain rather than the often unrealistic expectation of eliminating all pain (Wicksell, Melin, & Olsson, 2007)

PAIN MANAGEMENT FOR OUTPATIENTS

Families need guidance in managing their children's pain, including mutually agreed-upon treatment goals using pharmacologic and nonpharmacologic approaches with a follow-up plan and means to contact the health care providers who are involved in their child's pain management (Simons, Logan, Chastain, & Cerullo, 2010; Slater, De Lima, Campbell, Lane, & Collins, 2010; Wicksell et al., 2007). Contact information needs to be provided, especially for uncontrolled pain or management of analgesic-related adverse effects. Assisting the patient and the family in determining limits and responsibilities may be necessary even within the most functional of families and is often best accomplished through written plans of care.

Written Pain Management Plans

A therapeutic alliance is made by systematically outlining pain management options, actively involving the patient and family, and describing the responsibilities of the individual child and his parents in the form of a document signed by the child and parent (when the patient is a minor). Such documents serve as an agreement on the part of the child or adolescent regarding the need for compliance with all aspects of the treatment plan, including the need to take only medications prescribed by this specialized group and other issues involving safekeeping of the medications (Anghelescu, Oakes, & Popenhagan, 2006; Passik & Kirsh, 2005). See Figure 11.1 for the document used by this author for each patient cared for by the pain management service, establishing clear expectations on what can be offered to reduce pain followed by the child's and parents' responsibilities.

Discussing such a document can be therapeutic as each party accepts a role in the plan. Adolescents, in particular, need supervision and close support when opioid use is indicated with the need of health care providers to help patients and families determine limits and responsibilities when having opioids in their homes (Slater et al., 2010).

Ongoing Evaluation of the Treatment Plan

Diaries offer a method of recording patterns of pain along with the use of analgesics and their effectiveness (Maikler, Broome, Bailey, & Lea, 2001). The author's pain management service requires the use of pain diaries that outline the schedule for all prescribed medications along with when and how to contact the pain management service for unrelieved pain and adverse effects. See Figure 11.2 for an example.

By including the expertise of multiple disciplines, the pain management plan will:

- Provide optimal analgesia (pain relief) with the fewest side effects,
- Ensure practical and safe medication administration by families,
- Allow for patterns of pain to be addressed (e.g., recognizing episodic increases in pain and having a plan for PRN [as needed] doses), and
- Allow for normal developmental activities for the child within the context of the medical disease or chronic pain syndrome.

Form 4574
St. Jude Children's Research Hospital
332 N. Lauderdale St.
Memphis, Tennessee 38105-2794
Rev. 06/07

PAIN MANAGEMENT SERVICE

Your child has been referred to the Pain Management Service to help relieve his or her pain.

What is the Pain Management Service? The Pain Management Service includes doctors, nurses, psychologists, physical therapists, and pharmacists. This group will work with you, your child and your primary doctor to help relieve your child's pain by having you come to the Pain Clinic when you are outpatient or coming to your room each day when you are inpatient.

The Pain Management Service may use one or several approaches to deal with pain.

1. Pain medications are sometimes called analgesics. More than one analgesic at a time may be prescribed. However, you should not add an analgesic without first checking with a member of the Pain Management Services. The medicines prescribed may include

    • Opioids (narcotics)
    • Anti-inflammatory medicines, and
    • Medications to treat nerve pain.

    Please refer to the Medication Cards for more information about the pain medicine that you are taking. As with all types of medicines, they can cause side effects. If these symptoms occur, notify the Pain Management Service so they can adjust the dosage, change to another medicine, or add another drug to lessen the side effects.

2. Psychosocial techniques can give you a sense of control over the pain. If recommended, you will be given detailed instructions about how to use these techniques. Some techniques frequently used include the following:

    • Relaxation—to alleviate anxiety and reduce muscle tension
    • Distraction—to learn how to focus on something other than the pain
    • Guided imagery—to concentrate on images to relax
    • Play therapy—to provide an outlet for emotions and learn how to cope with pain

3. Physical therapy techniques may help reduce the pain of a specific site. These techniques will also help keep you active, independent, and strong. If recommended, you will be given a detailed program of activities which may include the following:

    • Exercises—to strengthen weak muscles, loosen stiff muscles, increase blood flow, or help with balance.
    • Massage—to decrease swelling, help with relaxation or loosen scar tissue
    • Orthotics (braces)—to support painful or weak joints, immobilize an injury, stretch a tight muscle
    • Transcutaneous electrical nerve stimulation (TENS) unit—for certain types of pain such as neuropathic pain
    • Heat or cold therapy—to decrease swelling or inflammation, loosen tight muscles

Figure 11.1 ▒ An example of a pain management agreement.
Copyright 2007 by St. Jude Children's Research Hospital, Memphis, TN. Used with permission.

How can I help? To provide consistent and safe pain management, we expect you to do the following:

- Follow all parts of the treatment plan developed by the Pain Management Service.
- Store medicines safely. Do not give your pain medicines to anyone else.
- Take pain medications exactly as prescribed by the Pain Management Service.
- Notify the Pain Management Service immediately about any side effects. (See below for details on how to contact us.)
- Call the Pain Management Service if you feel that a change in the dose or timing of your medication is needed. Do not change your regimen without asking us.
- Keep all appointments with the Pain Management Service and be on time. If your visit will be delayed for a reason you cannot prevent, please call the Pain Management Service physician or clinical nurse specialist (901-495-3300) to see if it is in your best interest to delay your appointment time.
- Expect frequent re-evaluation of the pain problem. It is necessary to monitor the pain and make necessary adjustments in the treatment plan. Appointments will be at least once every two weeks. You may be asked to maintain telephone contact even more frequently.
- Expect to pick up your medications at the hospital. Only in extreme situations will we mail medications to your home. You will receive no more than a four-week supply of any mailed medications.
- **Bring all bottles of medication that the Pain Management Service prescribes to each clinic appointment.** This will enable us to give you refills.
- You might be asked to keep a written record of when additional medications are taken to help decrease the pain.
- Discuss any over-the-counter or complimentary medicine with the Pain Management Service before using them.
- Do not drink alcohol or use any recreational substances while taking opioids.
- **Remember, as long as the Pain Management Service is prescribing pain medications, no other health care provider should be writing orders for refills or changing your pain medication plan. No changes should be made such as changing the dose of the pain medicines or adding any new pain medicines unless a member of the Pain Management Service is contacted.**
- When it is no longer necessary for your child to be followed by the Pain Management Service, we will tell you and your primary St Jude doctor will then manage any pain he may have.
- Opioids may cause dizziness and drowsiness. Opioids may impair your ability to drive a car or operate heavy machinery, so do not participate in these activities if you are sleepy, drowsy, dizzy, or not alert after you take opioids.

Be sure to ask questions related to our recommendations. It is important that you understand the plan. Call the Pain Management Service physician or clinical nurse specialist for any questions or concerns:

- During normal business hours, call 901-495-4032 and the secretary will contact a member of the Pain Management Service to return your call as soon as possible.
- During other hours, call 901-495-3300 and ask the operator to page the Pain Management Service physician on-call. Please remain on the telephone line until the physician connects with the call.

Please sign here to indicate your have received this information:

_____   _____   _____

Patient   Parent (if the patient is a minor)   Date

_____

Pain Management Service Member

June 2007 © St Jude Children's Research Hospital

Figure 11.1 ▦ *(Continued)*

Charting Doses While Taking Oramorph SR® (Long-acting Morphine)

Patient Name: _____ Parent/guardian:_____ Date:_____

Morphine is an opioid (narcotic) used to treat pain. If your child needs ongoing pain relief, the doctor may prescribe Oramorph SR® (a long-acting form of morphine). Follow the dosages for Oramorph SR® as written below. Give the doses to your child as close to 12 hours apart as you can. Because of a risk for overdose, Oramorph SR® tablets should not be chewed, crushed, or cut. For pain that comes on quickly, the doctor will prescribe another pain medicine called _____. Most often, this medicine will relieve pain within 30 minutes for a period of 2–4 hours. For this reason, it is called "immediate-release" or "fast-acting." Your child may take _____ (number of tablets/capsules/ml) of this fast-acting drug every_____ hours. Use the chart below to record the number of fast-acting doses. If your child still has pain even when taking the pain medicines as written below, call the Pain Management Service (Pain Team).

Date(s)	Oramorph SR® dose(s):	Number of _____ doses taken of the fast-acting (give mg if they are different strengths)	Other medicines to take	More information

Remember: As long as the Pain Team prescribes these medicines, no one else should write orders for refills or change your child's pain medicine plan without talking to the Pain Team staff. After you pick up refills of these medicines, you should have enough of each drug to last until your child's next Pain Clinic visit.

See the handout "Patient Medication: Morphine" for more details about side effects and special guidelines for this drug. Please call the Pain Team if you have concerns about:

- How well these medicines control your child's pain,
- Any side effects of these drugs, or
- How to give these pain medicines.

If your child has been taking opioids for more than a few days, he should be tapered off the drugs to prevent side effects: stomach cramping, jitters, sweating, and diarrhea. If your child has any of these symptoms, call the Pain Team right away.

To reach the Pain Team staff, please follow these guidelines:

- Monday–Friday, during normal clinic hours, call 595-4622 and ask to speak to the Pain Clinic Nurse or Pain Clinical Nurse Specialist. If you are in the hospital, dial 4622. If you are outside the Memphis area, call toll-free 1-866-2STJUDE (1-866-278-5833), extension 4622.
- Weekends, holidays, and after hours, call 595-3300 and ask the operator to page the Pain Team doctor.
- If you speak to another doctor about pain issues, please remind the doctor that the St. Jude Pain Team is working with your child.

Please bring this sheet of paper and all pain medicines to each clinic visit. The chart will help the Pain Team know how well these drugs are working and if your child needs refills.

Figure 11.2 ▓ An example of a pain diary.
Copyright 2005 by St. Jude Children's Research Hospital, Memphis, TN. Used with permission.

Clinical Pearl	When the escalation of pain is disproportional to the child's source of pain, health care providers need to consider these questions:

- Is the analgesia regimen easy to understand and follow?
- Is the child taking all the analgesics as prescribed (e.g., does the analgesic plan cover the types of pain in adequate doses for age, weight, medical, or surgical condition)?
- Is there a problem with drug delivery (e.g., the patient is not absorbing the medication [e.g., a fentanyl patch is loose or the patient vomits oral doses] or the pump is not infusing the medication as prescribed)?
- Could the source of pain be becoming more serious (e.g., the tumor growing, new metastasis, infection, swelling, tight cast, or blocked wound drain)?

In summary, the American Academy of Pediatrics emphasizes the responsibilities of health care providers to expand their knowledge about pain management, use appropriate assessment tools and techniques, anticipate painful experiences, and intervene accordingly with evidence-based approaches (American Academy of Pediatrics, 2001). Collaborating with health care providers who have diverse skills and, most important, the passion and professional commitment to improve care through evidence-based assessment tools, effective analgesics, innovative drug delivery systems, and teaching children nonpharmacologic techniques that can reduce suffering throughout life defines multidisciplinary approaches to pain management (Berde & Solodiuk, 2003; Simons et al., 2010; Slater et al., 2010).

REFERENCES

American Academy of Pediatrics. (2001). The assessment and management of acute pain in infants, children, and adolescents. *Pediatrics, 108*(3), 793–797.

Anghelescu, D., Oakes, L., & Popenhagan, M. (2006). Management of pain due to cancer in neonates, children, and adolescents. In O. A. de Leon-Casasola (Ed.), *Cancer pain: Pharmacologic, interventional, and palliative care approaches* (pp. 509–521). Philadelphia, PA: Elsevier.

Berde, C. B., & Solodiuk, J. (2003). Multidisciplinary programs for management of acute and chronic pain in children. In N. L. Schechter, C. B. Berde, & M. Yaster (Eds.), *Pain in infants, children, and adolescents* (2nd ed., pp. 471–486). Philadelphia, PA: Lippincott Williams & Wilkins.

Connelly, M., & Schanberg, L. (2006). Latest developments in the assessment and management of chronic musculoskeletal pain syndromes in children. *Current Opinion in Rheumatology, 18*(5), 496–502.

Maikler, V. E., Broome, M. E., Bailey, P., & Lea, G. (2001). Children's and adolescents' use of diaries for sickle cell pain. *Journal of the Society of Pediatric Nurses, 6*(4), 161–169.

Oakes, L. L., Anghelescu, D. L., Windsor, K. B., & Barnhill, P. D. (2008). An institutional quality improvement initiative for pain management for pediatric cancer inpatients. *Journal of Pain and Symptom Management, 35*(6), 656–669.

Passik, S. D., & Kirsh, K. L. (2005). Managing pain in patients with aberrant drug-taking behaviors. *Journal of Supportive Oncology, 3*(1), 83–86.

Simons, L. E., Logan, D. E., Chastain, L., & Cerullo, M. (2010). Engagement in multidisciplinary interventions for pediatric chronic pain: Parental expectations, barriers, and child outcomes. *Clinical Journal of Pain, 26*(4), 291–299.

Slater, M. E., De Lima, J., Campbell, K., Lane, L., & Collins, J. (2010). Opioids for the management of severe chronic nonmalignant pain in children: A retrospective 1-year practice survey in a children's hospital. *Pain Medicine, 11*(2), 207–214.

Stinson, J., & Bruce, E. (2009). Chronic pain in children. In A. Twycross, S. J. Dowden, & E. Bruce (Eds.), *Managing pain in children: A clinical guide* (pp. 145–170). Oxford, United Kingdom: Wiley-Blackwell.

Wicksell, R. K., Melin, L., & Olsson, G. L. (2007). Exposure and acceptance in the rehabilitation of adolescents with idiopathic chronic pain—a pilot study. *European Journal of Pain, 11*(3), 267–274.

12

Role of Parents

The effects of pain on children have been acknowledged in recent years. However, the distress of pain also affects the parents as well. While most families receive accurate information about their child's condition and its required treatments, few families receive concrete information about the factors that attenuate or exacerbate pain (Cohen, Bernard, Greco, & McClellan, 2002; McCarthy & Kleiber, 2006). The author's institution provides general information to all parents as illustrated in Figure 12.1. (More specific information regarding medications, nonpharmacologic interventions, and other pain-relieving strategies can be found in the patient education section of the Appendix.)

ROLE OF PARENTS DURING PROCEDURES

Studies reveal that parents, regardless of culture and other socioeconomic backgrounds, are the greatest source of strength for children facing a painful procedure (Broome & Huth, 2003; Jones, Qazi, & Young, 2005), with most parents preferring to remain present and to participate or soothe their child even for highly invasive procedures (Polkki, Pietila, Vehvilainen-Julkunen, Laukkala, & Ryhanen, 2002). Excluding parents from observing invasive procedures has

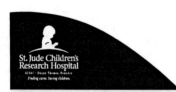

Do you know...

An educational series for patients and their families

What you can do to help your child in pain

About pain

A child with cancer or other diseases treated at St Jude will likely have pain at times. The pain can keep him from being active, from sleeping well, from enjoying family and friends, and even from eating. Pain can also make him feel afraid or depressed. When your child hurts, it is important that he feels a sense of control over the pain. Fortunately, the more you know about pain, the better you will be able to help your child. It is important for you to understand the kind of pain he is having, what influences the pain, and the best way to help him cope with the pain. Rather than allowing him to feel helpless, you can help him learn skills that will help reduce his pain.

If your child is feeling pain, it is very important that you tell his doctor or nurse as soon as possible. With treatment, most pain can be reduced easily. If his doctor is having a hard time relieving the pain, a special group of people at St Jude, the Pain Management Service, can help. They can be called at any time, day or night, to help treat the pain.

What causes pain?

Pain can have many different causes. Most cancer pain comes when a tumor presses on bones, nerves, or body organs. Treatment of an illness can cause pain as well. Your child may also have pain that has nothing to do with his illness or its treatment. Like everyone else, he can get headaches, muscle strains, and other aches and pains. You should check with your child's doctor or nurse about what to do for your child for these everyday aches and pains before giving him additional medicines.

- Pain related to a procedure, treatment or tests such as IVs, injections, and lumbar punctures (spinal taps). It is usually localized to the site of the procedure. If your child is having a procedure such as the insertion of a needle into a vein, an injection, or a lumbar puncture (spinal tap), ask your doctor or nurse about the use of numbing cream.

- Pain related to the cancer or its treatment: Pain from a tumor pushing on body parts can be reduced by using medications called analgesics. If your child needs to have surgery or if he has side effects from the chemotherapy or radiation therapy, your child's doctor or nurse will tell you which medications will work best for the type of pain your child is having. If your child describes his pain using terms such as "tingling", "shooting", or "like needles," his doctor may prescribe specific medicines to reduce pain involving the nerves.

This document is not intended to take the place of the care and attention of your personal physician or other professional medical services. Our aim is to promote active participation in your care and treatment by providing information and education. Questions about individual health concerns or specific treatment options should be discussed with your physician.

Figure 12.1 ▮ Parent education regarding their children's pain. Copyright 2003 by St. Jude Children's Research Hospital, Memphis, TN. Used with permission.

Do you know... continued

What *you* can do to help your child in pain

Assessing pain

If your child is in pain, he may do one of the following:

- Complain of pain
- Cry, moan, be irritable or withdraw quietly
- Be restless or not want to move at all
- Hold or guard the area of discomfort
- Not eat or drink as much as usual
- Have difficulties sleeping or sleeping too much to avoid the pain

Your doctor and nurse will ask your child to tell how much they are hurting by using one of three methods:

1. The FACES pain scale:

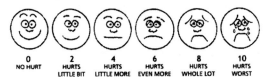

0	2	4	6	8	10
NO HURT	HURTS LITTLE BIT	HURTS LITTLE MORE	HURTS EVEN MORE	HURTS WHOLE LOT	HURTS WORST

From Wong D. L., Hockenberry-Eaton, M., Wilson D., Winkelstein M.L., Schwartz P.: Wong's Essentials of Pediatric Nursing, ed. 6, St. Louis, 2001, p.1301. Copyrighted by Mosby, Inc. Reprinted by permission.

2. If your child is old enough, he may be asked to rate his pain from 0 to 10 without the FACES pain scale.

3. If your child is too young to rate his pain, your doctor or nurse will use a scale (called the FLACC) as they watch for behaviors that might mean your child is in pain.

You know your child better than anyone, so tell the doctor or nurse if your child is acting differently than normal. Talk to your child about what he is feeling and thinking.

- Your child's **thoughts** about what he hears are important. ("I was told this will hurt the last time so it will hurt this time.")
- The **beliefs** he has learned influence what he tells you about his pain. ("I'm a big boy and big boys don't cry!")
- **Emotions** influence the amount of pain. ("Where's my Mommy? I'm scared without my Mommy!")
- **Attitudes** from other people play a role. ("It's expected to hurt at least some.")

Be careful not to reinforce negative thoughts, beliefs, emotions and attitudes. Some helpful responses to your child's pain are to:

- Inform your child about what is happening to him, if he wants to know about it.
- Acknowledge the pain; *do not* minimize or deny it.

This document is not intended to take the place of the care and attention of your personal physician or other professional medical services. Our aim is to promote active participation in your care and treatment by providing information and education. Questions about individual health concerns or specific treatment options should be discussed with your physician.

Figure 12.1 ▓ *(Continued)*

Do you know... continued

What *you* can do to help your child in pain

- Make physical contact with your child. Hold his hand or give him a hug.
- If possible, remain with your child until the pain is controlled.
- Talk about the positive steps that are being taken to reduce his pain.
- Help your child do something to make the pain go away.
- Keep your own anxiety under control and remain calm.
- Support your child's way of coping.

Treating cancer pain

Pain treatments work differently for different people. You need to fully understand how your child's medications should be taken and that you follow those directions very carefully. Because some actions can lead to serious or even dangerous results:

- Do not give him more medicine than is prescribed by the doctor;
- Do not give it to him more frequently than is prescribed;
- Do not stop it abruptly without your doctor's advice;
- Do not crush pills that cannot be crushed, cut or chewed; and
- Do not add any other medications or herbal remedies without first talking to the doctor.

Your child may not get the pain relief he needs from just using medicines. Surgery, radiation therapy and other treatments can be used to give even more pain relief. It is very important that you tell his doctor or nurse how he feels and whether or not the treatments are helping. Sometimes patients worry that their doctor or nurse will think that they are complaining, but this is not true. Your child's doctor and nurse need this information so they can find the right pain medicine and treatments for your child.

Here are some things to help make the pain go away. These techniques may not be a substitute for pain medication, but they can help the pain medicines work better.

Technique	How it works	Examples
Relaxation	• Relieves anxiety • Reduces muscle tightness • Good for episodes of brief and/or severe pain	• Deep breathing (try soap bubbles or party blowers) • Muscle relaxation • Meditation • Soothing music or nature sounds
Distraction	• Focus attention on something other than pain	• Counting, singing, praying • Watching television or movies (especially comedies), talking to family, listening to someone read, playing video games

Figure 12.1 ▨ *(Continued)*

Do you know... continued

What *you* can do to help your child in pain

Reframing/ Thought Stopping	• Evaluate negative thoughts and images and replace them with more positive ones	• "I've had similar pain, and it got better" • "I'm strong. I can do this!"
Imagery/ Hypnosis	• Concentrate on the image of a positive experience or situation or a favorite memory	• Ask your child to be very specific in describing the details of the imagined experience (colors, sounds, smells, tastes, feelings)
Modeling	• Learn from someone else's successes	• Have your child observe another child managing his pain and anxiety by staying calm and talking through his coping techniques.
Heat*	• Increases blood flow	• Warm baths or towels. Consult your physician before using heating pads.
Cold*	• Helps pain from inflammation, swelling, acute injury procedural pain	• Ice packs, crushed ice in a towel
Massage*	• Increases flow of body fluids • Gently stretches tissues • Helps tissue pain and edema	• Use gliding strokes over the skin • *Do not* push solid parts under the skin or massage directly on the painful area
Exercise*	• Strengthens muscles • Loosens stiff joints • Increases blood flow • Helps with most types of pain	• Walking, biking

* consult your doctor or nurse before using these techniques

Common questions parents ask

Do infants and children feel pain?

Yes. The belief that they do *not* experience pain is *not* true. Even though they are unable to talk about it, infants and children *do* feel pain. Therefore, they need to be treated with the same care and concern given to adults in pain.

Do children always admit to having pain?

No. If children are experiencing pain they may be afraid to tell someone about it.

Figure 12.1 ▧ *(Continued)*

Do you know... continued

What *you* can do to help your child in pain

Can children really tell us if the treatment of their pain is working well?

Yes, children are the experts of their own pain. Even very young children can tell us when they are in pain and how much they are hurting.

Will my child become "addicted" to the pain medication?

No, except in very rare cases. Some parents and children worry about becoming "addicted" or "hooked" if they take pain medications. Drug addiction means that a person is taking a drug to get a mental "high" instead of relief from real pain. However, patients with cancer take pain medicine to relieve pain so that they can be as active and comfortable as possible. The truth is addiction is very rare when medicine is taken for pain control.

If my child takes large doses of pain medicine now, will it stop working later when he really needs it?

No, the medicine will not stop working. Sometimes, however, your child's body might get used to the medicine, which is called "tolerance." If this happens, your child will need to be prescribed more pain medicines, but this will *not* cause any harm to him.

Can't my child just "tough it out"? What about the old saying, "No pain, no gain"?

It is unacceptable for a child ever to be in pain. Being sick and having to undergo treatment is difficult and scary enough for anyone. Untreated pain does *not* make them "tough" or help them to build character.

What can I do to help my child with his pain?

- Be calm and have a positive attitude that his doctors and nurses will reduce the pain as much as possible. However, you should *not* say "this won't hurt at all."
- Control your own anxiety and do *not* show negative cues such as gasping, flinching, and cringing.
- Do *not* scold or punish your child for not cooperating.
- Avoid helping to hold your child down during a procedure. Instead, hold his hand or offer ways to distract him from the procedure.

Can I stop giving the pain medicine to my child if his pain goes away?

No, you need to check with your child's medical team. Gradually stopping pain medicines helps avoid side effects. The slow decrease is important because the body has become used to the medicine much like your body gets used to nicotine or caffeine. Gradually stopping the medicine will allow time for the body to get used to not having the medicine. It does not mean your child is addicted to the medicine.

Questions?

If you have any questions or concerns, please call 595-3300 and ask for your primary clinic. If you are calling after hours or on the weekend, you can ask for the doctor on-call. Outside Memphis, dial toll-free 1-866-2STJUDE (1-866-278-5833) and press 0.

This document is not intended to take the place of the care and attention of your personal physician or other professional medical services. Our aim is to promote active participation in your care and treatment by providing information and education. Questions about individual health concerns or specific treatment options should be discussed with your physician.

Figure 12.1 ▦ *(Continued)*

been the traditional and outdated approach based on fears of parental interference or views that it is better for parents not to see. This restriction is perceived by many parents as a major source of anxiety during a time when they believe their presence is critical to their child's course of recovery. However, awareness of how parents can most effectively help their child is important and should be considered by asking, "How can we include parents in the procedure and allow the child the support he needs?"

Preparing for the Procedure
Preparing the Child

Parents are fairly accurate in predicting how distressed their children will be about an upcoming procedure because of their knowledge of their children's usual pattern of reactions. The parents' confidence in their ability to comfort their children's distress and acceptance of the nonpharmacologic intervention that will be provided influence the responses of all involved in the procedure (McCarthy & Kleiber, 2006).

Preparing the Parent

Assessing the relationship between parents and their children and the potential for a parent to enhance or interfere with his or her child's ability to cope during a procedure is the first step in preparing the parent. Even a young child can be quite perceptive of his or her parent's apprehensions or distress. If the parent is anxious, this will increase his or her child's level of anxiety as well. Because of this, health care providers should encourage parents to be positive about the experience. The effect of parental presence on children's pain and distress during a procedure depends on the parent's own anxiety level, parent–child interactions, and the parent's ability to help the child cope effectively. Certain parental behaviors are associated with children coping well, and other behaviors are linked with poor coping and distress (Blount, Piira, Cohen, & Cheng, 2006). Often, parental anxiety may arise from the parents' own distress at not knowing how to assist their children most effectively.

Parents need information about what will take place during the procedure, including what circumstances would prompt their being asked to leave the child during the procedure. Critical to their being effective in supporting their child is the need to describe and reach consensus on what the role of the parents will be during the procedure. The best approach is an individualized one, giving parents the option to remain present but not pressuring them to stay.

During the Procedure

Reassurance is commonly used by parents and staff and, although meant to decrease the child's distress, may actually increase it, which is perplexing and counterintuitive. Researchers have found (Chambers, Craig, & Bennett, 2002; Cohen et al., 2002; McMurtry, Chambers, McGrath, & Asp, 2010; McMurtry, McGrath, Asp, & Chambers, 2007; Windich-Biermeier, Sjoberg, Dale, Eshelman, & Guzzetta, 2007) the following:

- Parental pain-promoting language, such as reassurance, empathy, apologizing for the pain (e.g., "I am so sorry you have to go through this"), and even mildly rebuking (e.g., "If you move, they will have to do the procedure again"), increases children's reports of pain.
- Parental pain-reducing language (i.e., distraction, humor, reassurance, and encouraging coping behaviors) decreases children's reports of pain. Reassurance is defined as "procedure-related comments that are directed toward the child with the intent of reassuring the child about his or her condition or the course of the procedure." Distraction is defined as "talk that does not pertain to the treatment procedure or the child's illness."
- Criticizing, threatening, apologizing, giving control over to the child, catastrophizing, and becoming agitated are associated with increased distress.

Parents may benefit from training in effective methods to help children cope through the use of distraction, such as watching television, reading, looking at books, or playing with small toys (Cavender, Goff, Hollon, & Guzzetta, 2004; Kleiber, Craft-Rosenberg, & Harper, 2001; McCarthy & Kleiber, 2006; Windich-Biermeier et al., 2007).

Having parents at the bedside will require some level of monitoring parents to determine whether they need support. If parents become distressed during the procedure, they need to be redirected to calm the child or be escorted out of the room with no shame implied.

PARENTAL ROLE FOR INPATIENT CARE

Not much is known about parents' perceptions of the nature, timing, adequacy, and understanding of information given to them regarding options for their children's postoperative pain control. Recent research indicated that parent understanding of the risks and benefits of postoperative pain management is quite variable and often insufficient (Tait, Voepel-Lewis, Snyder, & Malviya, 2008). Another study concluded that parents need more guidance in the use of nonpharmacologic methods of surgical pain relief and emotional support during their child's hospitalization (Polkki et al., 2002).

PARENTAL ROLE FOR OUTPATIENT CARE

Parents, not health care providers, are the providers of pain management for children who have minor injuries or surgical procedures in which hospital admission is not required. Few studies have examined children's postoperative pain management in the home. Studies of parents' management of children's pain following short stay and day surgery revealed that even when parents recognized that their children were in pain, most gave inadequate doses of analgesics to control the pain (Finley, McGrath, Forward, McNeill, & Fitzgerald, 1996; Fortier, MacLaren, Martin, Perret-Karimi, & Kain, 2009; Huth & Broome, 2007; Rony, Fortier, Chorney, Perret, & Kain, 2010; Sutters et al., 2010). Research efforts should be directed at the discrepancy between high ratings of postoperative pain provided by parents and the low dosing of analgesics they use for their children.

Medication Instruction

Because parents are in charge of the medicines the infants and children need on an outpatient basis, it is important that they have a sufficient amount of accurate information, both verbally and in a written format to match their literacy level. Content should include the following:

▨ The types and rationale for the analgesics and other medications in the event of adverse effects, such as laxatives to prevent opioid-induced constipation
▨ Adverse effects of each medication
▨ Written instructions on
  ● The dose to give as tablets or liquid
  ● How to give each medication (e.g., whether it can be cut into pieces)
  ● When to give a dose and what to do if a dose is missed or vomited
▨ Careful attention to which medicines are to be given at a scheduled time whether the child is having pain or not and which medicines to give if pain relief is needed (e.g., as needed [PRN] doses for break-through pain)
▨ Instructions to not increase, decrease, or discontinue a scheduled medicine without talking to a health care provider
▨ How to contact the health care providers with concerns about un-controlled pain (i.e., the pain is uncontrolled before the instructions indicate the next PRN dose can be given)
▨ Which adverse effects are to be reported immediately to the health care provider and which ones can be reported at the next visit with the health care provider
▨ How to securely store medications
▨ To check with the health care provider before giving any over-the-counter medications
▨ Signs and symptoms of opioid withdrawal and what actions to take if they occur (e.g., use PRN opioid dose)

Controlled-Release Opioids

For controlled-release preparations, parents should be told they cannot be chewed or broken, which could cause overdoing by becoming an immediate-release preparation. However, for one form of controlled-release morphine (Kadian), approval has been given for opening the capsule and emptying the contents into soft food that can be swallowed without chewing. Parents should be clear that controlled-release opioids are not to be given as a PRN dose because it will take hours to attain an analgesic effect.

In summary, parents and children overwhelmingly prefer to have parents remain present as much as possible. Nurses should advocate parental involvement in their children's care even in the most technical and intimidating environments, such as the pediatric intensive care unit (PICU).

Parental presence during their children's procedures is a well-researched topic. However, continued research that examines factors influencing parental participation in pain relief measures for inpatient and outpatient pain is needed.

REFERENCES

Blount, R. L., Piira, T., Cohen, L. L., & Cheng, P. S. (2006). Pediatric procedural pain. *Behaviour Modification, 30*(1), 24–49.

Broome, M. E., & Huth, M. M. (2003). Nursing management of the child in pain. In N. L. Schechter, C. B. Berde, & M. Yaster (Eds.), *Pain in infants, children, and adolescents* (2nd ed., pp. 417–433). Philadelphia, PA: Lippincott Williams & Wilkins.

Cavender, K., Goff, M. D., Hollon, E. C., & Guzzetta, C. E. (2004). Parents' positioning and distracting children during venipuncture. Effects on children's pain, fear, and distress. *Journal of Holistic Nursing, 22*(1), 32–56.

Chambers, C. T., Craig, K. D., & Bennett, S. M. (2002). The impact of maternal behavior on children's pain experiences: An experimental analysis. *Journal of Pediatric Psychology, 27*(3), 293–301.

Cohen, L. L., Bernard, R. S., Greco, L. A., & McClellan, C. B. (2002). A child-focused intervention for coping with procedural pain: Are parent and nurse coaches necessary? *Journal of Pediatric Psychology, 27*(8), 749–757.

Finley, G. A., McGrath, P. J., Forward, S. P., McNeill, G., & Fitzgerald, P. (1996). Parents' management of children's pain following 'minor' surgery. *Pain, 64*(1), 83–87.

Fortier, M. A., MacLaren, J. E., Martin, S. R., Perret-Karimi, D., & Kain, Z. N. (2009). Pediatric pain after ambulatory surgery: Where's the medication? *Pediatrics, 124*(4), e588–e595.

Huth, M. M., & Broome, M. E. (2007). A snapshot of children's postoperative tonsillectomy outcomes at home. *Journal for Specialists in Pediatric Nursing, 12*(3), 186–195.

Jones, M., Qazi, M., & Young, K. D. (2005). Ethnic differences in parent preference to be present for painful medical procedures. *Pediatrics, 116*(2), e191–e197.

Kleiber, C., Craft-Rosenberg, M., & Harper, D. C. (2001). Parents as distraction coaches during IV insertion: A randomized study. *Journal of Pain and Symptom Management, 22*(4), 851–861.

McCarthy, A. M., & Kleiber, C. (2006). A conceptual model of factors influencing children's responses to a painful procedure when parents are distraction coaches. *Journal of Pediatric Nursing, 21*(2), 88–98.

McMurtry, C. M., Chambers, C. T., McGrath, P. J., & Asp, E. (2010). When "don't worry" communicates fear: Children's perceptions of parental reassurance and distraction during a painful medical procedure. *Pain, 150*, 52–58.

McMurtry, C. M., McGrath, P. J., Asp, E., & Chambers, C. T. (2007). Parental reassurance and pediatric procedural pain: A linguistic description. *Journal of Pain, 8*(2), 95–101.

Polkki, T., Pietila, A. M., Vehvilainen-Julkunen, K., Laukkala, H., & Ryhanen, P. (2002). Parental views on participation in their child's pain relief measures and recommendations to health care providers. *Journal of Pediatric Nursing, 17*(4), 270–278.

Rony, R. Y., Fortier, M. A., Chorney, J. M., Perret, D., & Kain, Z. N. (2010). Parental postoperative pain management: Attitudes, assessment, and management. *Pediatrics, 125*(6), e1372–e1378.

Sutters, K. A., Miaskowski, C., Holdridge-Zeuner, D., Waite, S., Paul, S. M., Savedra, M. C., . . . Mahoney, K. (2010). A randomized clinical trial of the efficacy of scheduled dosing of acetaminophen and hydrocodone for the management of postoperative pain in children after tonsillectomy. *Clinical Journal of Pain, 26*(2), 95–103.

Tait, A. R., Voepel-Lewis, T., Snyder, R. M., & Malviya, S. (2008). Parents' understanding of information regarding their child's postoperative pain management. *Clinical Journal of Pain, 24*(7), 572–577.

Windich-Biermeier, A., Sjoberg, I., Dale, J. C., Eshelman, D., & Guzzetta, C. E. (2007). Effects of distraction on pain, fear, and distress during venous port access and venipuncture in children and adolescents with cancer. *Journal of Pediatric Oncology Nursing, 24*(1), 8–19.

VI

Special Treatment Considerations for Pain Including Impact on the Family

13

Needle-Related Procedures

Medical procedures, often including needles, are understandable sources of pain and distress for children. Common childhood painful medical procedures (e.g., immunizations, blood tests, and laceration repairs) along with minor everyday pain experiences, such as falls, bumps, and cuts, compose most of the typical child's pain events. Healthy newborns experience needle-related pain in their first hours of life (e.g., heel lances to obtain blood for routine metabolic screening and vitamin K injections). It is a common belief by health care providers that infants with neurological impairment have less risk of pain than unimpaired infants; however, these infants undergo more frequent painful procedures (Breau et al., 2006). Infants who are hospitalized in the first 2 weeks of life can experience an average of 14 invasive and painful procedures per day at a time when the infant is transitioning from the protective intrauterine environment (Anand et al., 2006; Yamada et al., 2008). For infants and children who suffer a serious illness or injury, brief diagnostic and therapeutic procedures are often a necessary part of medical care, as listed in Table 13.1.

Table 13.1 ▦ *Common Medical Procedures and Recommended Interventions*

Procedure	Recommended Interventions
IM or SC injections Venipuncture for laboratory tests PIV placement Subcutaneous reservoirs or ports access Wound suture Arterial line insertion PICC line insertion	Nonpharmacologic interventions, LAs via needleless systems
Wound and laceration suturing	SC buffered local anesthetics, nonpharmacologic interventions
Heel lancing	Oral sucrose, nonnutritive sucking, holding, feeding with breast milk
BMA Lumbar puncture Chest tube placement Central line	SC local anesthetics, nonpharmacologic interventions, possible systemic sedation and analgesia

Abbreviations: BMA, bone marrow aspiration; IM, intramuscular; LAs, local anesthetics; PICC, peripherally inserted central catheter; PIV, peripheral intravenous; SC, subcutaneous.
Source: From Dahlquist, Busby, et al., 2002; Dahlquist, Pendley, Landthrip, Jones, & Steuber, 2002; Spagrud et al., 2008; Weissman, Aranovitch, Blazer, & Zimmer, 2009; Windich-Biermeier, Sjoberg, Dale, Eshelman, & Guzzetta, 2007.

Clinical Pearl	Heel lancing has long been used for blood sampling for infants who lack vascular access. Although technically simple and considered a "minor" procedure, it produces bruising and inflammation. The pain associated with heel lancing followed by squeezing the invasive site has been the stimulus to examine the need to consider venipuncture as the preferred method of blood sampling for neonates (Shah & Ohlsson, 2007). Children who experienced frequent heel lances as infants display increased distress during the skin cleansing process prior to an injection, leading to the conclusion that infants may learn that a nonpainful stimulus is followed by a painful stimulus (Taddio, Shah, Gilbert-MacLeod, & Katz, 2002).

INTERVENTIONS TO REDUCE PAIN ASSOCIATED WITH NEEDLES

Medical procedures need to be completed with the lowest possible level of pain and anxiety by selecting suitable pharmacologic and nonpharmacologic interventions. Although analgesics and anesthetics will reduce needle-related pain, nonpharmacologic techniques are essential to control the anxiety and other emotions related to the procedures (Windich-Biermeier, Sjoberg, Dale, Eshelman, & Guzzetta, 2007). The use of multidisciplinary approaches, especially having the input of the child life specialist, is optimal (Zempsky & Cravero, 2004). Often, combining techniques and medications appears to be synergistic in reducing pain. Interventions such as positioning and facilitated tucking, the use of nonnutritive sucking (pacifiers), kangaroo care, breastfeeding (Shah, Aliwalas, & Shah, 2006; Weissman, Aranovitch, Blazer, & Zimmer, 2009), and oral sucrose have been shown to provide clearly measurable, although often incomplete, relief of pain (Chermont, Falcao, de Souza Silva, de Cassia Xavier Balda, & Guinsburg, 2009). (For nonpharmacologic techniques, see Chapters 8–10, and for the role of the family in supporting the children during needle-related procedures, see Chapter 12.)

Local Anesthetics

Indications

Analgesia for reducing pain related to any needle insertion is described in Table 13.1.

Dosage

Maximum safe doses for age and weight are recommended and should be strictly followed (Dowden, 2009). Dosing guidelines for infiltration anesthesia with lidocaine (Xylocaine) (Greco & Berde, 2005):

- < 6 months of age: 4 mg/kg
- ≥ 6 months of age: 5 mg/kg

Forms and Administration

Subcutaneous Infiltration. Lidocaine is the most commonly administered local anesthetic (LA) for dermal procedures. Lidocaine was originally administered by using a small needle to puncture the skin with infiltration below the stratum corneum, and children feared the needle prior to the infiltration and the burning sensation of the LA. Providing painless infiltration will require buffering it with bicarbonate, warming the lidocaine before use, and injecting it slowly with a small-gauge needle (Zempsky & Cravero, 2004).

Needleless Systems. More recent administration of LAs via needleless systems is widely available and is much more appealing to children. These systems, described in detail in Table 13.2, include the following:

- Creams with lidocaine (LMX4) or with a combination of lidocaine and prilocaine (EMLA [eutectic mixture of local anesthetic]) (Fetzer, 2002; Kaur, Gupta, & Kumar, 2003; Luhmann, Hurt, Shootman, & Kennedy, 2004). Because of passive absorption through the skin, advance planning by health care providers is necessary to allow effective application time.
- Iontophoresis drug delivery systems, which use a small external electric current to facilitate delivery of lidocaine (Squire, Kirchhoff, & Hissong, 2000).
- Lidocaine and tetracaine (Synera) integrated into a controlled heat-aided drug delivery patch to facilitate absorption (Sethna et al., 2005).
- J-tip syringe, a single-use sterile, needle-free injection device with a self-contained compressed carbon dioxide gas cartridge that forces medication through a micro-orifice at a high velocity through the skin and into the underlying subcutaneous tissues, found useful for reducing the pain from peripheral intravenous (PIV) needle insertions (Spanos et al., 2008). This system can deliver LA with minimal skin trauma and petechiae in children with bleeding tendencies (Jimenez, Bradford, Seidel, Sousa, & Lynn, 2006; Lysakowski, Dumont, Tramer, & Tassonyi, 2003; Wolf, Stoddart, Murphy, & Sasada, 2002; Zempsky, Robbins, Richards, Leong, & Schechter,

Table 13.2 ■ *Needleless Systems in Providing Local Anesthetics for Needle-Related Pain*

System	Ingredients	Minimal Preparation Time for Effective Analgesia	Comments
EMLA	2.5% lidocaine and 2.5% prilocaine	60–90 min	■ Use with caution for infants younger than 3 months because of possible methemoglobinemia associated with metabolism of prilocaine ■ Not effective for heel lancing or finger sticks ■ Vasoconstriction decreasing vein visibility ■ May be applied by parent
LMX4	4% lidocaine	30 min	■ Available over the counter ■ May be applied by parent
Synera	Lidocaine (70 mg) and tetracaine (70 mg)	20–30 min	■ Not approved for parent application
Numby Stuff	Lidocaine topical solutions, usually 1% or 2%	20 min	■ Tingling and potential skin burns may make this less acceptable ■ Do use on broken skin ■ Electrode application to contoured skin areas is difficult ■ Not approved for parent application
Needle-free lidocaine injection device (J-tip)	1% buffered lidocaine	1 min	■ Creates a disconcerting "pop" when activated ■ Local hyperemia and minor bleeding ■ Not approved for parent application

Abbreviation: EMLA, eutectic mixture of local anesthetic.
Source: From American Pain Society, 2008; Ellis, Sharp, Newhook, & Cohen, 2004; Kleiber, Sorenson, Whiteside, Gronstal, & Tannous, 2002; Zempsky & Cravero, 2004.

2008) and has been found to be cost-effective when providing needleless injections of lidocaine in a busy emergency department (ED) compared with lidocaine creams or iontophoresis (Pershad, Steinberg, & Waters, 2008).

■ Laser-assisted delivery of LAs, which uses a pulse of radiant energy to remove the stratum corneum of the skin to shorten the time for drug penetration. However, more research is needed regarding the dose and safety of this system, especially for children younger than 3 years or with immunosuppression (Koh, Harrison, Swanson, Norvell, & Coomber, 2007).

Adverse Effects

Adverse effects can occur from either an excessive dose of the LA in the intended route or accidental injection of the LA into the general circulation, resulting in high plasma concentrations of the drug that can affect the cardiac and central nervous systems (i.e., vasodilation, hypotension, and seizures) (Berde et al., 2005).

Subcutaneous Administration. For infants and small children, the inability to aspirate blood into a syringe does not always mean the needle has missed a vessel, because veins may collapse on aspiration.

EMLA. For prilocaine, which is a component of EMLA, methemoglobinemia is an additional risk for infants.

Vapocoolants

A considerably less expensive method to reduce pain via vapocoolants, such as fluorocarbon, was considered to provide effective pain relief for immunizations. However, because the duration of action is shorter than the necessary time for adequate skin cleansing, vapocoolants are no longer recommended as effective relief for IV placement (Costello, Ramundo, Christopher, & Powell, 2006; Reis, Roth, Syphan, Tarbell, & Holubkov, 2003; Zempsky & Cravero, 2004).

Sucrose

Indications

Sucrose has been found to be safe and effective for healthy and full-term infants for minor procedures (Stevens, Yamada, & Ohlsson, 2004; Tsao, Evans, Meldrum, Altman, & Zeltzer, 2008). Reduction of pain and distress (e.g., decreased heart rate and behavioral indicators such as crying) has been demonstrated for infants up to 4 months old, especially in combination with nonnutritive sucking or topical anesthetics, for single invasive procedures, such as immunizations, heel lancing, suctioning, nasogastric tube insertion, IV insertion, and lumbar punctures (Akman, Ozek, Bilgen, Ozdogan, & Cebeci, 2002; Franck, 2000; Hatfield, Gusic, Dyer, & Polomano, 2008; Lefrak et al., 2006; Lindh, Wiklund, Blomquist, & Hakansson, 2003; Zempsky & Cravero, 2004). The underlying mechanism of sucrose and nonnutritive sucking are currently not well understood, but are believed to be mediated by both endogenous opioid and nonopioid systems (Gradin & Schollin, 2005; Taddio, Shah, Shah, & Katz, 2003; Tsao et al., 2008).

Dosage and Administration

Health care providers should use the smallest amount of sucrose that provides pain relief, as the optimal dose has not yet been established (Anderson & Palmer, 2006). The peak onset of action seems to be in 2 minutes with a duration of effect from 5 to 10 minutes (Taddio et al., 2003). More research is needed to determine whether efficacy is prolonged by providing boost doses during the procedure (Stevens et al., 2004). Mixed findings have been reported regarding the use of sucrose in preterm and ill infants (Tsao et al., 2008). The use of sucrose in combination with other nonpharmacologic interventions such as kangaroo care as well as other pharmacologic interventions requires further study (Anderson & Palmer, 2006).

Breast Milk

Several mechanisms by which breast milk or breastfeeding may provide analgesic effects have been offered, including the presence of a comforting person, the physical sensation (skin-to-skin contact with the comforting person), the diversion of attention with the sweetness of the breast milk, and the higher concentrations of tryptophan (a precursor of melatonin in the breast milk) (Shah et al., 2006).

Intravenous Sedation and Analgesia

For some procedures, such as bone marrow aspirations, biopsies, and lumbar punctures, intravenous administration of sedatives and analgesics may be indicated. The goals are to prevent feeling noxious stimuli, to permit the maintenance of spontaneous ventilation, and to produce residual postprocedure analgesia with minimal side effects. However, the risk–benefit ratio needs to be considered, including the need to have specific conditions met (e.g., appropriate hours of nothing by mouth [NPO] status or lack of upper respiratory tract illnesses) to reduce the complications associated with this method of reducing needle-related pain. Anesthesia-trained clinicians (e.g., anesthesiologists, nurse anesthetists, or intensivists) provide doses of short-acting agents (e.g., propofol and fentanyl) while monitoring and protecting the patient's airway. These procedures involve specific skills and equipment outside the scope of this book.

THE MEDICAL PROCEDURE

Planning for the Procedure

Health care providers need to determine which strategies, discussed previously, are most appropriate for the procedure being performed (see Table 13.1 for recommendations for various procedures). Factors to consider when determining the plan include the child's age, the procedure being performed, the complexity of the child's underlying medical condition, and the child's ability to understand his role in holding still. Planning for the procedure can be enhanced by the health care provider answering the following questions:

■ Why is the procedure being performed? Is it essential? Could it be delayed and combined with a pending procedure that requires sedation?

- How will the procedure be performed?
- Where will the procedure be performed?
- Who are the key health care providers to be present?
- What is the expected intensity and duration of the pain?
- How frightening will it be? How important is it that the child remain still during the procedure? The use of physical restraint should be avoided as much as possible. If it is necessary, it will require child–parent agreement.
- How do the parents think the child will react? How do the parents think they themselves will react?
- What can the parents do to help?

As to where the procedure should be conducted, some health care providers think it is best to avoid performing procedures in the child's bed to maintain the image of the bed being a safe space. In contrast, other experts conclude that children find it more comforting to be in a familiar place (Bruce, 2009).

Preparation for the Procedure

Children have the right to know what is happening to them so they can feel more in control. Preparation, even for the most emergent procedure, needs to be done with age-appropriate explanations. A warm smile and a slow, respectful approach are particularly important to reduce a frightened child's perception of the health care provider as a threat. Include the parents by asking them what helps their children feel better (see Chapter 12).

Clinical Pearl	Preparation requires a delicate balance of providing just the right amount of information, not enough to scare the child, but adequate to prepare them for their role in successful completion of the procedure.
	• The younger the child, the briefer the explanation needs to be, in small bits and closer to the time of the procedure. Older children benefit from more notification in advance to allow them time to prepare themselves.

(Continued)

(Continued)

■ Information needs to be provided as to why, how, where, and what to expect, including any sensations they may feel, especially the degree of pain they will feel (i.e., "this will feel like a prick or poke"). False information, such as "this will not hurt at all," is not helpful and teaches the child to be distrustful, leading to more fear of subsequent procedures.

■ Avoid words that can increase anxiety and misunderstanding, such as "cut," "shot," "stretcher," "dye," and "put to sleep."

■ Describe what noises they may hear and what machines or materials they might see or use, including oxygen. If time permits, have the child act out the procedure, a technique called *medical play* (See Chapter 8).

■ Explain what will be done to reduce the pain and what the child's role will be.

During the Procedure

The health care provider is to control the environment, promoting relaxation, and facilitating coping behaviors. Offer distractions, which should have been discussed during planning for the procedure (Windich-Biermeier et al., 2007). Parents should not be asked to hold their child in a restraining manner, but in a comfortable position.

Even young children may be assigned a small "job," such as holding the tape, pouring saline on the dressing, or removing the old dressing. By being active participants in their care, children feel more in control rather than feeling controlled by their pain.

Choices can be offered to the child whenever possible. For example, "Should we start with the burn dressing or the central line dressing change?" "What color do you want the cast to be?" Other helpful strategies include the following:

■ Not forcing the child to lie down if he does not want to, unless it is necessary for the procedure.

■ Avoiding stressors, such as monitors with beeping noises.

■ For PIV insertion, avoiding the arm of the preferred hand to facilitate thumb sucking.

▓ Allowing comfort items, such as favorite blankets or stuffed animals.
▓ Allowing the child to count down from 5 or 10 for short procedures such as injections.

Continually offer positive feedback to the child, such as "you are doing great" and "we are almost finished."

Postprocedure

After a distressing procedure, nurses should encourage children to express their feelings about pain. Medical play with dolls is a way for younger children to work through what has happened to them. Older children may want to draw pictures.

THE IMPACT OF UNRELIEVED PROCEDURAL PAIN

Children who are offered and supported with appropriate interventions have positive viewpoints, with increased levels of self-control and a sense of achievement and skills they can carry throughout life. Unfortunately, many children who are not adequately prepared or offered even the simplest of interventions to reduce pain develop greater levels of anxiety in anticipation of repeated painful procedures. If children are underprepared and distressed during procedures, fragmented and distorted recall can easily become exaggerated memories of the pain experienced, resulting in increased distress during subsequent procedures (Kleiber, Sorenson, Whiteside, Gronstal, & Tannous, 2002). Even children who appear to have low levels of distress tend to have distorted negative recall of the procedures (Chen, Zeltzer, Craske, & Katz, 2000). Hospitalized children who have a greater quantity of invasive procedures have more medical fears and more posttraumatic stress disorder symptoms 6 months after discharge (Rennick, Johnston, Dougherty, Platt, & Ritchie, 2002). Thus, the experiences that children have during painful medical procedures, whether perceived as positive or negative, are likely to play a significant role in shaping responses to pain in the future.

Many effective methods to reduce procedural pain are available and are mandated by various professional health care organizations (American Academy of Pediatrics, 2001; Oncology Nursing Society, 2004). However, many barriers, particularly knowledge about available products, concerns about their cost, and knowledge of how to use them as part of the routine of the procedures, seem to thwart health care providers in using these interventions (Ellis, Sharp, Newhook, & Cohen, 2004). One study looked at the advantage of each regarding cost of the product plus costs associated with time in the ED with outcomes, including pain score reductions, concluding that the J-tip syringe system appeared to offer the most cost-effective option to pediatric ED health care providers (Pershad et al., 2008). More research is needed to develop strategies to overcome barriers in reducing needle-related pain and anxiety. The quest continues for affordable, rapid-acting, cutaneous analgesics that do not cause pain and produce no significant local or systemic toxicity (Houck & Sethna, 2005; Spanos et al., 2008).

REFERENCES

Akman, I., Ozek, E., Bilgen, H., Ozdogan, T., & Cebeci, D. (2002). Sweet solutions and pacifiers for pain relief in newborn infants. *Journal of Pain, 3*(3), 199–202.

American Academy of Pediatrics. (2001). The assessment and management of acute pain in infants, children, and adolescents. *Pediatrics, 108*(3), 793–797.

American Pain Society. (2008). *Principles of analgesic use in the treatment of acute pain and cancer pain.* Glenview, IL: Author.

Anand, K. J., Aranda, J. V., Berde, C. B., Buckman, S., Capparelli, E. V., Carlo, W., . . . Walco, G. A. (2006). Summary proceedings from the neonatal pain-control group. *Pediatrics, 117*(3), S9–S22.

Anderson, B. J., & Palmer, G. M. (2006). Recent pharmacological advances in paediatric analgesics. *Biomedicine & Pharmacotherapy, 60*(7), 303–309.

Berde, C. B., Jaksic, T., Lynn, A. M., Maxwell, L. G., Soriano, S. G., & Tibboel, D. (2005). Anesthesia and analgesia during and after surgery in neonates. *Clinical Therapeutics, 27*(6), 900–921.

Breau, L. M., McGrath, P. J., Stevens, B., Beyene, J., Camfield, C., Finley, G. A., . . . Ohlsson, A. (2006). Judgments of pain in the neonatal intensive care setting: A survey of direct care staffs' perceptions of pain in infants at risk for neurological impairment. *Clinical Journal of Pain*, *22*(2), 122–129.

Bruce, E. (2009). Management of painful procedures. In A. Twycross, S. J. Dowden, & E. Bruce (Eds.), *Managing pain in children: A clinical guide* (pp. 201–218). Oxford, United Kingdom: Wiley-Blackwell.

Chen, E., Zeltzer, L. K., Craske, M. G., & Katz, E. R. (2000). Children's memories for painful cancer treatment procedures: Implications for distress. *Child Development*, *71*(4), 933–947.

Chermont, A. G., Falcao, L. F., de Souza Silva, E. H., de Cassia Xavier Balda, R., & Guinsburg, R. (2009). Skin-to-skin contact and/or oral 25% dextrose for procedural pain relief for term newborn infants. *Pediatrics*, *124*(6), e1101–1107.

Costello, M., Ramundo, M., Christopher, N. C., & Powell, K. R. (2006). Ethyl vinyl chloride vapocoolant spray fails to decrease pain associated with intravenous cannulation in children. *Clinical Pediatrics (Philadelphia)*, *45*(7), 628–632.

Dahlquist, L. M., Busby, S. M., Slifer, K. J., Tucker, C. L., Eischen, S., Hilley, L., & Sulc, W. (2002). Distraction for children of different ages who undergo repeated needle sticks. *Journal of Pediatric Oncology Nursing*, *19*(1), 22–34.

Dahlquist, L. M., Pendley, J. S., Landthrip, D. S., Jones, C. L., & Steuber, C. P. (2002). Distraction intervention for preschoolers undergoing intramuscular injections and subcutaneous port access. *Health Psychology*, *21*(1), 94–99.

Dowden, S. J. (2009). Palliative care in children. In A. Twycross, S. J. Dowden, & E. Bruce (Eds.), *Managing pain in children: A clinical guide* (pp. 171–200). Oxford, United Kingdom: Wiley-Blackwell.

Ellis, J. A., Sharp, D., Newhook, K., & Cohen, J. (2004). Selling comfort: A survey of interventions for needle procedures in a pediatric hospital. *Pain Management Nursing*, *5*(4), 144–152.

Fetzer, S. J. (2002). Reducing venipuncture and intravenous insertion pain with eutectic mixture of local anesthetic: A meta-analysis. *Nursing Research*, *51*(2), 119–124.

Franck, L. (2000). Environmental and behavioral strategies to prevent and manage neonatal pain. In K. J. Anand, B. Stevens, & P. J. McGrath (Eds.),

Pain in infants (2nd ed., Vol. 10, pp. 203–216). Amsterdam, The Netherlands: Elsevier.

Gradin, M., & Schollin, J. (2005). The role of endogenous opioids in mediating pain reduction by orally administered glucose among newborns. *Pediatrics, 115*(4), 1004–1007.

Greco, C., & Berde, C. (2005). Pain management for the hospitalized pediatric patient. *Pediatric Clinics of North America, 52*(4), 995–1027.

Hatfield, L. A., Gusic, M. E., Dyer, A. M., & Polomano, R. C. (2008). Analgesic properties of oral sucrose during routine immunizations at 2 and 4 months of age. *Pediatrics, 121*(2), e327–334.

Houck, C. S., & Sethna, N. F. (2005). Transdermal analgesia with local anesthetics in children: Review, update, and future directions. *Expert Review of Neurotherapeutics, 5*(5), 625–634.

Jimenez, N., Bradford, H., Seidel, K. D., Sousa, M., & Lynn, A. M. (2006). A comparison of a needle-free injection system for local anesthesia versus EMLA for intravenous catheter insertion in the pediatric patient. *Anesthesia and Analgesia, 102*(2), 411–414.

Kaur, G., Gupta, P., & Kumar, A. (2003). A randomized trial of eutectic mixture of local anesthetics during lumbar puncture in newborns. *Archives of Pediatrics and Adolescent Medicine, 157*(11), 1065–1070.

Kleiber, C., Sorenson, M., Whiteside, K., Gronstal, B. A., & Tannous, R. (2002). Topical anesthetics for intravenous insertion in children: A randomized equivalency study. *Pediatrics, 110*(4), 758–761.

Koh, J. L., Harrison, D., Swanson, V., Norvell, D. C., & Coomber, D. C. (2007). A comparison of laser-assisted drug delivery at two output energies for enhancing the delivery of topically applied LMX-4 cream prior to venipuncture. *Anesthesia and Analgesia, 104*(4), 847–849.

Lefrak, L., Burch, K., Caravantes, R., Knoerlein, K., DeNolf, N., Duncan, J., . . . Toczylowski, K. (2006). Sucrose analgesia: Identifying potentially better practices. *Pediatrics, 118*(Suppl. 2), S197–202.

Lindh, V., Wiklund, U., Blomquist, H. K., & Hakansson, S. (2003). EMLA cream and oral glucose for immunization pain in 3-month-old infants. *Pain, 104*, 381–388.

Luhmann, J., Hurt, S., Shootman, M., & Kennedy, R. (2004). A comparison of buffered lidocaine versus ELA-Max before peripheral intravenous catheter insertions in children. *Pediatrics, 113*(3), e217–220.

Lysakowski, C., Dumont, L., Tramer, M. R., & Tassonyi, E. (2003). A needle-free jet-injection system with lidocaine for peripheral intravenous cannula insertion: A randomized controlled trial with cost-effectiveness analysis. *Anesthesia and Analgesia, 96*(1), 215–219.

Oncology Nursing Society. (2004). Access device guidelines: Recommendations for nursing practice and education. *National Guideline Clearinghouse*. Retrieved from www.guideline.gov

Pershad, J., Steinberg, S. C., & Waters, T. M. (2008). Cost-effectiveness analysis of anesthetic agents during peripheral intravenous cannulation in the pediatric emergency department. *Archives of Pediatrics & Adolescent Medicine, 162*(10), 952–961.

Reis, E. C., Roth, E. K., Syphan, J. L., Tarbell, S. E., & Holubkov, R. (2003). Effective pain reduction for multiple immunization injections in young infants. *Archives of Pediatrics and Adolescent Medicine, 157*(11), 1115–1120.

Rennick, J. E., Johnston, C. C., Dougherty, G., Platt, R., & Ritchie, J. A. (2002). Children's psychological responses after critical illness and exposure to invasive technology. *Journal of Developmental and Behavioral Pediatrics, 23*(3), 133–144.

Sethna, N. F., Verghese, S. T., Hannallah, R. S., Solodiuk, J. C., Zurakowski, D., & Berde, C. B. (2005). A randomized controlled trial to evaluate S-Caine patch for reducing pain associated with vascular access in children. *Anesthesiology, 102*(2), 403–408.

Shah, P. S., Aliwalas, L. I., & Shah, V. (2006). Breastfeeding or breast milk for procedural pain in neonates. *Cochrane Database Systematic Reviews, 3*, CD004950.

Shah, V., & Ohlsson, A. (2007). Venepuncture versus heel lance for blood sampling in term neonates. *Cochrane Database Systematic Reviews, 4*, CD001452.

Spagrud, L. J., von Baeyer, C. L., Ali, K., Mpofu, C., Fennell, L. P., Friesen, K., & Mitchell, J. (2008). Pain, distress, and adult–child interaction during venipuncture in pediatric oncology: An examination of three types of venous access. *Journal of Pain and Symptom Management, 36*(2), 173–184.

Spanos, S., Booth, R., Koenig, H., Sikes, K., Gracely, E., & Kim, I. K. (2008). Jet injection of 1% buffered lidocaine versus topical ELA-Max for anesthesia before peripheral intravenous catheterization in children: A randomized controlled trial. *Pediatric Emergency Care, 24*(8), 511–515.

Squire, S. J., Kirchhoff, K. T., & Hissong, K. (2000). Comparing two methods of topical anesthesia used before intravenous cannulation in pediatric patients. *Journal of Pediatric Health Care, 14*(2), 68–72.

Stevens, B., Yamada, J., & Ohlsson, A. (2004). Sucrose for analgesia in newborn infants undergoing painful procedures. *Cochrane Database Systematic Reviews*, *3*, CD001069.

Taddio, A., Shah, V., Gilbert-MacLeod, C., & Katz, J. (2002). Conditioning and hyperalgesia in newborns exposed to repeated heel lances. *Journal of the American Medical Association*, *288*(7), 857–861.

Taddio, A., Shah, V., Shah, P., & Katz, J. (2003). Beta-endorphin concentration after administration of sucrose in preterm infants. *Archives of Pediatrics & Adolescent Medicine*, *157*(11), 1071–1074.

Tsao, J. C., Evans, S., Meldrum, M., Altman, T., & Zeltzer, L. K. (2008). A review of CAM for procedural pain in infancy: Part I. Sucrose and nonnutritive sucking. *Evidence-based Complementary and Alternative Medicine*, *5*(4), 371–381.

Weissman, A., Aranovitch, M., Blazer, S., & Zimmer, E. Z. (2009). Heel lancing in newborns: Behavioral and spectral analysis assessment of pain control methods. *Pediatrics*, *124*(5), e921–926.

Windich-Biermeier, A., Sjoberg, I., Dale, J. C., Eshelman, D., & Guzzetta, C. E. (2007). Effects of distraction on pain, fear, and distress during venous port access and venipuncture in children and adolescents with cancer. *Journal of Pediatric Oncology Nursing*, *24*(1), 8–19.

Wolf, A. R., Stoddart, P. A., Murphy, P. J., & Sasada, M. (2002). Rapid skin anaesthesia using high-velocity lignocaine particles: A prospective placebo-controlled trial. *Archives of Disease in Childhood*, *86*(4), 309–312.

Yamada, J., Stinson, J., Lamba, J., Dickson, A., McGrath, P. J., & Stevens, B. (2008). A review of systematic reviews on pain interventions in hospitalized infants. *Pain Research & Management*, *13*(5), 413–420.

Zempsky, W. T., & Cravero, J. P. (2004). Relief of pain and anxiety in pediatric patients in emergency medical systems. *Pediatrics*, *114*(5), 1348–1356.

Zempsky, W. T., Robbins, B., Richards, P. T., Leong, M. S., & Schechter, N. L. (2008). A novel needle-free powder lidocaine delivery system for rapid local analgesia. *The Journal of Pediatrics*, *152*(3), 405–411.

14

Critical Illness

Discomfort, including pain and anxiety, is an almost universal consequence of critical illness. Providing effective analgesia for critically ill infants and children requires addressing both their physical and psychological comfort levels. Consensus guidelines regarding analgesia and sedation have been published for critically ill children (Playfor et al., 2007) as well as for infants (Anand et al., 2006).

SOURCES OF PAIN

Underlying Medical Illness or Injury

For both infants in a neonatal intensive care unit (NICU) and children in a pediatric intensive care unit (PICU), the medical diagnosis requiring their admission to these units itself is often painful (e.g., cardiac surgery or trauma).

Intermittent Medical Procedures

The frequent need for invasive procedures, such as the insertion of intravenous (IV) needles, chest tubes, arterial catheters, and heel lances, although life-saving, is both painful and anxiety-provoking for critically ill patients. Nasogastric tubes involve some degree of

247

discomfort as well. In many instances, especially if an endotracheal tube (ETT) and mechanical ventilation are a part of the medical treatment, continuous analgesia and sedation infusions are required to minimize the emotional distress and to prevent the accidental removal of such life-saving devices.

Environment of Pediatric Intensive Care Unit and Neonatal Intensive Care Unit

PICU and NICU surroundings and routines are stressful for infants and children, who, along with the frequent sources of pain, suffer from sleep deprivation mixed with the sensory overstimulation of bright lights and unfamiliar noises from imposing medical devices. At best, parental contact is limited, with unnatural barriers (e.g., parents may not be able to hold their child or participate in his or her care) adding to the child's distress.

Clinical Pearl

Other related symptoms that can exacerbate pain, which are found in critically ill children, include the following:

- Anxiety—a sustained state of apprehension in response to a real or perceived threat associated with motor tension, autonomic activity, and vigilant scanning for a source of comfort and reassurance of safety.
- Agitation—the excessive, often nonpurposeful, motor activity associated with internal tension and accompanied by anxiety, panic, depression, delusions, hallucinations, and delirium. Causes of agitation include hypoxia, adverse reactions to or withdrawal from medications, metabolic disorders, sepsis, sleep deprivation, and reactions to unfamiliar environments.
- Delirium—the state of reduced ability to respond to external stimuli, usually manifested as disorganized thinking (rambling and incoherent speech), decreased level of consciousness, and altered sensory perception, such as hallucinations, disorientation, and altered levels of psychomotor activity. Agitation can be a symptom of delirium.

PAIN ASSESSMENT

Infants and children who are critically ill have less ability to verbalize or move to indicate their pain because of neurological deficits associated with their illness or injury. When ventilatory support is required, pain management is even more of a challenge because of the need for analgesia and sedation to provide comfort and tolerance to the actions of the ventilator. At times, critically ill patients will need neuromuscular blocking agents (NMBAs) to further facilitate mechanical ventilation. These agents do not have sedative or analgesic properties and are not intended to be used without concomitant use of opioids and sedatives. The biggest challenge to the health care provider is the fact that these patients will be pharmacologically paralyzed and will not be able to move to indicate any form of distress. Use of pain assessment scales becomes impossible, and the health care provider, most often the bedside nurse, must rely on physiological signs and parental input to determine whether their patients are having pain or its related symptoms while being offered life-sustaining complex technologies. The judgment of the bedside nurse is essential.

Several approaches to pain assessment of the critically ill child have been established, but published research support for each approach for critically ill infants and children is limited.

PHYSIOLOGICAL INDICATORS OF PAIN

Physiological signs of increased pain include an increase in heart rate, blood pressure, and respiratory rate, as well as changes in facial expression and pupil size, the presence of tears, or diaphoresis (Ramelet, Abu-Saad, Rees, & McDonald, 2004). Neonates may respond somewhat differently with an increase or decrease in heart rate. These measures have the same limitations as the behavioral methods, particularly, the difficulty in determining changes related to pain versus other forms of distress. Changes in physiological indicators generally occur acutely, and, with time, these changes become less dramatic and noticeable as adaption to the source of stress takes place, sometimes within minutes of the painful stimulus. As a result, health care providers cannot depend on these signs as concrete markers for pain. Additionally, the challenge to health care providers is to know whether these indicators are caused by pain or are from other symptoms, such as anxiety, agitation, or delirium. Physical pain needs to be ruled out as a contributing factor, often with a trial of analgesics to determine if a reduction in agitation occurs following an analgesic. If increased pain is ruled out, the need to identify the medical cause of the distress (e.g., hypoxia) or agitation (e.g., fear of the intensive care unit [ICU] environment) and increasing the sedative dose are necessary.

BEHAVIORAL INDICATORS FOR PAIN

This method may be useful for critically ill children who are able to move to demonstrate some degree of discomfort. Health care providers need to be aware that behavioral tools are more likely to help with recognition of acute pain and distress, such as immediate post-operative pain or procedurally related pain, but lead to underrating more persistent pain.

The COMFORT Scale

Specifically designed and validated for infants and children up to 17 years of age, the COMFORT scale (see Figure 14.1) has been used to measure global behavioral distress, such as pain in critically ill patients in NICU and PICU, including those requiring mechanical ventilation (Ambuel, Hamlett, Marx, & Blumer, 1992; Bear & Ward-Smith, 2006; Carnevale & Razack, 2002; van Dijk, Peters, van Deventer, & Tibboel, 2005; Wong, McIntosh, Menon, & Franck, 2003). This scale was originally developed as an eight-item (six behavioral and two physiological items) assessment of physiological distress, including pain (Ambuel et al., 1992). Developers of the COMFORT scale recommended 2 hours of formal training,

COMFORT behavior © *scale*

Date

Time

Observer

Patient sticker

Please place a mark

Alertness
- Deeply asleep (eyes closed, no response to changes in the environment) ☐ 1
- Lightly asleep (eyes mostly closed, occasional responses) ☐ 2
- Drowsy (child closes his/her eyes frequently, less responsive to the environment) ☐ 3
- Awake and alert (child responsive to the environment) ☐ 4
- Awake and hyper-alert (exaggerated responses to environmental stimuli) ☐ 5

Calmness/Agitation
- Calm (child appears serene and tranquil) ☐ 1
- Slightly anxious (child shows slight anxiety) ☐ 2
- Anxious (child appears agitated but remains in control) ☐ 3
- Very anxious (child appears very agitated, just able to control) ☐ 4
- Panicky (severe distress with loss of control) ☐ 5

Respiratory response
(score only in mechanically ventilated children)
- No spontaneous respiration ☐ 1
- Spontaneous and ventilator respiration ☐ 2
- Restlessness or resistance to ventilator ☐ 3
- Actively breathes against ventilator or coughs regularly ☐ 4
- Fights ventilator ☐ 5

Crying
(score only in spontaneously breathing children)
- Quiet breathing, no crying sounds ☐ 1
- Occasional sobbing or moaning ☐ 2
- Whining (monotonous sound) ☐ 3
- Crying ☐ 4
- Screaming or shrieking ☐ 5

Physical movement
- No movement ☐ 1
- Occasional, (three or fewer) slight movements ☐ 2
- Frequent, (more than three) slight movements ☐ 3
- Vigorous movements limited to extremities ☐ 4
- Vigorous movements including torso and head ☐ 5

Muscle tone
- Muscles totally relaxed; no muscle tone ☐ 1
- Reduced muscle tone; less resistance than normal ☐ 2
- Normal muscle tone ☐ 3
- Increased muscle tone and flexion of fingers and toes ☐ 4
- Extreme muscle rigidity and flexion of fingers and toes ☐ 5

Facial tension
- Facial muscles totally relaxed ☐ 1
- Normal facial tone ☐ 2
- Tension evident in some facial muscles (not sustained) ☐ 3
- Tension evident throughout facial muscles (sustained) ☐ 4
- Facial muscles contorted and grimacing ☐ 5

Total score ☐

VAS (Visual Analogue Scale)
Put a mark on the line below to indicate how much pain you think the child has at **this very moment.**

no pain |————————————————| worst pain   VAS score ☐

Details medication

Details child's condition

Type of assessment
(before or after medication or standard assessment)
Mean arterial blood pressure and heart rate are not included in this version of the COMFORT Scale.

Figure 14.1 ■ COMFORT Scale.
From H. M. Koot, J. B. de Boer, and M. van Dijk. Copyright Dutch version: version 4, November 2003. Used with permission.

with the health care provider observing 3 minutes for each assessment (Ambuel et al., 1992). Later, clinical research led other researchers to modify the scale, renaming it as COMFORT-B with the removal of two physiological items (mean arterial pressure and heart rate), which were cumbersome to score in PICU patients who often have non-pain-related hemodynamic conditions (Carnevale & Razack, 2002; Ista, van Dijk, Tibboel, & de Hoog, 2005). Other researchers have looked at how the COMFORT-B scale could be used in nonventilated children, replacing the "respiratory response" item with a "crying" scoring determination (Gjerstad, Wagner, Henrichsen, & Storm, 2008; van Dijk et al., 2000).

The Neonatal Pain, Agitation, and Sedation Scale

The Neonatal Pain, Agitation, and Sedation Scale (N-PASS) was developed in response to the need for a tool to assess infant pain as well as sedation level for infants cared for in NICU (Hummel, Lawlor-Klean, & Weiss, 2010). See Chapter 2 for more details.

The FLACC Scale

One recent study has been published using the FLACC in the ICU setting with 29 adults and 8 children (Voepel-Lewis, Zanotti, Dammeyer, & Merkel, 2010). Initial results for reliability and validity for this tool have been demonstrated with minor modification of the cry category to facilitate scoring of intubated patients (e.g., "silent cry") and with the addition of descriptors indicating pain (e.g., breath holding and splinting). See Chapter 2 for more details.

ACKNOWLEDGMENT OF PAIN BY ASSUMING PAIN IS PRESENT

When patients are deeply sedated or pharmacologically paralyzed with NMBA (e.g., vecuronium [Norcuron]), the use of behavioral scales is not possible because of the patients' total lack of ability to demonstrate via behaviors or to verbalize pain. Without a means to score pain intensity, health care providers must rely on physiological indicators (Razmus & Wilson, 2006) and are to assume that pain is present because of the patients' risk of discomfort (e.g., with an ETT). This method of pain assessment does not attempt to quantify the pain, but instead is based on the assumption that pain is present, indicating the need for vigilance by health care providers to ensure optimal analgesia and other comfort measures for these most vulnerable of critically ill patients (Pasero & McCaffery, 2002). This method of pain assessment mandates that patients receive ongoing opioid infusions with the addition of sedatives to control related symptoms. Frequent reassessment for physiological signs of increased pain (or anxiety or agitation) is required to determine the need for further titration of the infusions.

OTHER RELATED ASSESSMENT METHODS

Sedation Assessment Scales

Sedation scales designed for the ongoing assessment of the purposeful provision of sedation are available but not often used in the clinical setting, as most are cumbersome and time consuming. However, sedation scales could guide health care providers in the titration of sedatives and provide a means of communicating a sedation goal for health care providers between shifts. As described in the previous section of this chapter, the COMFORT and N-PASS scales are available for such use. Another scale, the State Behavioral Scale for infants and young children supported with mechanical ventilation, has been recently developed with the need for replication and validation by other clinical researchers (Curley, Harris, Fraser, Johnson, & Arnold, 2006). Other sedation scales developed for critically ill adults but reportedly used for children in PICU are the Motor Activity Assessment Scale (Devlin et al., 1999) and Richmond Agitation-Sedation Scale (Schieveld et al., 2009; Sessler et al., 2002).

Bispectral Index

Given the difficulties involved in the subjective assessment of the level of sedation during deep sedation or during the administration of NMBAs, there are clearly potential benefits in having a more objective measurement of sedation using neurophysiological techniques, such as the Bispectral Index Score (BIS) or auditory evoked potentials. The BIS value is a continuous measure that assesses a child's level of consciousness by processing electroencephalographic data obtained using a noninvasive sensor placed on the forehead, which may assist the health care provider in preventing oversedation or undersedation when moderate to deep sedation is desired during mechanical ventilation. Used in conjunction with clinical assessment of the child's comfort, some studies have shown correlation of BIS values to increasing depth of sedation and consciousness using subjective sedation assessment scales in pediatric studies (Hutchins, 2008; Playfor et al., 2007). Technical limitations in the critical care environment with electrical interference and muscle activity may falsely elevate BIS scores. In summary, inconsistent correlation of BIS scores to COMFORT scores has been insufficient to support the routine use of PICU sedation assessment (Playfor et al., 2007).

Agitation Scales

The scales described for use in determining sedation levels in critically ill patients can be used to determine the presence or level of agitation. The University of Michigan PICU recently developed a scale to assist health care providers in differentiating pain from agitation in pediatric patients. The scale is known as the ACAT Agitation Scale, an acronym for the categories of assessment: activity, consolability, alertness, and threat to safety (Fraser & Merkel, 2009; see Table 14.1).

Nurses are challenged to sort out what the causes may be in agitated infants and children so they can provide the appropriate interventions. Even when research-based tools are available for health

Table 14.1 ■ *PICU ACAT Agitation Scale*

	Scoring			
	0	1	2	3
Activity Restlessness/ squirming	Calm	Intermittent squirming	Persistent attempts to move; restless and squirming	Excessive movement and pulling at tubes
Consolability Ability to console	No interven- tion needed	Easy to console with voice or touch	Difficult to console (short period < 5 minutes)	Inconsolable
Alertness Ability to follow instructions	Yes, without reinforce- ment	Yes, with reinforce- ment	Inconsistent, requiring frequent reinforcement	Does not follow instructions; confused
Threat to Safety Risk for harm or self- extubation	Calm and tolerates ventilation	Distressed at times; calms when stimulus is removed; unsafe at times; tolerates ventilation most of the time	Intermittently unsafe to be left alone; recovers after ETT suctioning	High threat of safety and risk of self-harm; high risk of self- extubation; fighting ventilation

Instructions: Observe more than 15–30 minutes and determine each subscore. Subscores are not to be added together. If the child's behavior meets 2 of the 4 categories, select the score that describes "threat to safety." If the patient's behavior is persistently scored 2 or 3 despite interventions, delirium should be considered.

Abbreviation: ETT, endotracheal tube.

care providers to use, the reality in a busy ICU is that pain assess-ment has to be practical. PICU nurses need assessment tools that are appropriate, have minimal administrative time, and easy to apply to a wide age range of children. Most important, these tools need to be readily available at the patient's bedside and designed to be used quickly with little formal training.

PHARMACOLOGIC MANAGEMENT

The pharmacokinetics and pharmacodynamics of analgesics and sedatives are significantly altered in critically ill patients, requiring careful attention to individualizing the regimen for specific pa-tients. Drug toxicity may be a problem in critically ill patients, es-pecially those with renal or hepatic compromise, who are more likely to exhibit decreases in clearance resulting in longer dura-tions of action from accumulation of the medication and its me-tabolites. The response to a dose of medication varies greatly not only among patients but also over time within an individual pa-tient because of tolerance to the beneficial effects, leading to recep-tor down-regulation and competitive drug interactions, as well as changes in pH, serum albumin, autonomic activity, or renal and liver function (Tobias, 2003).

Opioids

The key to safe and effective administration is titration under close observation, even when critically ill patients have protected airways via the ETT and are provided mechanical ventilations. The oral route is often not feasible in the PICU setting, so the IV route is preferred. When analgesics are prescribed as PRN (as needed) regimens, health care providers are to be reminded that critically ill children have ill-nesses or technology that may preclude them from being able to communicate their discomfort, which may cause them to reexperi-ence pain before another dose is administered. Continuous infusions of opioids are preferred to avoid large variations in plasma concentrations and to maintain continuous pain relief. Fentanyl (Sublimaze) is often the opioid of choice because of its less frequent adverse effects (e.g., less associated with histamine-related vasodilation and hypotension). See Chapter 4 for more details.

Because patients are often not able to use the bolus button of a patient-controlled analgesia pump, the nurse is frequently determined to be the best one to give rapid pain control to provide care that must be delivered with little advance warning (e.g., suctioning an ETT or inserting catheters or chest tubes emergently).

Providing nurse-controlled analgesia (NCA) with a bolus from a pump in a timely manner as soon as pain is assessed avoids the time-consuming and suboptimal process of the nurse leaving the bedside to obtain a dose from a locked cabinet. NCA should be limited to hospital units in which the nurse-to-patient ratio provides the time to be nearby to press the bolus button when the child is in pain (Oakes, 2008). Recent guidelines have been issued regarding "authorized" nurses providing bolus doses with specific education, monitoring, and quality assurance activities to maximize patient safety (Wuhrman et al., 2007).

Sedatives

For both infants and children, adequate pain control may preclude the need for other sedatives. However, if agitation persists or if the patient requires mechanical ventilation, benzodiazepines (i.e., midazolam [Versed] or lorazepam [Ativan]) and barbiturates (e.g., pentobarbital [Nembutal]) are commonly used as first-line sedative agents. Proper selection and administration of sedatives require knowledge of their comparative effects, characteristics, and limitations. Ideally, the goal is to have the child be free from pain and anxiety, able to tolerate medical procedures such as suctioning, and able to be aroused easily from light sleep, enabling effective neurological assessment.

Clinical Pearl

The goals of analgesics and sedatives are as follows:

- Alleviate anxiety or distress
- Improve comfort
- Facilitate medical procedures
- Promote sleep
- Prevent later memory of particularly distressing interventions
- Tolerate having an ETT
- Enable safe and effective ventilation
- Reduce oxygen consumption
- Control intracranial pressure

NONPHARMACOLOGIC INTERVENTIONS

For children who are more aware of their surroundings, refer to Chapter 8 with the assistance of a child life specialist whenever available. Touch is one of the most effective means of communication that health care providers can encourage between family members and their children, even with the most critically ill. For immobile patients, basic comfort measures are always necessary, including the following:

- Positioning for comfort in a neutral alignment with all parts of the body supported and the joints slightly flexed
- Frequent position changes to allow self-calming behaviors, such as sucking the thumb
- Attention to mouth, eye, and skin care
- Prevention of pulling of the numerous tubes
- Attention to possible muscle cramps, itching, and thirst (e.g., mouth care)

Health care providers can increase patient comfort by reducing the lights and noise in the patient's environment as much as possible. Health care providers need to obtain parental input for information on how to mimic their child's activity and sleep schedule and should include parental assistance in their child's care as much as possible. By clustering care and interventions, nurses can advocate, whenever possible, a routine for children, including protected periods as "safe times" during which caregivers cannot intrude except for emergencies, conveying to children that they have some control over what is happening to them.

TREATMENT CHALLENGES

Withdrawal of Opioids and Sedatives

If opioids and sedatives are used for control of pain and distress during ventilation for more than a few days, careful consideration must be given at the time of removing the source of distress (e.g., ETT) to ensure withdrawal syndromes do not occur as mediations are discontinued. Many of the signs and symptoms of abstinence are the same regardless of the drug involved. The time of onset will vary, depending on the half-life of the drug, which needs to be considered if the infusion was used for 7 days or longer (Playfor et al., 2007). Patients receiving opioids and sedatives regularly for more than 5 days can develop some degree of physical dependence with a distressing withdrawal syndrome if the drug is suddenly antagonized, stopped, or markedly reduced in dose (Anand et al., 2010). See Chapter 4 for details on opioid discontinuance and withdrawal syndrome, a process called "weaning." Pain control should always be a priority over the weaning plan. In the case of additional pain during weaning, the weaning process should be stopped and analgesics should be added, taking into consideration the patient's opioid tolerance.

Opioid Weaning Regimens

Weaning strategies using oral methadone and transdermal or oral clonidine are quite variable, and the health care provider needs to consider the length of exposure, type of opioid, practitioner bias and preference, and whether there is ongoing pain with a continued need for opioids (American Pain Society [APS], 2008). No standard regimen has been published in the literature. For either methadone (Dolophine) or clonidine (Catapres) regimens, the goal should be a patient who is not agitated or distressed and can sleep but is not overly sedated. Patients can benefit from institutions developing standardized approaches for such discontinuance of opioids and benzodiazepines (Berens et al., 2006).

Methadone (Dolophine)

Health care providers can convert the opioid daily cumulative dose to methadone and give orally or via nasogastric tube. Because of methadone's prolonged half-life, plasma levels of the drug will decline slowly days after the last oral dose, allowing gradual weaning. One prospective randomized trial of a 5-day versus 10-day weaning regimen using oral methadone showed minimal differences in critically ill opioid-tolerant children, suggesting a 5-day weaning can be done effectively (Berens et al., 2006). One recent guideline on how to use methadone to successfully wean opioids based on short term (7 to 14 days) versus long term (more than 14 days) has been published (Anand et al., 2010).

Clonidine (Catapres)

The central nervous system effects of clonidine produce mild sedation and a sense of well-being and calmness that also help ameliorate the symptoms of withdrawal. Clonidine should be started at 2 mcg/kg/day and increased slowly as needed to a maximum of 10 mcg/kg/day. It is important to measure heart rate and blood pressure regularly as it may cause bradycardia and hypotension. Adolescents can be weaned off the drug in 2 weeks as it is reduced by 0.1 to 0.2 mg each day. For infants and children, the reduction is to be limited to 0.05 mg every 3 days (Newcorn et al., 1998).

Sedative Weaning Regimens

Clinical features of benzodiazepine withdrawal differ marginally from those of opioid withdrawal (Ista, van Dijk, Gamel, Tibboel, & de Hoog, 2007). In addition to symptoms found with opioid withdrawal syndrome, severe anxiety, confusion, perceptual disorders, depression, facial grimacing, choreoathetoid movements, dyskinetic movements of the mouth, myoclonus, ataxia, poor visual tracking, and opisthotonos have been reported after abrupt discontinuance of benzodiazepines (Dominguez et al., 2006; Ista, van Dijk, de Hoog, Tibboel, & Duivenvoorden, 2009; Playfor et al., 2007). Experts recommend for patients on continuous benzodiazepines for more than 5 to 9 days, health care providers are to decrease the dose no more than 10% each day (Cunliffe, McArthur, & Dooley, 2004; Playfor et al., 2007; Tobias, 2003).

Withdrawal Scoring Systems

When reducing opioids and sedatives, a scoring system should be used to alert health care providers to their patients suffering any withdrawal symptoms, with recommended actions to take to provide comfort. In the 1970s, a scoring system for neonatal abstinence from opioids was developed for newborns of addicted mothers to capture any signs and symptoms of neonatal abstinence (Kron, Finnegan, Kaplan, Litt, & Phoenix, 1975). Recently, more attention has focused on developing similar withdrawal assessment tools for infants and children, including the Withdrawal Assessment Tool-1 (Franck, Harris, Soetenga, Amling, & Curley, 2008) and the Sophia Observation Withdrawal Symptom Scale (Ista et al., 2009). These tools and others have varying degrees of support for bedside use for consistently identifying withdrawal in infants and children who often cannot offer verbal confirmation of their symptoms. Many tools are still too lengthy and cumbersome for busy bedside health care providers to use often. Optimally, health care providers would have a validated tool with a cutoff to define clinical withdrawal to aid them in decision making to alter the weaning plan.

In summary, adequate analgesia and relief of anxiety are to be provided to even the sickest child, and the discomfort of withdrawal syndromes should be relieved as patients recover from their critical illness or injury. As the knowledge advances in how infants and children can be supported with technology and skills of various critical care health care providers, we must be mindful of the need to include the caring aspect and that of also responding to individual patients' cues and considering the effects of unrelieved pain on their future lives.

REFERENCES

Ambuel, B., Hamlett, K. W., Marx, C. M., & Blumer, J. L. (1992). Assessing distress in pediatric intensive care environments: The COMFORT scale. *Journal of Pediatric Psychology, 17*(1), 95–109.

American Pain Society. (2008). *Principles of analgesic use in the treatment of acute pain and cancer pain.* Glenview, IL: Author.

Anand, K. J., Aranda, J. V., Berde, C. B., Buckman, S., Capparelli, E. V., Carlo, W., . . . Walco, G. (2006). Summary proceedings from the neonatal pain-control group. *Pediatrics, 117*(3), S9–S22.

Anand, K. J., Wilson, D. F., Berger, J., Harrison, R., Meert, K. L., Zimmerman, J., . . . Eunice Kennedy Shriver National Institute of Child Health and Human Development Collaborative Pediatric Critical Care Research Network. (2010). Tolerance and withdrawal from prolonged opioid use in critically ill children. *Pediatrics, 125*(5), e1208–1225.

Bear, L. A., & Ward-Smith, P. (2006). Interrater reliability of the COMFORT Scale. *Pediatric Nursing, 32*(5), 427–434.

Berens, R. J., Meyer, M. T., Mikhailov, T. A., Colpaert, K. D., Czarnecki, M. L., Ghanayem, N. S., . . . Weisman, S. J. (2006). A prospective evaluation of opioid weaning in opioid-dependent pediatric critical care patients. *Anesthesia & Analgesia, 102*(4), 1045–1050.

Carnevale, F. A., & Razack, S. (2002). An item analysis of the COMFORT scale in a pediatric intensive care unit. *Pediatric Critical Care Medicine, 3*(2), 177–180.

Cunliffe, M., McArthur, L., & Dooley, F. (2004). Managing sedation withdrawal in children who undergo prolonged PICU admission after discharge to the ward. *Paediatric Anaesthesia, 14*(4), 293–298.

Curley, M. A., Harris, S. K., Fraser, K. A., Johnson, R. A., & Arnold, J. H. (2006). State Behavioral Scale: A sedation assessment instrument for infants and young children supported on mechanical ventilation. *Pediatric Critical Care Medicine, 7*(2), 107–114.

Devlin, J. W., Boleski, G., Mlynarek, M., Nerenz, D. R., Peterson, E., Jankowski, M., . . . Zarowitz, B. J. (1999). Motor Activity Assessment

Scale: A valid and reliable sedation scale for use with mechanically ventilated patients in an adult surgical intensive care unit. *Critical Care Medicine*, *27*(7), 1271–1275.

Dominguez, K. D., Crowley, M. R., Coleman, D. M., Katz, R. W., Wilkins, D. G., & Kelly, H. W. (2006). Withdrawal from lorazepam in critically ill children. *Annals of Pharmacotherapy*, *40*(6), 1035–1039.

Franck, L. S., Harris, S. K., Soetenga, D. J., Amling, J. K., & Curley, M. A. (2008). The Withdrawal Assessment Tool-1 (WAT-1): An assessment instrument for monitoring opioid and benzodiazepine withdrawal symptoms in pediatric patients. *Pediatric Critical Care Medicine*, *9*(6), 573–580.

Fraser, E., & Merkel, S. (2009). *Management of sedation and agitation in critically ill children*. Paper presented at the meeting of the American Society of Pain Management Nursing 19th National Conference Pediatric Pain Management Workshop, Jacksonville, FL.

Gjerstad, A. C., Wagner, K., Henrichsen, T., & Storm, H. (2008). Skin conductance versus the modified COMFORT sedation score as a measure of discomfort in artificially ventilated children. *Pediatrics*, *122*(4), e848–853.

Hummel, P., Lawlor-Klean, P., & Weiss, M. G. (2010). Validity and reliability of the N-PASS assessment tool with acute pain. *Journal of Perinatology*, *30*(7), 474–478.

Hutchins, L. (2008). Bispectral index monitoring. In J. Verger & R. Lebet (Eds.), *AACN Procedure manual for pediatric acute and critical care* (pp. 1237–1242). St. Louis, MO: Saunders Elsevier.

Ista, E., van Dijk, M., de Hoog, M., Tibboel, D., & Duivenvoorden, H. J. (2009). Construction of the Sophia Observation withdrawal Symptoms-scale (SOS) for critically ill children. *Intensive Care Medicine*, *35*(6), 1075–1081.

Ista, E., van Dijk, M., Gamel, C., Tibboel, D., & de Hoog, M. (2007). Withdrawal symptoms in children after long-term administration of sedatives and/or analgesics: A literature review. "Assessment remains troublesome." *Intensive Care Medicine*, *33*(8), 1396–1406.

Ista, E., van Dijk, M., Tibboel, D., & de Hoog, M. (2005). Assessment of sedation levels in pediatric intensive care patients can be improved by using the COMFORT "behavior" scale. *Pediatric Critical Care Medicine*, *6*(1), 58–63.

Kron, R. E., Finnegan, L. P., Kaplan, S. L., Litt, M., & Phoenix, M. D. (1975). The assessment of behavioral change in infants undergoing narcotic withdrawal: Comparative data from clinical and objective methods. *Addictive Diseases, 2*(1–2), 257–275.

Newcorn, J. H., Schulz, K., Harrison, M., DeBellis, M. D., Udarbe, J. K., & Halperin, J. M. (1998). Alpha 2-adrenergic agonists. Neurochemistry, efficacy, and clinical guidelines for use in children. *Pediatric Clinics of North America, 45*(5), 1099–1022.

Oakes, L. (2008). Patient controlled analgesia. In J. Verger & R. Lebet (Eds.), *AACN procedure manual for pediatric acute and critical care* (pp. 1269–1279). St. Louis, MO: Saunders Elsevier.

Pasero, C., & McCaffery, M. (2002). Pain in the critically ill. *American Journal of Nursing, 102*(1), 59–60.

Playfor, S., Jenkins, I., Boyles, C., Choonara, I., Davies, G., Haywood, T., . . . United Kingdom Paediatric Intensive Care Society Sedation, Analgesia and Neuromuscular Blockade Working Group. (2007). Consensus guidelines for sustained neuromuscular blockade in critically ill children. *Paediatric Anaesthesia, 17*(9), 881–887.

Ramelet, A. S., Abu-Saad, H. H., Rees, N., & McDonald, S. (2004). The challenges of pain measurement in critically ill young children: A comprehensive review. *Australian Critical Care, 17*(1), 33–45.

Razmus, I., & Wilson, D. (2006). Current trends in the development of sedation/analgesia scales for the pediatric critical care patient. *Paediatric Anaesthesia, 32*(5), 435–441.

Schieveld, J. N., van der Valk, J. A., Smeets, I., Berghmans, E., Wassenberg, R., Leroy, P. L., . . . van Os, J. (2009). Diagnostic considerations regarding pediatric delirium: A review and a proposal for an algorithm for pediatric intensive care units. *Intensive Care Medicine, 35*(11), 1843–1849.

Sessler, C. N., Gosnell, M. S., Grap, M. J., Brophy, G. M., O'Neal, P. V., Keane, K. A., . . . Elswick, R. K. (2002). The Richmond Agitation-Sedation Scale: Validity and reliability in adult intensive care unit patients. *American Journal of Respiratory and Critical Care Medicine, 166*(10), 1338–1344.

Tobias, J. (2003). Pain management for the critically ill child in the PICU. In N. L. Schechter, C. B. Berde, & M. Yaster (Eds.), *Pain in infants, children, and adolescents* (2nd ed., pp. 807–840). Philadelphia, PA: Lippincott Williams & Wilkins.

van Dijk, M., de Boer, J. B., Koot, H. M., Tibboel, D., Passchier, J., & Duivenvoorden, H. J. (2000). The reliability and validity of the COM-FORT scale as a postoperative pain instrument in 0 to 3-year-old infants. *Pain, 84*(2–3), 367–377.

van Dijk, M., Peters, J. W., van Deventer, P., & Tibboel, D. (2005). The COMFORT Behavior Scale: A tool for assessing pain and sedation in infants. *American Journal of Nursing, 105*(1), 33–36.

Voepel-Lewis, T., Zanotti, J., Dammeyer, J. A., & Merkel, S. (2010). Reliability and validity of the face, legs, activity, cry, consolability behavioral tool in assessing acute pain in critically ill patients. *American Journal of Critical Care, 19*(1), 55–61.

Wong, C. M., McIntosh, N., Menon, G., & Franck, L. (2003). The pain (and stress) in infants in neonatal intensive care unit. In N. L. Schechter, C. B. Berde, & M. Yaster (Eds.), *Pain in infants, children, and adolescents* (2nd ed., pp. 669–692). Philadelphia, PA: Lippincott Williams & Wilkins.

Wuhrman, E., Cooney, M. F., Dunwoody, C. J., Eksterowicz, N., Merkel, S., & Oakes, L. L. (2007). Authorized and unauthorized ("PCA by Proxy") dosing of analgesic infusion pumps: Position statement with clinical practice recommendations. *Pain Management Nursing, 8*(1), 4–11.

15

Terminal Illness

Children with terminal illness experience discomfort from the cumulative effects of progressive disease, invasive procedures, and psychological distress (Friedrichsdorf & Kang, 2007). The fear of inadequate pain control places an enormous emotional burden on an already distressed child and family, further exacerbating their pain. Achieving the goal of providing adequate analgesia while avoiding excessive sedation and adverse side effects can be challenging for health care providers. Even in leading pediatric hospitals in the United States, 89% of children dying of cancer experience pain, as reported by their parents in after-death interviews (Wolfe et al., 2000). This study further emphasized that parental and health care provider assessment of children's pain and other symptoms may differ. After efforts were made to improve palliative care for children in the same study setting, symptom distress, including pain, was reduced. These results were attributed to creating an environment that fostered an improvement in overall end-of-life care (Wolfe et al., 2008).

PRINCIPLES OF PALLIATIVE CARE

Ideally, palliative care is instituted at the time of diagnosis of a potentially life-threatening illness or injury and continues regardless of whether a child receives curative treatment directed at the disease

(Casillas & Zeltzer, 2010; Hinds & Oakes, 2010; Zernikow, Michel, Craig, & Anderson, 2009). Control of pain and other symptoms, as well as psychological, social, and spiritual problems is paramount. The goal is to provide the best possible quality of life for patients and their families, which is consistent with their values, regardless of the location of the patient (American Academy of Pediatrics, 2000). When a child is likely to have only few months to live, health care providers are to consider referring the child to a hospice organization prepared to take care of children and provide in-home support of a family as the child dies.

Clinical Pearl	*Palliative care* refers to the broader range of care as defined by the World Health Organization (WHO) and emphasizes the need to consider the child's body, mind, and spirit, along with support for the family, for diseases that are not always responsive to curative treatment (World Health Organization [WHO], 1998). *Hospice care*, delivered either in the home or in a residential hospice facility, is a subpart of palliative care focusing on the care needed at the end of life. A hospice refers to an organization of health care providers and volunteers who support the child and family during the final days of the child's life by assisting with symptom control, respite for the family caregivers, and bereavement care and follow-up after their child dies (Dowden, 2009).

PAIN ASSESSMENT

Health care providers need to be especially alert for pain at the end of life for children who have cancer because of possible compression of nerves and bone metastatic lesions, invasive infections, pathological fractures, gastritis, constipation, cystitis, and muscle spasticity. Self-report of pain will not be possible near death, necessitating the input of parents in determining whether optimal pain management has been provided. Although physical pain is the usual focus, health care providers are to be attuned to other related symptoms, including anxiety, depression, helplessness, hopelessness, sadness, and anger, all of which can have a considerable impact on pain intensity.

PHARMACOLOGIC MANAGEMENT

Although opioids are the mainstay for relieving pain at the end of life, nonsteroidal anti-inflammatory drugs (NSAIDS) and coanalgesics are often useful (Friedrichsdorf & Kang, 2007; Hewitt, Goldman, Collins, Childs, & Hain, 2008). In developing the pain management plan for a terminally ill child, health care providers are to consider the following (Dowden, 2009; Hooke, Hellsten, Stutzer, & Forte, 2002; Zernikow, Michel, Craig, & Anderson, 2009):

- The cause of the pain
- The ability of the child to take oral medications
- The need to anticipate the need for vascular access (i.e., peripherally inserted central catheter and Hickman catheters) as the child's ability to swallow diminishes
- The balance of risk versus benefit of medications causing liver and renal toxicity
- Treatments that can be practical in the home with parental administration using the simplest route preferred by the child and parents
- The need to match the analgesic delivery schedule to the pattern of pain (i.e., continuous delivery for persistent pain with a bolus dose for periods of exacerbation)
- Severe uncontrolled pain as a medical emergency, usually requiring immediate provision of intravenous (IV) doses of opioids
- Avoiding all unnecessary painful procedures

Clinical Pearl   Intractable pain, pain that is resistant to standard analgesia regimens, may require the use of tunneled epidural, intrathecal, and nerve block infusions for weeks for some children, particularly those with cancer (Baker, Lee, Regnard, Crack, & Callin, 2004; Dowden, 2009). For children with impairment of coagulation, the risk of epidural hematoma may be outweighed by potential benefits of epidural analgesia. Low-dose ketamine (Ketalar) infusions may also be considered useful for controlling severe neuropathic pain (Anghelescu & Oakes, 2005; Friedrichsdorf & Kang, 2007; Paice, 2010).

NONPHARMACOLOGIC MANAGEMENT

Nonpharmacologic interventions need to be included for children who are terminally ill (Dowden, 2009; Friedrichsdorf & Kang, 2007). The provision of music and art therapy, journaling, guided imagery, clown therapy, medical play, clinical hypnosis, massage, relaxation, controlled breathing, yoga, acupuncture, and biofeedback have all been reported to be effective (Grégoire & Frager, 2006; Kelly, 2007; Poltorak & Benore, 2006; Russell & Smart, 2007). See Chapters 8–10 for details.

BARRIERS TO TREATMENT

The ethical duty of a health care provider is to relieve pain by administering sufficient doses of analgesic medications to alleviate pain, despite the possibility of life-shortening and expected side effects (American Society of Pain Management Nursing [ASPMN], 1998). If death occurs as a result of providing appropriate doses of an opioid (i.e., opioid-induced respiratory depression), the health care provider did not perform euthanasia, which is the deliberate intent to terminate a patient's life (Dowden, 2009).

A small group of children with terminal illnesses will not have their severe pain controlled even with massive doses of opioids and appropriate use of coanalgesics. These children may require sedation along with the provision of analgesia, using a range of agents, including benzodiazepines, barbiturates, or other sedatives (Goldman, Frager, & Pomietto, 2003). The option of sedating a child as a method of providing analgesia is controversial, even when there seems to be no acceptable means to provide analgesia while preserving alertness, and is best performed by a health care provider skilled in palliative care (Paice, 2010).

PARENT EDUCATION AND HOME MANAGEMENT

Multiple factors may play a role in preventing adequate pain relief at the end of life. Health care providers are to be alert for parents' misconceptions about the use of opioids, specifically the risk of respiratory depression, sedation, or addiction, especially as the need arises to rapidly escalate doses of opioid infusions. Individual dose requirements of opioids at the end of life are highly variable, with most children requiring opioids via the IV route (Drake, Frost, & Collins, 2003) and reported dosages as high as 518 mg/kg/hr of morphine (Collins, Grier, Kinney, & Berde, 1995). A more recent study of children in their last week of life, looking at morphine-equivalent doses, found that they required a range of 0.25 to 24.5 mg/kg/day, with a mean dose of 1.88 mg/kg/day (Drake et al., 2003). Patient-controlled analgesia management in the home is optimal for parents to use to provide an immediate IV dose for severe pain (Schiessl, Gravou, Zernikow, Sittl, & Griessinger, 2008).

Care of a terminally ill child may be provided in the home with hospice support tailored to the child's needs and the family's ability to provide care. Seamless care between the child's medical team and home is achieved when hospice staff members have specialized knowledge and skills required to provide optimal symptom management to children. Ongoing reassurance of parents and the child may be necessary, including the following (Dowden, 2009; Friedrichsdorf & Kang, 2007; Hain, Miser, Devins, & Wallace, 2005):

- Saving opioids until the pain is worse is unnecessary.
- The child is not a drug addict.
- Opioids are best for severe pain.
- The correct dose of an opioid is the dose that relieves the pain.
- Inadequate doses of analgesia will prevent adequate sleep for the child and the parents.

Pediatric end-of-life care requires frequent reassessment of pain and its related symptoms. This care can be provided in the home with adequate support of terminally ill children and their parents, along with available health care providers who have expertise in pain management.

REFERENCES

American Academy of Pediatrics. (2000). Committee on bioethics and committee on hospital care. Palliative care for children. *Pediatrics*, *106*, 351–357.

American Society of Pain Management Nursing. (1998). *ASPMN position statement on end of life care*. Retrieved from www.aspmn.org

Anghelescu, D. L., & Oakes, L. L. (2005). Ketamine use for reduction of opioid tolerance in a 5-year-old girl with end-stage abdominal neuroblastoma. *Journal of Pain and Symptom Management, 30*(1), 1–3.

Baker, L., Lee, M., Regnard, C., Crack, L., & Callin, S. (2004). Evolving spinal analgesia practice in palliative care. *Palliative Medicine, 18*(6), 507–515.

Casillas, J., & Zeltzer, L. K. (2010). Cancer pain in children. In S. M. Fishman, J. C. Ballantyne, & J. P. Rathmell (Eds.), *Bonica's management of pain* (4th ed., pp. 669–680). Philadelphia, PA: Wolters Kluwer/Lippincott Williams & Wilkins.

Collins, J. J., Grier, H. E., Kinney, H. C., & Berde, C. B. (1995). Control of severe pain in children with terminal malignancy. *Journal of Pediatrics, 126*(4), 653–657.

Dowden, S. J. (2009). Palliative care in children. In A. Twycross, S. J. Dowden, & E. Bruce (Eds.), *Managing pain in children: A clinical guide* (pp. 171–200). Oxford, United Kingdom: Wiley-Blackwell.

Drake, R., Frost, J., & Collins, J. J. (2003). The symptoms of dying children. *Journal of Pain and Symptom Management, 26*(1), 594–603.

Friedrichsdorf, S. J., & Kang, T. I. (2007). The management of pain in children with life-limiting illnesses. *Pediatric Clinics of North America, 54*(5), 645–672.

Goldman, A., Frager, G., & Pomietto, M. (2003). Pain and palliative care. In N. L. Schechter, C. B. Berde, & M. Yaster (Eds.), *Pain in infants, children, and adolescents* (2nd ed., pp. 539–562). Philadelphia, PA: Lippincott Williams & Wilkins.

Grégoire, M. C., & Frager, G. (2006). Ensuring pain relief for children at the end of life. *Pain Research & Management, 11*(3), 163–171.

Hain, R. D., Miser, A., Devins, M., & Wallace, W. H. (2005). Strong opioids in pediatric palliative medicine. *Paediatric Drugs, 7*(1), 1–9.

Hewitt, M., Goldman, A., Collins, G. S., Childs, M., & Hain, R. (2008). Opioid use in palliative care of children and young people with cancer. *Journal of Pediatrics, 152*(1), 39–44.

Hinds, P. S., & Oakes, L. (2010). End-of-life decision making in pediatric oncology. In B. Ferrell & N. Coyle (Eds.), *Oxford textbook of palliative nursing* (3rd ed., pp. 1049–1063). New York, NY: Oxford University Press.

Hooke, C., Hellsten, M. B., Stutzer, C., & Forte, K. (2002). Pain management for the child with cancer in end-of-life care: APON position paper. *Journal of Pediatric Oncology Nursing, 19*(2), 43–47.

Kelly, K. M. (2007). Complementary and alternative medicines for use in supportive care in pediatric cancer. *Support Care Cancer, 15*(4), 457–460.

Paice, J. A. (2010). Pain at the end of life. In B. Ferrell & N. Coyle (Eds.), *Oxford textbook of palliative nursing* (3rd ed., pp. 161–185). New York, NY: Oxford University Press.

Poltorak, D. Y., & Benore, E. (2006). Cognitive-behavioral interventions for physical symptom management in pediatric palliative medicine. *Child & Adolescent Psychiatric Clinics of North America, 15*(3), 683–691.

Russell, C., & Smart, S. (2007). Guided imagery and distraction therapy in paediatric hospice care. *Paediatric Nursing, 19*(2), 24–25.

Schiessl, C., Gravou, C., Zernikow, B., Sittl, R., & Griessinger, N. (2008). Use of patient-controlled analgesia for pain control in dying children. *Support Care Cancer, 16*(5), 531–536.

Wolfe, J., Grier, H. E., Klar, N., Levin, S. B., Ellenbogen, J. M., Salem-Schatz, S., . . . Weeks, J. C. (2000). Symptoms and suffering at the end of life in children with cancer. *New England Journal of Medicine, 342*(5), 326–333.

Wolfe, J., Hammel, J. F., Edwards, K. E., Duncan, J., Comeau, M., Breyer, J., . . . Weeks, J. C. (2008). Easing of suffering in children with cancer at the end of life: Is care changing? *Journal of Clinical Oncology, 26*(10), 1717–1723.

World Health Organization. (1998). *Cancer pain relief and palliative care in children*. Geneva, Switzerland: Elsevier.

Zernikow, B., Michel, E., Craig, F., & Anderson, B. J. (2009). Pediatric palliative care: Use of opioids for the management of pain. *Paediatric Drugs, 11*(2), 129–151.

VII

Managing Common Pain Conditions

16

Postoperative and Trauma-Related Pain

POSTOPERATIVE PAIN

Children may undergo surgical procedures ranging from relatively minor operations, such as circumcision, to major ones involving the thorax, abdomen, cranium, pelvis, or extremities. Over the past 3 decades, attention to postoperative pain in children has made significant improvement. In 1983, the clinical practice of giving analgesics to children was reported as only 31% (Mather & Mackie, 1983). However, more recent studies continue to indicate the reluctance of nurses in providing prescribed analgesics because of insufficient knowledge about pain management and lack of consideration of its relief as a priority (Pölkki, Pietilä, & Vehviläinen-Julkunen, 2003; Twycross, 2007).

IMPACT OF UNRELIEVED POSTOPERATIVE PAIN

Postoperative pain leads to the reluctance of children to use their chest and abdominal muscles, resulting in ineffective coughing and clearing of secretions, contributing to atelectasis and pneumonia. Other potential consequences of unrelieved pain are related to a reluctance to ambulate (Joshi & Ogunnaike, 2005), increasing the risk of other postoperative complications (e.g., ileus, nausea, vomiting, thromboembolism, and venostasis).

Adequate assessment and aggressive pain management regimens aim to reduce postoperative organ dysfunction, promote earlier hospital discharge, and enhance rehabilitation (American Pain Society [APS], 2008). Common features across all types of postoperative pain will be described in the next two sections of this chapter, followed by reviews of management of specific surgical procedures common to childhood.

ASSESSMENT CHALLENGES FOR POSTOPERATIVE PAIN

Although self-report scales may be validated to use in children as young as 4 years, relating pain intensity is much less reliable soon after arrival in the postanesthesia care unit (PACU) while still under the influence of anesthesia (Bringuier et al., 2009). Health care providers need to be aware that behavioral tools may pick up anxiety associated with surgery rather than pain, with risk of overmedicating with analgesics. More research is needed in developing a reliable and valid tool to measure postoperative anxiety and its related effects on postoperative pain (Bringuier et al., 2009). Other challenges health care providers face are related to differentiating the many sources of pain to provide appropriate treatment approaches. For example, after abdominal surgery, a child may report "pain in my tummy." However, it is important to ask more probing questions to determine if the pain is from the incision, which is best treated with opioids, or from gas pain, which is best managed by activity to expel gas.

PHARMACOLOGIC MANAGEMENT FOR POSTOPERATIVE PAIN

Specific details, including dosages of medications and interventions are described in Chapters 3–7.

Preemptive Analgesia

Painful stimuli produce changes in the spinal cord that, in turn, influence the response to further stimuli (see Chapter 1). Preemptive analgesia, defined as providing analgesic delivery prior to the onset of noxious stimuli, is proposed to limit sensitization of the nervous system in response to stimuli, with the goal of reducing subsequent pain. The hypothesis is that this strategy prevents or reduces the *memory* of pain transmitted from the peripheral nervous system to the spinal cord and brain. The benefit of preemptive analgesia has been well established in animal studies (Ong, Lirk, Seymour, & Jenkins, 2005). However, results from adult clinical studies using local anesthetic wound infiltrations, epidural infusions, nonsteroidal anti-inflammatory drugs (NSAIDs), and other medications have not consistently demonstrated efficacy at reducing postoperative pain (Ong et al., 2005) or determining the optimal dose of proposed medications (i.e., gabapentin and pregabalin) (Dauri et al., 2009; Tiippana, Hamunen, Kontinen, & Kalso, 2007).

Multimodal Postoperative Regimens

Postoperative pain regimens involve varying combination of opioids, NSAIDs, epidural or peripheral nerve block infusions, and coanalgesics for children (Verghese & Hannallah, 2005) as well as for newborns and infants (Anand et al., 2006). The multimodal approach is useful by taking advantage of the medication's synergistic effects while minimizing the occurrence of adverse effects by lowering the dose of some of the components of the regimen (American Society of Anesthesiologists, 2004; Kehlet & Wilmore, 2002). For example, for children recovering from orthopedic surgeries, the combination of acetaminophen (Tylenol) or an NSAID can reduce postoperative morphine requirements by 30% compared with single drug administration (Hiller, Meretoja, Korpela, Piiparinen, & Taivainen, 2006).

However, repeated doses of NSAIDs should be used with caution, especially for children undergoing certain types of surgeries where bleeding is of major concern, such as in those patients undergoing tonsillectomy (Greco & Berde, 2005). The use of NSAIDs for tonsillectomy surgery continues to generate debate despite frequent use in some institutions. A Cochrane review concluded that NSAIDs did not cause any increase in hemorrhage requiring a reexploration in the operating room (Cardwell, Siviter, & Smith, 2005). Results of one study was included in this review in which preemptive use of an NSAID (ketoprofen [Orudis]) did not indicate preoperative use was of benefit in terms of reducing pain or opioid consumption (Kokki & Salonen, 2002). Of concern was that two patients (5%) had to return to the operating room for postoperative bleeding.

Use of gabapentin (Neurontin) and pregabalin (Lyrica) in reducing postoperative pain has been described in systematic reviews for adults undergoing gynecological, abdominal, neurosurgical, musculoskeletal, thoracic, neck, and breast procedures (Dauri et al., 2009) and in one recent study of children who underwent spinal fusion procedures (Rusy et al., 2010). Conclusions of such studies support the synergistic analgesic effects as helpful in decreasing pain intensity and lowering opioid consumption compared with placebo treatment groups. However, head-to-head comparisons of various combinations of actual medications (e.g., NSAID–opioid regimen versus gabapentin–opioid combination) have not clearly determined which regimen is optimal in providing relief of postoperative pain.

NONPHARMACOLOGIC MANAGEMENT FOR POSTOPERATIVE PAIN

Use of cognitive-behavioral and cognitive techniques to reduce postoperative pain in hospitalized children have also demonstrated efficacy, specifically guided imagery, distraction (Huth, Broome, & Good, 2004; Pölkki, Pietilä, Vehviläinen-Julkunen, Laukkala, & Kiviluoma, 2008), and music therapy (Nilsson, Kokinsky, Nilsson, Sidenvall, & Enskär, 2009). Physical approaches used to relieve pain from surgery, including transcutaneous nerve stimulation, have been found to be effective in reducing postoperative pain (Rakel & Frantz, 2003). Specific details about nonpharmacologic approaches are described in Chapters 8–10.

COMMON SURGICAL PROCEDURES

Circumcision

Circumcision is reported to be one of the most common elective surgical procedures performed on infants in the United States (American Academy of Pediatrics Task Force on Circumcision, 1999). Although respected professional organizations support the use of analgesia during newborn circumcision (American Academy of Pediatrics Task Force on Circumcision, 1999; American College of Obstetricians and Gynecologists [ACOG], 2001; American Society of Pain Management Nursing [ASPMN], 2001), the procedure is often performed without analgesia because of differing perceptions among clinicians as to whether newborns experience pain during circumcision (Razmus, Dalton, & Wilson, 2004).

Dorsal penile block is the best method to reduce pain as supported in a Cochrane review (Brady-Fryer, Wiebe, & Lander, 2004). Sucrose alone does not adequately reduce pain (Kaufman, Cimo, Miller, & Blass, 2002). The effects of combining sucrose or other interventions, such as tactile stimulation, or use of lidocaine creams (LMX4) seem to be additive (Kaufman et al., 2002; Lehr et al., 2005; Razmus et al., 2004; Tsao, Evans, Meldrum, Altman, & Zeltzer, 2008).

Orthopedic Procedures

Orthopedic surgery is among the most painful of surgeries (Lamontagne, Hepworth, & Salisbury, 2001) because of the significant muscular and skeletal tissue damage and reconstruction that are required and which cause both nociceptive and neuropathic pain (Marchettini, Formaglio, & Lacerenza, 2001). Specific postoperative pain syndromes after orthopedic surgery have been described, and the efficacy of various multimodal analgesic techniques have been examined, including peripheral nerve block infusions (Chiaretti & Langer, 2005; Kost-Byerly, 2002; Verghese & Hannallah, 2005).

Surgical correction of scoliosis often requires an opioid infusion, usually with patient-controlled analgesia or epidural (Gauger et al., 2009). For children with pectus excavatum, minimally invasive surgery can be provided, consisting of placing a preformed convex steel bar under the sternum through bilateral thoracic incisions and then forcibly turning the bar over to elevate the sternum (Nuss procedure). Initial postoperative days can be characterized by severe pain. Therefore, use of epidural infusions followed by administration of intravenous (IV) and oral opioids should be provided per the individual's specific needs (Cucchiaro, Adzick, Rose, Maxwell, & Watcha, 2006).

Other Major Surgeries

Postoperative pain management following thoracic, abdominal, and pelvic procedures often includes an epidural infusion. The use of epidural analgesia has been found to be associated with fewer postoperative pneumonias compared with systemic analgesia with opioids because of less sedative effect of opioids when administered via the epidural route than when given intravenously (Golianu & Hammer, 2005; Ingelmo et al., 2007; Popping, Elia, Marret, Remy, & Tramer, 2008). The administration of opioids should not be avoided because of concerns for decreased gut motility because unrelieved pain also has significant postoperative complications, such as the patient being reluctant to ambulate or to take deep breaths, increasing the risk of atelectasis.

TRAUMA-RELATED PAIN

Patients with trauma arrive with many symptoms that require rapid evaluation for effective treatment. The medical history of the child is often unknown to the emergency department (ED) staff, further challenging the health care provider in selecting effective pain-reducing interventions. Children in severe pain need immediate triage for pain assessment and pain interventions via IV route whenever possible, or consider intranasal fentanyl (Sublimaze) if IV access is not available (Finn & Harris, 2010). No evidence exists to support health care providers who hesitate to use analgesics for fear of masking symptoms or clouding mental status in order to treat the child with an injury (Zempsky & Cravero, 2004). Pain evaluation is an important part of triage but limited experience is available using validated scales in the ED (Bailey, Bergeron, Gravel, & Daoust, 2007).

Although delaying an emergency procedure while waiting is not advisable, health care providers working in ED triage areas during this phase of trauma management need to prepare the child for any potential needle-related procedures, including applying lidocaine creams or using a more immediate topical anesthesia (see Chapter 13; Zempsky & Cravero, 2004). For pharmacological management of trauma-related pain, see Chapters 3–7.

Minor Trauma

As part of laceration repair, clinicians need to minimize pain and anxiety. Several topical anesthetic/vasoconstrictor preparations, such as lidocaine, epinephrine, and tetracaine, can be compounded by pharmacies and available to apply as a liquid preparation, providing excellent wound anesthesia in 20 to 30 minutes (Zempsky & Cravero, 2004). The use of distraction techniques is effective in reducing situational anxiety in older children and lowering parental perception of pain distress in younger children (Sinha, Christopher, Fenn, & Reeves, 2006). See Chapters 8–10 for nonpharmacologic interventions.

Acute Musculoskeletal Injuries

Strains and sprains are frequent complaints among children presenting to the ED for care, with management often provided by cold therapy, elevation, and immobilization. Ibuprofen (Motrin) and other NSAIDs may not be effective analgesics for children with these injuries, and stronger analgesics may be required (Tanabe, Ferket, Thomas, Paice, & Marcantonio, 2002). Distraction techniques can be an effective adjunct to analgesia for children with musculoskeletal pain in the ED and should be made available.

Burns

Burns are associated with severe pain at rest as well as related to wound care, with dressing changes often described as excruciatingly painful despite the administration of the maximum allowable dose of opioids. IV morphine and intranasal fentanyl are given for dressing changes (Borland, Bergesio, Pascoe, Turner, & Woodger, 2005). Some studies have looked at the use of morphine to prevent posttraumatic stress disorder symptoms in preschool children with burns (Stoddard et al., 2009). Additional attention has been noted regarding the need for effective nonpharmacologic interventions during dressing changes (Miller, Rodger, Bucolo, Greer, & Kimble, 2010).

Amputation

Phantom pain syndrome, following an amputation from trauma or elective surgery, occurs when the child continues to have pain appearing to come from where the affected amputated limb had previously been painful. Possible damage to the nerve endings in the surgical stump with subsequent abnormalities in the regrowth of nerves at the stump is associated with severe neuropathic pain, which can be very challenging to treat. No clear, effective regimen has been found, but coanalgesics and methadone (Dolophine) are often used but not proven in clinical trials when compared with placebo (Casillas & Zeltzer, 2010). Use of clinical hypnosis aimed at altering the metabolic activity in pain perception areas of the brain as well as massage and acupuncture has been recommended (Casillas & Zeltzer, 2010).

> **Clinical Pearl**
>
> ▪ Phantom limb sensations are described as itchy or just "feeling my leg is still there, swinging in the wheelchair."
> ▪ Phantom limb pain is described as pain or severe itching, burning, cramping, and shooting pain usually beginning within days of the loss of the limb and gradually decreases in frequency and duration over time.
> ▪ Phantom pain is more severe if pain was present prior to amputation (Casillas & Zeltzer, 2010).

Pain management practices for children in ED have indicated that suboptimal dosages of analgesia continue to be the practice of many ED health care providers because of inadequate training in assessment and management of pain (Rupp & Delaney, 2004). A systematic approach to pain management and anxiolysis, including staff education and protocol development, can have a positive effect on providing comfort to children (Santervas et al., 2009; Zempsky & Cravero, 2004). A systemwide approach to pain management with awareness woven into all aspects of postoperative- and trauma-related pain is recommended for health care providers to consider for all children.

REFERENCES

American Academy of Pediatrics Task Force on Circumcision. (1999). Circumcision policy statement. *Pediatrics, 103*(3), 686–693.

American College of Obstetricians and Gynecologists. (2001). ACOG Committee Opinion. Circumcision. Number 260. *Obstetrics and Gynecology, 98*(4), 707–708.

American Pain Society. (2008). *Principles of analgesic use in the treatment of acute pain and cancer pain.* Glenview, IL: Author.

American Society of Anesthesiologists. (2004). Practice guidelines for acute pain management in the perioperative setting: An updated report by the American Society of Anesthesiologists Task Force on Acute Pain Management. *Anesthesiology, 100*(6), 1573–1581.

American Society of Pain Management Nursing. (2001). *Neonatal circumcision pain relief* (Position Statement). Retrieved from www.aspmn.org

Anand, K. J., Aranda, J. V., Berde, C. B., Buckman, S., Capparelli, E. V., Carlo, W., . . . Walco, G, A. (2006). Summary proceedings from the neonatal pain-control group. *Pediatrics, 117*(3), S9–S22.

Bailey, B., Bergeron, S., Gravel, J., & Daoust, R. (2007). Comparison of four pain scales in children with acute abdominal pain in a pediatric emergency department. *Annals of Emergency Medicine, 50*(4), 379–383.

Borland, M. L., Bergesio, R., Pascoe, E. M., Turner, S., & Woodger, S. (2005). Intranasal fentanyl is an equivalent analgesic to oral morphine in paediatric burns patients for dressing changes: A randomised double blind crossover study. *Burns, 31*(7), 831–837.

Brady-Fryer, B., Wiebe, N., & Lander, J. A. (2004). Pain relief for neonatal circumcision. *Cochrane Database of Systematic Reviews, 4,* CD004217.

Bringuier, S., Picot, M. C., Dadure, C., Rochette, A., Raux, O., Boulhais, M., & Capdevila, X. (2009). A prospective comparison of postsurgical behavioral pain scales in preschoolers highlighting the risk of false evaluations. *Pain, 145,* 60–68.

Cardwell, M., Siviter, G., & Smith, A. (2005). Non-steroidal anti-inflammatory drugs and perioperative bleeding in paediatric tonsillectomy. *Cochrane Database of Systematic Reviews, 2,* CD003591.

Casillas, J., & Zeltzer, L. K. (2010). Cancer pain in children. In S. M. Fishman, J. C. Ballantyne, & J. P. Rathmell (Eds.), *Bonica's management of pain* (4th ed., pp. 669–680). Philadelphia, PA: Wolters Kluwer/Lippincott Williams & Wilkins.

Chiaretti, A., & Langer, A. (2005). Prevention and treatment of postoperative pain with particular reference to children. *Advances and Technical Standards in Neurosurgery, 30,* 225–271.

Cucchiaro, G., Adzick, S. N., Rose, J. B., Maxwell, L., & Watcha, M. (2006). A comparison of epidural bupivacaine-fentanyl and bupivacaine-clonidine in children undergoing the Nuss procedure. *Anesthesia and Analgesia, 103*(2), 322–327.

Dauri, M., Faria, S., Gatti, A., Celidonio, L., Carpenedo, R., & Sabato, A. F. (2009). Gabapentin and pregabalin for the acute postoperative pain management. A systematic-narrative review of the recent clinical evidences. *Current Drug Targets, 10*(8), 716–733.

Finn, M., & Harris, D. (2010). Intranasal fentanyl for analgesia in the paediatric emergency department. *Emergency Medicine Journal, 27*(4), 300–301.

Gauger, V. T., Voepel-Lewis, T. D., Burke, C. N., Kostrzewa, A. J., Caird, M. S., Wagner, D. S., & Farley, F. A. (2009). Epidural analgesia compared with intravenous analgesia after pediatric posterior spinal fusion. *Journal of Pediatric Orthopaedics, 29*(6), 588–593.

Golianu, B., & Hammer, G. B. (2005). Pain management for pediatric thoracic surgery. *Current Opinion in Anesthesiology, 18*(1), 13–21.

Greco, C., & Berde, C. (2005). Pain management for the hospitalized pediatric patient. *Pediatric Clinics of North America, 52*(4), 995–1027.

Hiller, A., Meretoja, O. A., Korpela, R., Piiparinen, S., & Taivainen, T. (2006). The analgesic efficacy of acetaminophen, ketoprofen, or their combination for pediatric surgical patients having soft tissue or orthopedic procedures. *Anesthesia and Analgesia, 102*(5), 1365–1371.

Huth, M. M., Broome, M. E., & Good, M. (2004). Imagery reduces children's postoperative pain. *Pain, 110*(1–2), 439–448.

Ingelmo, P. M., Gelsumino, C., Acosta, A. P., Lopez, V., Gimenez, C., Halac, A., . . . Fumagalli, R. (2007). Epidural analgesia in children: Planning, organization and development of a new program. *Minerva Anestesiologica, 73*(11), 575–585.

Joshi, G. P., & Ogunnaike, B. O. (2005). Consequences of inadequate postoperative pain relief and chronic persistent postoperative pain. *Anesthesiology Clinics of North America, 23*(1), 21–36.

Kaufman, G. E., Cimo, S., Miller, L. W., & Blass, E. M. (2002). An evaluation of the effects of sucrose on neonatal pain with 2 commonly used circumcision methods. *American Journal of Obstetrics and Gynecology, 186*(3), 564–568.

Kehlet, H., & Wilmore, D. W. (2002). Multimodal strategies to improve surgical outcome. *American Journal of Surgery, 183*(6), 630–641.

Kokki, H., & Salonen, A. (2002). Comparison of pre- and postoperative administration of ketoprofen for analgesia after tonsillectomy in children. *Paediatric Anaesthesia, 12*(2), 162–167.

Kost-Byerly, S. (2002). New concepts in acute and extended postoperative pain management in children. *Anesthesiology Clinics of North America, 20*(1), 115–135.

Lamontagne, L. L., Hepworth, J. T., & Salisbury, M. H. (2001). Anxiety and postoperative pain in children who undergo major orthopedic surgery. *Applied Nursing Research, 14*(3), 119–124.

Lehr, V. T., Cepeda, E., Frattarelli, D. A., Thomas, R., LaMothe, J., & Aranda, J. V. (2005). Lidocaine 4% cream compared with lidocaine

2.5% and prilocaine 2.5% or dorsal penile block for circumcision. *American Journal of Perinatology, 22*(5), 231–237.

Marchettini, P., Formaglio, F., & Lacerenza, M. (2001). Iatrogenic painful neuropathic complications of surgery in cancer. *Acta Anaesthesiologica Scandinavica, 45*(9), 1090–1094.

Mather, L., & Mackie, J. (1983). The incidence of postoperative pain in children. *Pain, 15*(3), 271–282.

Miller, K., Rodger, S., Bucolo, S., Greer, R., & Kimble, R. M. (2010). Multi-modal distraction. Using technology to combat pain in young children with burn injuries. *Burns, 36*(5), 647–658.

Nilsson, S., Kokinsky, E., Nilsson, U., Sidenvall, B., & Enskär, K. (2009). School-aged children's experiences of postoperative music medicine on pain, distress, and anxiety. *Paediatric Anaesthesia, 19*(12), 1184–1190.

Ong, C. K., Lirk, P., Seymour, R. A., & Jenkins, B. J. (2005). The efficacy of preemptive analgesia for acute postoperative pain management: A meta-analysis. *Anesthesia and Analgesia, 100*(3), 757–773.

Pölkki, T., Pietilä, A. M., & Vehviläinen-Julkunen, K. (2003). Hospitalized children's descriptions of their experiences with postsurgical pain relieving methods. *International Journal of Nursing Studies, 40*(1), 33–44.

Pölkki, T., Pietilä, A. M., Vehviläinen-Julkunen, K., Laukkala, H., & Kiviluoma, K. (2008). Imagery-induced relaxation in children's postoperative pain relief: A randomized pilot study. *Journal of Pediatric Nursing, 23*(3), 217–224.

Popping, D. M., Elia, N., Marret, E., Remy, C., & Tramer, M. R. (2008). Protective effects of epidural analgesia on pulmonary complications after abdominal and thoracic surgery: A meta-analysis. *Archives of Surgery, 143*(10), 990–999.

Rakel, B., & Frantz, R. (2003). Effectiveness of transcutaneous electrical nerve stimulation on postoperative pain with movement. *Journal of Pain, 4*(8), 455–464.

Razmus, I. S., Dalton, M. E., & Wilson, D. (2004). Pain management for newborn circumcision. *Pediatric Nursing, 30*(5), 414–417, 427.

Rupp, T., & Delaney, K. A. (2004). Inadequate analgesia in emergency medicine. *Annals of Emergency Medicine, 43*(4), 494–503.

Rusy, L. M., Hainsworth, K. R., Nelson, T. J., Czarnecki, M. L., Tassone, J. C., Thometz, J. G., . . . Weisman S. J. (2010). Gabapentin use in pediatric spinal fusion patients: A randomized, double-blind, controlled trial. *Anesthesia and Analgesia, 110*(5), 1393–1398.

Santervas, Y. F., Cotanda, C. P., Carretero, L. M., Garcia, V. L., Sainz de la Maza, V. T., & Cubells, C. L. (2009). Impact of a program to improve pain management in an emergency department. *European Journal of Emergency Medicine, 17*(2), 110–112.

Sinha, M., Christopher, N. C., Fenn, R., & Reeves, L. (2006). Evaluation of nonpharmacologic methods of pain and anxiety management for laceration repair in the pediatric emergency department. *Pediatrics, 117*(4), 1162–1168.

Stoddard, F. J., Jr., Sorrentino, E. A., Ceranoglu, T. A., Saxe, G., Murphy, J. M., Drake, J. E., . . . Tompkins, R. G. (2009). Preliminary evidence for the effects of morphine on posttraumatic stress disorder symptoms in one- to four-year-olds with burns. *Journal of Burn Care & Research, 30*(5), 836–843.

Tanabe, P., Ferket, K., Thomas, R., Paice, J., & Marcantonio, R. (2002). The effect of standard care, ibuprofen, and distraction on pain relief and patient satisfaction in children with musculoskeletal trauma. *Journal of Emergergency Nursing, 28*(2), 118–125.

Tiippana, E. M., Hamunen, K., Kontinen, V. K., & Kalso, E. (2007). Do surgical patients benefit from perioperative gabapentin/pregabalin? A systematic review of efficacy and safety. *Anesthesia and Analgesia, 104*(6), 1545–1556.

Tsao, J. C., Evans, S., Meldrum, M., Altman, T., & Zeltzer, L. K. (2008). A review of CAM for procedural pain in infancy: Part I. Sucrose and non-nutritive sucking. *Evidenced-based Complementary and Alternative Medicine, 5*(4), 371–381.

Twycross, A. (2007). Children's nurses' postoperative pain management practices: An observational study. *International Journal of Nursing Studies, 44*(6), 869–881.

Verghese, S. T., & Hannallah, R. S. (2005). Postoperative pain management in children. *Anesthesiology Clinics of North America, 23*(1), 163–184.

Zempsky, W. T., & Cravero, J. P. (2004). Relief of pain and anxiety in pediatric patients in emergency medical systems. *Pediatrics, 114*(5), 1348–1356.

17

Pain and Sickle-Cell Disease

Sickle-cell disease (SCD) is a genetic disorder associated with hemolysis and vaso-occlusion. In the United States, it affects primarily persons of African heritage and occurs approximately in 1 of 500 African American births (Dampier & Shapiro, 2003). It is estimated that between 72,000 and 98,000 people live with SCD in the United States today (Hassell, 2010). When deoxygenated, the abnormal hemoglobin (sickle hemoglobin) elongates, deforming the red blood cell (RBC) into a rigid "sickle" shape, causing early hemolysis and acute localized ischemia from vaso-occlusion of the microvasculature. This leads to acutely painful events called vaso-occlusive pain crises. Other complications of SCD include damage to major organs (e.g., brain, liver, kidneys, and lungs) and increased vulnerability to severe infections caused by the damage of the spleen (Platt, Eckman, Beasley, & Miller, 2002).

Although the presentation varies considerably with SCD, children have an average of 5 to 7 pain crises per year and require hospitalization 1 to 2 times each year for pain (Mitchell et al., 2007). The pain crises are triggered by many factors, including hypoxia, acidosis, dehydration, and infections. Treatment of SCD has typically focused on symptom control in the form of supportive care, consisting of hydration, warmth, and analgesia, and medications to prevent or reduce complications, such as penicillin for infections and hydroxyurea for vaso-occlusive crises. Although no definitive cure for SCD exists, bone marrow transplantation has cured many children with SCD, but this treatment has limitations because of the unavailability of matched siblings and associated toxicities (Panepinto et al., 2007). Gene therapy has not yet been tested in humans with SCD, but, if successful, it may become another alternative to curing this disease.

TYPES OF PAIN

Pain from SCD is generally classified as acute or chronic. Although the pain of SCD is primarily nociceptive in nature, health care providers are to recognize that pain may originate from many sources (e.g., muscles, bone, or visceral organs). Lack of understanding of the characteristics of SCD pain may contribute to mistrust and stigmatization of patients with SCD.

Clinical Pearl

The ABCs for managing sickle-cell pain are (Platt et al., 2002) as follows:

A. Assessment of the pain (use an age-appropriate pain assessment tool)
B. Believe the patient's level of pain
C. Complications or cause of pain (look for complications such as acute chest syndrome [ACS] or avascular necrosis of the femur)
D. Drugs and distraction
   - Pain medication (opioids and nonsteroidal anti-inflammatory drugs [NSAIDs], if no contraindications)
   - Distraction interventions (for age-appropriate distraction interventions, see Chapter 8).
E. Environment (rest in quiet area with privacy)
F. Fluids (hypotonic fluids)

Acute Pain

Acute pain remains the most common and most troubling symptom experienced by children with SCD and the most frequent reason families seek medical care, often in the emergency department (ED)

(Jacob et al., 2003). Its onset and severity are unpredictable and associated with life-threatening exacerbations of the disease. Most visits to the hospital and hematology clinics are for exacerbations of vaso-occlusive SCD pain in the back, chest, and extremities.

Generalized Acute Pain and Inflammation of Joints

Ischemic pain can occur in any part of the body that has nociceptors or peripheral nerves, but more often involves both long and flat bones as well as the adjacent soft tissues and joints. Children generally describe the pain as deep, intense, aching, and intolerable (Dampier & Shapiro, 2003). Severe SCD pain can be described as excruciating (e.g., "breaking all of my bones at the same time") (Platt et al., 2002). Each crisis typically lasts 4 to 5 days in young children but tends to last longer as the patient ages. It is not uncommon for an adult with SCD to have 2- to 3-week-long pain crisis.

Acute Hand-Foot Syndrome (Dactylitis)

This acute pain syndrome occurs most commonly in infants, manifesting between 6 months and 2 years of age, during which the protective effects of the large amounts of fetal hemoglobin present at birth have been lost as the abnormal sickle hemoglobin (HbS) becomes more prevalent (Greco & Berde, 2010). Symptoms include irritability, low-grade fever, refusal to walk, and painful dorsal swelling of the hands and feet.

Acute Chest Syndrome

ACS can result from any of several inciting events, most notably viral and bacterial pneumonia with in situ sickling of RBCs in the lung. Symptoms of ACS include chest pain, cough, fever, and hypoxia. Even with aggressive use of blood transfusions and antibiotics, this syndrome is a common cause of SCD-related mortality for patients of all ages (American Pain Society [APS], 1999).

Acute Abdominal Pain Syndromes

Because of the misshapen RBCs and their fragments damaging the spleen, splenic sequestration can occur and can be catastrophic in young children because of circulatory collapse (APS, 1999). Various other causes of abdominal pain need to be considered, including the possibility of bilirubin-containing gallstones from chronic hemolysis and subsequent cholelithiasis.

Priapism

Painful erections occur from sickling of RBCs in the sinusoids of the penis and may last for a few hours to a few days.

Chronic Pain

Chronic pain in SCD is associated with bone damage, such as avascular necrosis of the hips, shoulders, and knees, with some older patients requiring hip resurfacing and other joint operations (Ballas, 2010). Physical therapy is essential in reducing pain and maintaining function. Chronic damage to nerves can result from bone compression or injury from the inflammatory substances associated with pain crises and ultimately leads to the risk of neuropathic pain. Headaches and migraines are also a common problem for children with SCD. One study showing one third of the children with SCD have weekly occurrences of headaches (Palermo, Platt-Houston, Kiska, & Berman, 2005). Long-term effects of pain lead to the risk of chronic pain syndromes caused by the associated circulatory abnormalities of SCD.

RAPID ASSESSMENT DURING A PAINFUL EPISODE

Frequent acute pain episodes have been associated with increased mortality, and rapid evaluation is therefore critical not only to ensure prompt relief of pain, but also to assess for life-threatening complications. By delaying treatment, health care providers may delay their ability to diagnose and treat these potentially catastrophic events. The APS has published guidelines with recommendations to health care providers to provide initial analgesics within 15 to 20 minutes of the patient's arrival to an ED (APS, 1999).

The best question to ask the patient is, "Is this pain, how your pain from SCD usually feels?" If so, the patient can be treated with opioids. If not, a search for possible complications or other causes is necessary. Pain in the chest, head, or abdomen warrants a careful evaluation for complications and non-SCD causes. A detailed history and physical examination are important for identifying correctable precipitating factors, such as infection, dehydration, and severe anemia. Laboratory evaluation does not help in the diagnosis of pain episodes, but it does help to identify other mitigating factors, such as worsening anemia, infection, acidosis, and hypoxia.

PHARMACOLOGIC MANAGEMENT

SCD produces the only common pain syndrome in which opioids are considered the major therapy, which is initiated at a young age and continued throughout adult life (Ballas, 2010).

Mild to Moderate Pain Episodes

Many children have self-limited and reversible pain that can be typically managed at home with NSAIDs, acetaminophen (Tylenol), and oral opioids (Pence, Valrie, Gil, Redding-Lallinger, & Daeschner, 2007).

Severe Pain

Severe pain that lasts for hours will require medical care and, often, treatment with opioids in the ED. The APS guidelines recommend morphine to be given intravenously (IV) or subcutaneously if IV access cannot be obtained on the first attempt (APS, 1999). Intramuscular administration is not recommended because it is associated with unreliable absorption and the potential for muscle and soft tissue damage (Tanabe et al., 2007). See Chapter 4 for dosing recommendations. The standard of care includes initiating opioids in the ED (Greco & Berde, 2005; Jacob et al., 2005; Melzer-Lange, Walsh-Kelly, Lea, Hillery, & Scott, 2004). The APS guidelines recommend that titration of analgesics be continued until a clinically significant decrease in pain intensity is achieved or until side effects become problematic (APS, 1999). Multimodal therapy is beneficial, including ketorolac (Toradol) IV every 6 to 8 hours. See Chapter 3 for dosing guidelines.

Other related pharmacologic management includes hydration using hypotonic solutions to rehydrate the RBCs to reduce the tendency toward sickling, with subsequent pain relief. If venous access cannot be obtained, oral hydration should be used.

NONPHARMACOLOGIC MANAGEMENT

Children with SCD and their families have to cope with a chronic medical condition that causes psychological, social, and physical distress affecting their quality of life (Panepinto, O'Mahar, DeBaun, Loberiza, & Scott, 2005). As with other chronic pain conditions, nonpharmacologic interventions have been considered to be adjuncts to routine pharmacologic treatment for the management of SCD pain.

Cognitive-Behavioral Techniques

Cognitive-behavioral techniques complement current medical treatment, and studies of their efficacy have yielded encouraging results (Anie & Green, 2002; Christie & Wilson, 2005). See Chapter 8 for a further discussion about cognitive-behavioral techniques.

Physical Approaches

The physical approach for prevention of pain is to avoid extremes of temperatures, particularly extreme cold, which causes vasoconstriction of superficial blood vessels in the skin and muscles, promoting

SCD pain in those body sites (Dampier & Shapiro, 2003). However, if a pain crisis occurs, warm moist heat, including whirlpool baths to relieve leg pain, is often described as useful. Regular moderate exercise is helpful in maintaining muscle tone.

BARRIERS TO TREATMENT

Patients with SCD pain often encounter barriers to receiving appropriate care, including lack of continuity of care and perceived opioid addiction. Many health care providers believe that patients with SCD are opioid dependent and "drug seekers" despite a lack of data supporting this belief (Elander, Lusher, Bevan, Telfer, & Burton, 2004; Tanabe et al., 2007). This is complicated by the fact that young patients, especially adolescents with unrelieved pain, including those with SCD, develop certain learned behaviors, such as acting in an extreme manner as a result of thinking that otherwise "no one will believe I am having pain." They resort to exaggerated or manipulative pain behaviors, making those patients more vulnerable to misperceptions of substance dependence.

Follow-up studies evaluating how ED health care providers have used the APS guidelines for managing SCD pain (APS, 1999) have revealed conscious or subconscious delay in triage and administration of the initial analgesic. The triage nurse of an ED plays a critical role in determining how quickly patients with an acute pain episode will be evaluated by other health care providers.

PATIENT EDUCATION AND HOME MANAGEMENT

Once a child's pain is controlled in the hospital, clinic, or ED, the patient and parents are to be instructed on further use of NSAIDs and opioids with instructions on what to do if pain escalates or if fever or new symptoms develop.

The implications of long-term use of opioids are unknown but require ongoing supervision, especially for adolescents. Patients with SCD pain require a therapeutic alliance between themselves, their family, and their health care providers to avoid fragmented or episodic care. See Chapter 11 for an example of a formal and written "agreement for pain management services" outlining the commitment of the SCD medical team to provide effective analgesics, as well as the child's acceptance of his own responsibilities for medication compliance, safekeeping, and the use of appropriate nonpharmacologic interventions (Dampier & Shapiro, 2003).

IMPACT OF PAIN

Some children with SCD manage their disease and pain with minimal physical or psychosocial disruptions, but many children experience significant difficulties with sleeping, eating, and normal activities (Jacob et al., 2006), which further contribute to depression, anxiety, decreased social activities, and decreased school attendance (Mitchell et al., 2007). Children are burdened with the memories of past episodes of pain, and even when management is effective, they become well aware of the inevitability of future episodes of SCD pain. Prior experiences with pain treatment will affect how patients will cope with pain during future episodes.

In summary, it is critical that all health care providers recognize the potential serious physiological and psychosocial complications of inadequate pain relief for children with SCD and the importance of providing rapid assessment and pain control with the administration of effective analgesics in a timely manner (APS, 1999; Ballas, 2010; Dampier & Shapiro, 2003; Melzer-Lange et al., 2004; Platt et al., 2002).

REFERENCES

American Pain Society. (1999). *Guidelines for management of acute and chronic pain in sickle cell disease.* Glenview, IL: Author.

Anie, K. A., & Green, J. (2002). Psychological therapies for sickle cell disease and pain. *Cochrane Database of Systematic Reviews, 2,* CD001916.

Ballas, S. K. (2010). Pain and sickle cell disease. In S. M. Fishman, J. C. Ballantyne, & J. P. Rathmell (Eds.), *Bonica's management of pain* (4th ed., pp. 806–827). Philadelphia, PA: Wolters Kluwer/Lippincott Williams & Wilkins.

Christie, D., & Wilson, C. (2005). CBT in paediatric and adolescent health settings: A review of practice-based evidence. *Pediatric Rehabilitation, 8*(4), 241–247.

Dampier, C., & Shapiro, B. (2003). Management of pain in sickle cell disease. In N. L. Schechter, C. B. Berde, & M. Yaster (Eds.), *Pain in infants, children, and adolescents* (2nd ed., pp. 489–515). Philadelphia, PA: Lippincott Williams & Wilkins.

Elander, J., Lusher, J., Bevan, D., Telfer, P., & Burton, B. (2004). Understanding the causes of problematic pain management in sickle cell disease: Evidence that pseudoaddiction plays a more important role than genuine analgesic dependence. *Journal of Pain and Symptom Management, 27*(2), 156–169.

Greco, C., & Berde, C. (2005). Pain management for the hospitalized pediatric patient. *Pediatric Clinics of North America, 52*(4), 995–1027.

Greco, C., & Berde, C. (2010). Acute pain management in children. In S. M. Fishman, J. C. Ballantyne, & J. P. Rathmell (Eds.), *Bonica's management of pain* (4th ed., pp. 681–698). Philadelphia, PA: Wolters Kluwer/Lippincott Williams & Wilkins.

Hassell, K. L. (2010). Population estimates of sickle cell disease in the U.S. *American Journal of Preventive Medicine, 38*(Suppl. 4), S512–521.

Jacob, E., Beyer, J. E., Miaskowski, C., Savedra, M., Treadwell, M., & Styles, L. (2005). Are there phases to the vaso-occlusive painful episode in sickle cell disease? *Journal of Pain and Symptom Management, 29*(4), 392–400.

Jacob, E., Miaskowski, C., Savedra, M., Beyer, J. E., Treadwell, M., & Styles, L. (2003). Changes in intensity, location, and quality of vaso-occlusive pain in children with sickle cell disease. *Pain, 102*(1–2), 187–193.

Jacob, E., Miaskowski, C., Savedra, M., Beyer, J. E., Treadwell, M., & Styles, L. (2006). Changes in sleep, food intake, and activity levels during acute painful episodes in children with sickle cell disease. *Journal of Pediatric Nursing, 21*(1), 23–34.

Melzer-Lange, M. D., Walsh-Kelly, C. M., Lea, G., Hillery, C. A., & Scott, J. P. (2004). Patient-controlled analgesia for sickle cell pain crisis in a pediatric emergency department. *Pediatric Emergency Care, 20*(1), 2–4.

Mitchell, M. J., Lemanek, K., Palermo, T. M., Crosby, L. E., Nichols, A., & Powers, S. W. (2007). Parent perspectives on pain management, coping, and family functioning in pediatric sickle cell disease. *Clinical Pediatrics (Philadelphia), 46*(4), 311–319.

Palermo, T. M., Platt-Houston, C., Kiska, R. E., & Berman, B. (2005). Headache symptoms in pediatric sickle cell patients. *Journal of Pediatric Hematology/Oncology, 27*(8), 420–424.

Panepinto, J. A., O'Mahar, K. M., DeBaun, M. R., Loberiza, F. R., & Scott, J. P. (2005). Health-related quality of life in children with sickle cell disease: Child and parent perception. *British Journal of Haematology, 130*(3), 437–444.

Panepinto, J. A., Walters, M. C., Carreras, J., Marsh, J., Bredeson, C. N., Gale, R. P., . . . Non-Malignant Marrow Disorders Working Committee, Center for International Blood and Marrow Transplant Research. (2007). Matched-related donor transplantation for sickle cell disease: Report from the Center for International Blood and Transplant Research. *British Journal of Haematology, 137*(5), 479–485.

Pence, L., Valrie, C. R., Gil, K. M., Redding-Lallinger, R., & Daeschner, C. (2007). Optimism predicting daily pain medication use in adolescents with sickle cell disease. *Journal of Pain and Symptom Management, 33*(3), 302–309.

Platt, A., Eckman, J. R., Beasley, J., & Miller, G. (2002). Treating sickle cell pain: An update from the Georgia comprehensive sickle cell center. *Journal of Emergency Nursing, 28*(4), 297–303.

Tanabe, P., Myers, R., Zosel, A., Brice, J., Ansari, A. H., Evans, J., & Paice, J. A. (2007). Emergency department management of acute pain episodes in sickle cell disease. *Academic Emergency Medicine, 14*(5), 419–425.

18

Cancer and Pain

In the United States, approximately 15.4 children per 100,000 are diagnosed with cancer each year (National Cancer Institute). Remarkable improvements in treatment have led to an 80% survival rate across all childhood cancers, at least for those in developed countries, stimulating the need to ensure optimal symptom management (Casillas & Zeltzer, 2010; Yeh, Wang, Chiang, Lin, & Chien, 2009). Although the successful treatment of cancer is more frequently achieved in children than in adults, aggressive treatment often means enduring repetitive cycles of chemotherapy associated with painful side effects, as well as numerous invasive diagnostic and therapeutic procedures.

TYPES OF PAIN

Pain causes the most concern and fear for children with all types of malignancies, even more than the fear that they may not be cured of their disease (Ljungman, Gordh, Sorensen, & Kreuger, 2000; Moody, Meyer, Mancuso, Charlson, & Robbins, 2006). Of concern, research indicates that many children and their parents believe that pain is an unavoidable component of cancer treatment (Ljungman et al., 2000). The main source of pain is related to the treatment of the cancer (e.g., mucositis from chemotherapy) and from the significant number of medical procedures (e.g., lumbar punctures or surgeries). For instance, children with one of the most common pediatric cancers, acute lymphocytic leukemia, receive lumbar punctures as often as once a week to once every 3 months for the first year of their treatment, along with injections of growth factors to combat neutropenia, central line insertions, and bone marrow biopsies. This author has been forewarned by her patients to refrain from offering false reassurance such as "this will just be one stick." Patients have said, "Follow me around this week, and you will see how many sticks I will have." Because survivors of childhood cancers have reported symptoms of posttraumatic stress disorders induced by the memories of ineffective relief of pain during invasive procedures (Stuber et al, 1997), health care providers are to be aware of the need to minimize pain and the associated anxiety by referring to Chapter 13.

Assessment

Pain assessment is an ongoing process using age-appropriate pain scales as described in Chapter 2. Various nociceptive and neuropathic pain syndromes are included in Table 18.1. The reality that faces many health care providers caring for children with cancer is to consider many of the sources of pain as both nociceptive and neuropathic in nature. See Table 18.1.

PHARMACOLOGIC MANAGEMENT

Experts who care for pediatric oncology patients know that pain management is more complex than the World Health Organization (WHO) Ladder projects (Mercadante, 2004; Zernikow et al, 2006). Drug therapy is the mainstay of management of pain for all age groups, including neonates.

Nonsteroidal Anti-Inflammatory Drugs (NSAIDs)

Acetaminophen (Tylenol), NSAIDs, and salicylates are useful for mild to moderate pain either alone or in combination with opioids.

Table 18.1 ▓ *Types of Pain in Children With Cancer*

Disease Related	Treatment-Related
Tumor invasion of muscle, soft tissue, or bone Compression of central or peripheral nervous system structures	**Chemotherapy** • Mucositis, esophagitis, typhlitis • Peripheral neuropathies (vincristine, cyclosporine) • Myopathies (steroids) • Secondary infections (pneumonia, diarrhea)
Procedure Related Routine physical examination Venipuncture Injections (intramuscular or subcutaneous) Accessing subcutaneous reservoirs or ports Dressing and tape changes Suture removal Bone marrow aspiration and biopsy Lumbar puncture Postdural puncture headache Bony pain from marrow aspiration	**Radiation Therapy** • Mucositis, enteritis, proctitis • Dermatitis or burns • Plexopathies **Other Medicines** • Steroid-induced avascular necrosis, myalgias, arthralgias • Growth factor-induced bone pain
Surgery Related Acute postoperative Specific syndromes: post-thoracotomy, phantom limb	**Other Conditions** Graft-versus-host disease from stem cell transplantation Postherpetic neuralgia Usual childhood illnesses and injuries

Source: American Pain Society (APS), 2005; Anghelescu, Oakes, & Popenhagan, 2006.

Rectal administration typically is contraindicated in neutropenic or thrombocytopenic patients to avoid damage to rectal tissues that could lead to infection or rectal bleeding. Because NSAIDs have antipyretic action, they may be contraindicated for patients who are neutropenic to avoid masking fever as an early sign of infection (American Pain Society [APS], 2005). NSAIDs should be avoided in patients receiving high-dose methotrexate because of the potential for delayed clearance of the methotrexate (Litalien & Jacqz-Aigrain, 2001). All NSAIDs inhibit platelet aggregation and often are contraindicated in children with chemotherapy-induced thrombocytopenia. In summary, indications for NSAIDS for children with cancer are narrower than for children with other painful conditions because of the potential side effects, and they should be prescribed with caution (McNicol, Strassels, Goudas, Lau, & Carr, 2004). See Chapter 3 for more details about NSAIDs.

Opioids

Opioids are the mainstay for moderate to severe cancer pain because of their effectiveness, ease of titration, and favorable risk-to-benefit ratio (APS, 2005). Patient-controlled analgesia (PCA) pumps are particularly useful for treating cancer pain in order to titrate the dose of opioid to the source of pain, such as providing pain relief for a child with severe mucositis, which makes oral ingestion of opioids more difficult. See Chapter 4 for more details about opioids and PCA.

TREATMENT CHALLENGES

Treatment of cancer pain includes the need to control the source of pain, thus treating the cancer with tumor-specific approaches, including, when appropriate to the specific diagnosis, surgical resection, chemotherapy, and radiation therapy. Although different types of pain are considered individually, patients usually experience a mixture of two or more types.

Acute Pain
Treatment-Related Pain

The most frequent cause of pain for children undergoing chemotherapy and radiation therapy is mucositis. Mucositis is commonly described according to the WHO's grading system, ranging from grade I (mild) to grade IV (severe) (Casillas & Zeltzer, 2010), with opioids deemed essential for the patient's comfort. Adequate pain control is necessary for mouth-cleansing regimens to minimize the risk of infection. Topical agents, such as lidocaine (Xylocaine), can be provided in a "swish and spit" regimen to help decrease the pain as well. Children resist adequate mouth care regimens unless pain relief is optimal, usually requiring opioids. Opioid delivery via a PCA becomes essential, especially for grade III and IV mucositis, to provide ongoing pain relief with the ability to use the bolus from the PCA before mouth care.

Tumor-Related Pain

Tumor-related pain is generally not the most significant source except at the initial diagnosis, at the time of relapse, or during end-of-life care. Fortunately, many pediatric cancers respond rapidly to primary treatment (e.g., chemotherapy and radiation therapy), which reduces pain as the cancer cells are destroyed. Of note, a child with a brain tumor who presents with a headache needs careful evaluation to determine the source of pain, which may arise from a non-cancer-related source. On the other hand, the headache could be from increased intracranial pressure caused by the tumor or a ventricular peritoneal shunt failure, either of which requires emergent attention and treatment. Providing analgesic therapy for a patient who has a brain tumor and a headache is best done in collaboration with the oncology and neurosurgical services.

New Onset of Acute Pain

Although health care providers often conclude that sudden increases in pain, despite adequate opioid doses, indicate the development of opioid tolerance; the presence of any new acute pain may signal a new metastatic lesion, prompting the need for diagnostic imaging or other laboratory procedures.

Severe Nociceptive Pain

Severe pain from the following sources can be particularly difficult to control:

- Bone pain from tumors causing bony destruction.
- Visceral pain from tumors involving organ invasion with capsular wall stretching, organ compression, obstruction of intestines, tumor regrowth within the organ, or peritoneal cavity bleeding.

▓ Mixed neuropathic-nociceptive pain from direct invasion of tissues and organs as well as compression of nerves. For example, tumors in the pelvis can also cause lower extremity weakness and bladder and bowel dysfunction.

Along with escalating doses of opioids and judicious use of steroids and NSAIDs, chemotherapy and radiation therapy are used for pain relief by reducing the tumor size or slowing its rate of growth. When such cancer therapies are effective, health care providers need to increase assessment and downward titration of the opioid dose to match effective tumor reduction to avoid opioid side effects.

Neuropathic Pain

Children may experience neuropathic pain in the jaw, legs, hands, feet, and abdomen. When providing useful coanalgesics, which are generally only available in oral preparations, the challenge is to do so in spite of chemotherapy-induced nausea and mucositis (see Chapter 5). Once maximum doses of anticonvulsants and tricyclic antidepressants have been achieved, methadone (Dolophine) can be considered by health care providers experienced with its use (See Chapter 4).

Clinical Pearl

Health care providers should anticipate the need to aggressively treat neuropathic pain associated with cancer therapy, including the following:

▓ Chemotherapy, such as vincristine. Treatment of the pain needs to be done in collaboration with physical therapists because of the associated motor dysfunctions of the feet and hands.
▓ Cyclosporine or other agents used for a successful bone marrow transplant.
▓ Limb-sparing procedures or, if not possible, amputation with the associated phantom pain.

When escalating doses of opioids do not relieve pain caused by spinal cord compression or malignant lesions of the brachial or lumbosacral plexus, adding steroids, particularly dexamethasone, to the pain management regimen is useful. In extreme cases of nerve entrapment and excruciating pain, children may need neurodestructive procedures using phenol or alcohol.

Bone Pain from Leukemic Blast Infiltration

Often, the reluctance of a young child to walk normally is the presenting sign leading to a diagnosis of acute lymphocytic leukemia. The rapid growth of leukemic blasts within the bone marrow causes diffuse bone pain. Because the use of NSAIDs is often contraindicated during chemotherapy, opioids are the analgesic of choice. Fortunately, the bone pain will usually rapidly abate as the leukemic blasts respond to the chemotherapy, and subsequent rapid weaning from the opioids is the usual pattern. However, for children with relapsed leukemia that does not respond to steroids, chemotherapy, or radiation therapy, the escalation of the opioid doses, along with NSAIDs, if not contraindicated, is essential for adequate pain relief.

End-of-Life Management of Pain

Children who are dying of cancer may require rapid escalation of opioids to maintain control when tolerance occurs (Hooke, Hellsten, Stutzer, & Forte, 2002). Children dying with solid tumors are particularly likely to need high doses of opioids (Hewitt, Goldman, Collins, Childs, & Hain, 2008). The need to increase an opioid dose usually is not related to tolerance but rather to tumor growth, most rapidly during the final weeks of life, with reports as high as 518 mg/kg/hr of intravenous (IV) morphine or its equianalgesic equivalent (Collins, Grier, Kinney, & Berde, 1995). Intractable pain from increased tumor bulk that does not respond to increasing doses of opioids may require palliative chemotherapy or radiation therapy (Hewitt et al., 2008). These children may have severe neuropathic pain associated with tumor extension along the course of major nerves, requiring attempts to maximize the use of coanalgesics as described in Chapter 5. For more information about pain management during the terminal illness phase, refer to Chapter 15.

Chronic Pain

Literature relating to long-term pain management problems arising from cancer treatment in children is scant but includes chronic abdominal pain, avascular necrosis of various joints resulting from steroids as part of their chemotherapy regimen, neuropathic and mechanical pain after bone tumor resection, and other causes of pain. Children who undergo radiation or thoracic surgery may also develop scoliosis or other forms of musculoskeletal pain syndromes. Although the use of NSAIDs and nonpharmacologic interventions are the recommended strategy, some children require chronic opioids or long-term management with coanalgesics for neuropathic pain syndromes, such as those having phantom limb pain or neuropathy associated with nerve damage. As in all non-cancer-related chronic pain, experts believe chronic pain is best managed by a multidisciplinary team using multimodal interventions of analgesics, physical therapy, and nonpharmacologic techniques (Anghelescu, Oakes, & Popenhagen, 2006; Collins & Weisman, 2003).

Clinical Pearl

When children require a hematopoietic stem cell infusion, in the past known as a bone marrow transplant, they are at high risk for a unique pain syndrome called graft-versus-host disease (GVHD), which occurs when the host (recipient) cells appear foreign to the engrafted (donor) hematopoietic stem cells (Casillas & Zeltzer, 2010). GVHD occurs as either:

- Acute GVHD syndrome within the first 100 days of the stem cell infusion, causing dermatitis, enteritis, and hepatitis. Clinical manifestations include a diffuse skin rash, ranging

> from mild involvement of the palms of the hands and soles
> of the feet to severe bullous desquamation and skin slough-
> ing, and abdominal pain with diarrhea. Treatment is with
> opioids and coanalgesics as indicated.
> ▪ Chronic GVHD occurs 100 days or more after the stem
> cell infusion and is thought to be caused by an autoim-
> mune process that may result in scleroderma-type skin
> changes accompanied by joint stiffness, immobility, and
> chronic pain.

NONPHARMACOLOGIC MANAGEMENT

Adequate analgesic dosing needs to be complemented by practical nonpharmacologic approaches to ensure optimal pain relief for children with cancer (De Negri et al, 2006).

Cognitive-behavioral techniques complement current medical treatment, and studies of their efficacy have yielded encouraging results. Distraction with developmentally appropriate activities that are highly engaging and enjoyable have the potential to effectively reduce distress for children who have repeated needle sticks (Dahlquist et al, 2002). Research on how to integrate self-selected music to decrease distress related to radiation therapy is available (Clark et al, 2006). The use of humor therapy along with massage has been shown to effectively complement the necessary aggressive use of opioids for patients who remain inpatient for weeks for engraftment from a stem cell infusion (Phipps, 2002). Other evidence to support the use of clinical hypnosis, guided imagery, and acupuncture is available (Kelly, 2007).

In summary, caring for children with cancer requires health care providers to respond to various sources of pain, using medications that may need rapidly escalating doses, as well as engaging children in useful nonpharmacologic interventions within the context of various symptoms and aggressive treatment of their disease.

REFERENCES

American Pain Society (2005). *Guidelines for the management of cancer pain in adults and children*. Glenview, IL: Author.

Anghelescu, D., Oakes, L., & Popenhagan, M. (2006). Management of pain due to cancer in neonates, children, and adolescents. In O.A. de Leon-Casasola (Ed.), *Cancer pain: Pharmacologic, interventional, and palliative care approaches* (pp. 509–521). Philadelphia, PA: Elsevier.

Casillas, J., & Zeltzer, L. K. (2010). Cancer pain in children. In S. M. Fishman, J. C. Ballantyne, & J. P. Rathmell (Eds.), *Bonica's management of pain* (4th ed., pp. 669–680). Philadelphia, PA: Wolters Kluwer/ Lippincott Williams & Wilkins.

Clark, M., Isaacks-Downton, G., Wells, N., Redlin-Frazier, S., Eck, C., Hepworth, J. T., & Chakravarthy B. (2006). Use of preferred music to reduce emotional distress and symptom activity during radiation therapy. *Journal of Music Therapy, 43*(3), 247–265.

Collins, J., & Weisman, S. (2003). Management of pain in childhood cancer. In N. L. Schechter, C. B. Berde, & M. Yaster (Eds.), *Pain in infants, children, and adolescents* (2nd ed., pp. 517–538). Philadelphia, PA: Lippincott Williams & Wilkins.

Collins, J. J., Grier, H. E., Kinney, H. C., & Berde, C. B. (1995). Control of severe pain in children with terminal malignancy. *Journal of Pediatrics, 126*(4), 653–657.

Dahlquist, L. M., Busby, S. M., Slifer, K. J., Tucker, C. L., Eischen, S., Hilley, L., & Sulc, W. (2002). Distraction for children of different ages who undergo repeated needle sticks. *Journal of Pediatric Oncology Nursing, 19*(1), 22–34.

De Negri, P., Ivani, G., Tonetti, F., Tirri, T., Modano, P., & Reato, C. (2006). Management of procedure-related pain in children. In O. A. de Leon-Casasola (Ed.), *Cancer pain: Pharmacologic, interventional, and palliative care approaches* (pp. 523–528). Philadelphia, PA: Elsevier.

Hewitt, M., Goldman, A., Collins, G. S., Childs, M., & Hain, R. (2008). Opioid use in palliative care of children and young people with cancer. *Journal of Pediatrics, 152*(1), 39–44.

Hooke, C., Hellsten, M. B., Stutzer, C., & Forte, K. (2002). Pain management for the child with cancer in end-of-life care: APON position paper. *Journal of Pediatric Oncology Nursing, 19*(2), 43–47.

Kelly, K. M. (2007). Complementary and alternative medicines for use in supportive care in pediatric cancer. *Support Care Cancer, 15*(4), 457–460.

Litalien, C., & Jacqz-Aigrain, E. (2001). Risks and benefits of nonsteroidal anti-inflammatory drugs in children: A comparison with paracetamol. *Paediatric Drugs, 3*(11), 817–858.

Ljungman, G., Gordh, T., Sorensen, S., & Kreuger, A. (2000). Pain variations during cancer treatment in children: A descriptive survey. *Pediatric Hematology Oncology, 17*(3), 211–221.

McNicol, E., Strassels, S., Goudas, L., Lau, J., & Carr, D. (2004). Nonsteroidal anti-inflammatory drugs, alone or combined with opioids, for cancer pain: A systematic review. *Journal of Clinical Oncology, 22*(10), 1975–1992.

Mercadante, S. (2004). Cancer pain management in children. *Palliative Medicine, 18*(7), 654–662.

Moody, K., Meyer, M., Mancuso, C. A., Charlson, M., & Robbins, L. (2006). Exploring concerns of children with cancer. *Support Care Cancer, 14*(9), 960–966.

National Cancer Institute. *Age-adjusted SEER cancer incidence rates: 1975-2006.* Retrieved March 17, 2010, from http://seer.cancer.gov/csr/1975_2006/results_single/sect_28_table.02.pdf

Phipps, S. (2002). Reduction of distress associated with paediatric bone marrow transplant: Complementary health promotion interventions. *Pediatric Rehabilitation, 5*(4), 223–234.

Stuber, M. L., Kazak, A. E., Meeske, K., Barakat, L., Guthrie, D., Garnier, H., . . . Meadows, A. (1997). Predictors of posttraumatic stress symptoms in childhood cancer survivors. *Pediatrics, 100*(6), 958–964.

Yeh, C. H., Wang, C. H., Chiang, Y. C., Lin, L., & Chien, L. C. (2009). Assessment of symptoms reported by 10- to 18-year-old cancer patients in Taiwan. *Journal of Pain and Symptom Management, 38*(5), 738–746.

Zernikow, B., Smale, H., Michel, E., Hasan, C., Jorch, N., & Andler, W. (2006). Paediatric cancer pain management using the WHO analgesic ladder—results of a prospective analysis from 2265 treatment days during a quality improvement study. *European Journal of Pain, 10*(7), 587–595.

19

Chronic Pain

As many as 20% of children in the United States have chronic pain, which is pain that is persistent or recurring frequently for more than 3 months (American Pain Society [APS], 2001; Perquin et al., 2000) that impacts negatively on function and health-related quality of life. In severe cases, chronic pain can occur daily and can have a significant impact on the children and their families (Connelly & Schanberg, 2006; Hunfeld et al., 2001). The persistence of pain often becomes the central focus for families, distracting them from normal activities and roles, including parents having to miss work for trips to various health care providers, seeking to find a source and treatment for their children's persistent pain complaints.

> **Clinical Pearl**
> Health-related quality of life refers to an individual's perception of the impact a disease or condition has on his or her physical well-being, as well as social and psychological function domains. Children with chronic pain have a lower quality of life than healthy children (Schechter, Palermo, Walco, & Berde, 2010).

Chronic pain often occurs in children who otherwise look well, resulting in health care providers labeling them as "malingerers" or not really having pain. Appropriate laboratory and diagnostic imaging studies need to be completed to rule out an acute process that would require immediate medical intervention. A clinical examination and patient history are useful in identifying specific chronic pain syndromes. To establish a therapeutic relationship, the health care provider is to convey a sincere belief that the child really has pain. It is likely that the child and family have already received the message that the pain is not real and the child is just seeking attention. Various chronic pain conditions occur in children, with estimates of prevalence difficult to interpret because of inconsistent classifications and diagnostic difficulties (Schechter et al., 2010). In general, chronic pain overall is more prevalent in older children and adolescents (Anthony & Schanberg, 2007; Gold et al., 2009) and more common in girls than in boys (Anthony & Schanberg, 2007; Hunfeld et al., 2001; Lynch, Kashikar-Zuck, Goldschneider, & Jones, 2007).

Several of the more common chronic pain disorders with specific assessment and management considerations for each will be described in the next section. Common features across all pediatric chronic pain will then be reviewed later in this chapter in the section titled Approach to Pediatric Chronic Pain.

SPECIFIC CHRONIC PAIN CONDITIONS

Headache

One of most common conditions to affect children in developed countries is chronic headaches, occurring in up to 75% of children before the age of 15 years (Hershey, 2010; Schechter et al., 2010). The two most common types are migraine with or without aura and tension-type headaches or a blend of these two types, which often coexist in the early phases of the headaches. (Grazzi, 2004; Schechter et al., 2010). Health care providers need to refer to specific classification systems, such as that of the International Headache Society, for specific criteria used for diagnosis and management purposes (Hamalainen & Masek, 2003). However, in general, migraine headaches are described as a throbbing, more localized pain accompanied by nausea, vomiting, and photophobia that usually lasts several hours, with some children reporting the occurrence of auras preceding the headaches (visual images that are blurring, flickering changes in the visual field and flashing lights). Tension-type headaches are described as dull, diffuse, and persistent pain that may last for hours, days, months, or even years. A positive family history (especially maternal) seems to predispose children to headaches.

Assessment and Diagnosis

A detailed history is critical for the diagnosis and classification of headaches, which poses unique challenges when the child has difficulty describing the headaches or is too young to describe the headaches. Health care providers need to rule out possible serious neurological causes for the headaches, such as epilepsy, ophthalmologic or dental problems, sinusitis, brain tumors, or arteriovenous malformation, before implementing chronic pain strategies (Andrasik & Schwartz, 2006; Hamalainen & Masek, 2003). However, many children have headaches that are not from a diagnosable physical condition (Stinson & Bruce, 2009). Prompting the child to describe the headache in his own words and its associated signs and symptoms, such as visual changes, nausea, vomiting, and triggers for the headache, will provide useful information to determine the type of headache.

Treatment

Nonpharmacologic Techniques. Self-regulation strategies, such as relaxation, biofeedback, and cognitive-behavior techniques (CBT), have been found helpful in preventing and reducing headache pain (Grazzi, 2004; Hershey, 2010). In a review of randomized controlled trials with adolescents who suffer from recurrent tension headaches or migraines, therapist-assisted progressive relaxation was found to be effective (Andrasik & Schwartz, 2006; Larsson, Carlsson, Fichtel, & Melin, 2005). Initial support has been demonstrated in one trial using acupuncture to reduce headaches (Pintov, Lahat, Alstein, Vogel, & Barg, 1997). Allowing for adequate sleep, regular meal-times, and appropriate exercise can be helpful in reducing the frequency and intensity of headaches (Hamalainen & Masek, 2003). Treatment begins with identification and modification of obvious trigger and contributing factors, such as physical exertion, hunger, noise, traveling, and flashing lights (Andrasik & Schwartz, 2006; Kondev & Minster, 2003). For children who have headaches that seem to be related to specific foods, such as cheese, chocolate, or nuts, avoidance is the best solution.

Pharmacologic Interventions. The most effective medications are those that have a rapid onset of action and can be administered quickly. Acetaminophen (Tylenol), nonsteroidal anti-inflammatory drugs (NSAIDs), and nasal spray sumatriptan (Imitrex) are all effective symptomatic pharmacologic treatments for episodes of migraine in children (Damen et al., 2005; Grazzi, 2004). Further research in the use of tryptophan agents in children needs to be done, as well as consideration of how interventions not only reduce pain but also reduce days missed from school and other functional measures. Gabapentin (Neurontin), topiramate (Topamax), valproate (Depakote), and levetiracetam (Keppra) have demonstrated promising results for the prevention and treatment of migraine in children (Lewis et al., 2009), but since no well-controlled trials have been conducted, these agents cannot be formally recommended (Bakola, Skapinakis, Tzoufi, Damigos, & Mavreas, 2009; Golden, Haut, & Moshe, 2006).

Musculoskeletal Pain

Musculoskeletal pain includes pain of any joint, bone, or muscle and is generally divided into two groups. One group of children suffer pain from juvenile chronic arthritis (JCA), the most common chronic rheumatic condition in childhood, affecting approximately 285,000 children in North America (APS, 2002). Other children have musculoskeletal pain not related to arthritis, generally referred to as nonrheumatologic pain, which includes various syndromes also described in this section.

Juvenile Chronic Arthritis

Children with juvenile chronic arthritis (JCA) suffer from various joint deformities and destruction, osteoporosis, and growth abnormalities, causing pain and physical limitation. JCA represents a heterogenous group of arthritic conditions in which pain is described as mild to severe, corresponding to the degree of chronic inflammatory process. In contrast to adults, 30% to 50% of children go into remission after several years, depending on the subtype of arthritis (APS, 2002). Health care providers need to refer to specific classification systems, such as that of the American College of Rheumatology, for specific criteria used for diagnosis and management purposes (Kulas & Schanberg, 2003).

Assessment and Diagnosis. Most children with JCA experience pain, stiffness, and joint discomfort but differently from adults in that the pain seems to be less extensive and less intensive for most children (APS, 2002). Along with the clinical history and examination, laboratory studies, specifically a complete blood count and erythrocyte sedimentation rate, can be useful in tracking symptomatic flares in JCA. Causes of the flares are not clearly known but seem to be related to triggers such as infection, trauma, and psychosocial distresses (Kulas & Schanberg, 2003).

Nonpharmacologic Techniques. Physical approaches such as splinting, ice, heat, paraffin baths, and massage are all useful for adults, but no studies have been conducted clearly showing benefit for children with JCA (APS, 2002). Active exercise, including aerobic conditioning, may improve energy and increase the child's sense of well-being, thus indirectly reducing the pain of JCA (APS, 2002). Addressing coping strategies, eliminating stress when possible, and correcting misperceptions about JCA appear to help reduce the pain (Kulas & Schanberg, 2003), along with other nonpharmacologic strategies for pediatric chronic pain described in the next section of this chapter.

Pharmacologic Interventions. Control of JCA is essential for the treatment of pain and to lessen future problems with destruction of the joint (APS, 2002). Pain should not be ignored while waiting for the JCA treatment to take effect, because some of these agents may take months for their full benefit to be realized. The two mainstays of initial treatment are NSAIDS and intra-articular corticosteroid injection (APS, 2002). See Chapter 3.

Growing Pains

Recurrent nonarticular bilateral pains usually in the back of thighs, popliteal area, or calf lasting only 10 to 15 minutes, occurring late in the day or during the night are referred to as "growing pains." No clear etiology has been determined for this common complaint of school-age children (Connelly & Schanberg, 2006).

Assessment and Diagnosis. Because there is no diagnostic test, growing pains is a clinical diagnosis based on history and the lack of a persistent limp or symptoms during the day hours.

Nonpharmacologic Techniques. Massage, heat, and muscle stretching have been reported as useful for some children (Kulas & Schanberg, 2003). It is necessary for the health care provider to reassure parents and children that, although the pain is "real," no evidence has been found that children with growing pains develop more serious disorders, such as fibromyalgia (Uziel, Chapnick, Jaber, Nemet, & Hashkes, 2010), or that the pain is a sign of life-threatening disease, such as cancer.

Pharmacologic Interventions. Treatment is generally with NSAIDs (Kulas & Schanberg, 2003).

Juvenile Fibromyalgia Syndrome

Juvenile fibromyalgia syndrome (JFMS) is typically characterized as diffuse chronic musculoskeletal pain in at least three areas of the body with numerous tender points on palpation in the absence of an underlying specific etiology (Connelly & Schanberg, 2006; Kulas & Schanberg, 2003). Other common symptoms include sleep disturbances, chronic anxiety, tension, fatigue, and abdominal pain (Anthony & Schanberg, 2007; Kulas & Schanberg, 2003). Although many studies have attempted to determine if JFMS is linked to temperament, genetic predisposition, or family interactions, specific causal relationships have not been discerned (Anthony & Schanberg, 2007; Schechter et al., 2010).

Assessment and Diagnosis. Laboratory tests are normal but are often done to rule out other entities such as JCA. Although criteria have been set to diagnose adults with fibromyalgia, these criteria have not been validated in children (APS, 2005). Diagnosis of JFMS is difficult since a child will often exhibit few pain behaviors during physical examination yet verbalize their pain as "intense" or "unbearable" (Anthony & Schanberg, 2007). JFMS comprises vicious circles of pain, fatigue, insomnia, depressed mood, inactivity, and anxiety. Children with JFMS report moderate levels of pain that are higher than those reported by children with JCA (APS, 2005). Long-term follow-up studies of children with JFMS have shown conflicting results, some improving and others with school and social withdrawal patterns (APS, 2005).

Nonpharmacologic Techniques. The APS's recommendations include informing the child and family about the patterns of pain as related to mood and stress and use nonpharmacologic techniques to restore function, including the need for sleep and exercise, and to limit school absences (APS, 2005; Kulas & Schanberg, 2003). Using relaxation and distraction, adolescent girls were able to reduce both pain and disability and improve their coping skills (Kashikar-Zuck, Swain, Jones, & Graham, 2005). Not surprisingly, other researchers found that successful outcomes with CBT greatly depend on commitment by the patient and family regarding compliance (Connelly & Schanberg, 2006). Using aerobic exercise to minimize pain, improve sleep quality, enhance self-efficacy, and increase positive mood is also recommended (APS, 2005).

Pharmacologic Interventions. The use of NSAIDs, tricyclic antidepressants (TCAs), muscle relaxants, gabapentin (Neurontin), and pregabalin (Lyrica) has shown only moderate success for adults and has not been studied in children with JFMS (Kulas & Schanberg, 2003).

Complex Regional Pain Syndrome

Complex regional pain syndrome (CRPS) is a group of conditions associated with dysfunction of the autonomic nervous system, resulting in sensory changes and pain associated with abnormal skin color, temperature change, abnormal motor activity, and edema (Connelly & Schanberg, 2006; Greco & Berde, 2005; Stinson & Bruce, 2009; Wilder, 2003). Although the pathophysiology is not well defined, CRPS often follows a minor injury or traumatic event but with pain that is persistent and disproportionate to the initiating injury (Connelly & Schanberg, 2006). More common with lower limbs, the degree of dysfunction varies widely among patients. Left untreated, CRPS can lead to bone demineralization, muscle wasting, and joint contractures. CRPS is actually defined in terms of two types:

- CRPS Type 1 results from abnormalities in the processing of peripheral pain sensations with no clear nerve injury or lesion. This type was referred to in the past as *reflex sympathetic dystrophy.*
- CRPS Type 2 occurs as result of damage to a peripheral nerve. This type is also called *causalgia.*

Assessment and Diagnosis. Early recognition and treatment of CRPS is associated with the best chance at resolution. No laboratory findings or diagnostic imaging studies are indicative for CRPS. A physical examination and thorough medical history are needed to rule out other conditions, such as infection, stress fracture, and tumors. Clinical criteria for this syndrome have been defined as indicated in Table 19.1.

Nonpharmacologic Techniques. Intensive physical therapy, transcutaneous electrical nerve stimulation, and adjunctive CBT are recommended (Anthony & Schanberg, 2007; Connelly & Schanberg, 2006; Wilder, 2003).

Table 19.1 ▧ *Signs and Symptoms of Complex Regional Pain Syndrome*

Clinical criteria to meet the diagnosis of complex regional pain syndrome (CRPS) are the presence of the following:

▧ At least two neuropathic descriptors for the pain
▧ At least two of the physical signs of autonomic dysfunction

Neuropathic Pain Descriptors	Signs of Autonomic Dysfunction
Burning	Cyanosis
Dysesthesia	Mottling
Paresthesia	Hyperhidrosis
Mechanical allodynia	Extremity cooler than contralateral by 3° C
Hyperalgesia to cold	Edema

Source. From Wilder, 2003.

Pharmacologic Interventions. Use of coanalgesics, specifically TCAs and gabapentin, has been shown to be useful for CRPS (Wilder, 2003). If doses of these coanalgesics have been maximized or the child is not tolerating these medications and still has refractory pain, other interventions may be considered to facilitate the necessary aggressive physical therapy regimen, such as the following:

▧ Sympathetic blockade via infusion of local anesthetics (LA) to improve regional blood flow and reduce pain (Meier, Zurakowski, Berde, & Sethna, 2009; Wilder, 2003);
▧ Epidural nerve blockade via infusion of LAs (Wilder, 2003);
▧ Peripheral nerve blockade via continuous infusion of LAs (Dadure et al., 2005); or
▧ Spinal cord stimulators (Olsson, Meyerson, & Linderoth, 2008).

The above interventions are controversial, because these approaches can reinforce a passive rather than active role of the child unless physical therapy regimens are continued (Cepeda, Carr, & Lau, 2005; Greco & Berde, 2005).

Chronic Abdominal Pain

Once called recurrent abdominal pain, the current term defining persistent abdominal pain without obvious pathology is functional abdominal pain (FAP) (American Academy of Pediatrics [AAP] and North American Society for Pediatric Gastroenterology, 2005). Experts define FAP as three or more bouts of abdominal pain and associated gastrointestinal symptoms over a period of at least 3 months that are severe enough to interfere with normal activities (Scharff, Leichtner, & Rappaport, 2003; Stinson & Bruce, 2009). The age range for FAP tends to be school aged; however, FAP may evolve into irritable bowel syndrome (IBS) and other broader somatic concerns in adolescence and adulthood (Schechter et al., 2010).

Assessment and Diagnosis. The most common complaint is nonradiating pain lasting 1 to 3 hours around the umbilicus with altered bowel habits, pallor, sweating, nausea, and occasionally vomiting, and migraines have also been reported. Ruling out other causes of persistent abdominal pain by taking a careful history, health care providers are to explain to the child that, although the pain is real, there most likely is no underlying serious or chronic disease.

Clinical Pearl   Health care providers need to rule out any possible underlying pathological cause of the abdominal pain. Experts advise that an extensive workup (e.g., abdominal diagnostic imaging or an endoscopic examination) is rarely productive unless the medical history or physical examination reveals one of these "red flags" (Scharff et al., 2003):

- Weight loss
- Pain awakening the child at night
- Fevers
- Pain far from umbilicus
- Dysuria
- Guaiac-positive stools
- Anemia
- Elevated erythrocyte sedimentation rate

Nonpharmacologic Techniques. Although research for use of these techniques with children who have FAP is very limited, CBT such as biofeedback and stress management regimens have been found to be successful. Emphasis has been placed on parents to avoid reinforcement of "sick behaviors" and focus on rewarding healthy behaviors.

Pharmacologic Interventions. Time-limited use of medications (i.e., acid-reduction agents and smooth muscle relaxants) may help to decrease the frequency or severity of symptoms (AAP and North American Society for Pediatric Gastroenterology, 2005).

APPROACH TO PEDIATRIC CHRONIC PAIN

Common Assessment Strategies

Pain Diaries

Ongoing records of pain scores can help identify triggers and possible patterns of chronic pain (Connelly et al., 2010). Discussion of how the pain occurs for an individual child can prompt alterations in behavior and responses to pain, giving the child an increased sense of control (Hunfeld et al., 2001). However, pain diaries are to be used for short periods of time, only to gain an understanding of the pain. Prolonged use may be counterproductive by unduly focusing attention to the pain and subsequently increasing pain complaints (Schechter et al., 2010).

Assessment of Function

Because returning to normal function and activities is of paramount importance in treating chronic pain, various tools have been recommended to determine a baseline at the initiation of treatment as well as ongoing progress in treating the chronic pain. Such tools include a quality-of-life inventory (PedsQL) (Varni, Seid, & Kurtin, 2001) and the Bath Adolescent Pain Questionnaire (Eccleston et al., 2005). To obtain a full understanding of chronic pain, assessment tools need to be multidimensional and actually seek input of not only the child but also family members regarding the pain and its impact on the child's function, such as by using the Bath Adolescent Pain-Parent Impact Questionnaire (Jordan, Eccleston, McCracken, Connell, & Clinch, 2008).

Psychosocial Assessment

Because of the extensive underlying interrelationships of chronic pain to the biopsychosocial context of a child who seek medical intervention, health care providers are to consider the needed skills of a psychologist to administer and evaluate responses to standardized psychological tests to screen for mental health diagnoses, particularly anxiety, depression, and maladaptive coping behaviors. Other specific measures are beyond the scope of this book, but collaboration with a child psychologist is highly recommended.

Clinical Pearl

Clinical interviews should cover the developmental, behavioral, and social history of the child with chronic pain. Specifically, health care providers are to obtain (Eyckmans, Hilderson, Westhovens, Wouters, & Moons, 2010; Schechter et al., 2010) the following:

- History of early childhood
- Comprehensive school history
- History of peer and social relationships
- Family functioning

Consider interviewing the child and parents, and then, with permission, interview the child separately.

Treatment of Chronic Pain

Recognition by the health care provider that chronic pain is multifaceted, requiring the persistent use of individualized nonpharmacologic strategies with limited use of analgesics and coanalgesics, is key. For health care providers who focus on acute pain with reliance on pharmacologic strategies, this is a very different approach. If no associated etiology is established for the chronic pain, pharmacologic interventions alone are usually not effective. Rather than emphasizing pain control as the goal, the treatment plan needs to emphasize the renewed ability of the child to function in spite of the pain in an adaptive fashion while avoiding catastrophizing and fear-avoidance patterns common with chronic pain (Wicksell, Melin, & Olsson, 2007).

Successful treatment, defined as returning the child to normal function, will require a real multidisciplinary effort to:

- Establish goals, including the child returning to school and other normal daily activities even when having pain, as quickly as possible (Andrasik & Schwartz, 2006); and
- Facilitating adaptive problem solving, communication, and coping skills (Hunfeld et al., 2001; Merlijn et al., 2006). For example, families are encouraged to reduce or minimize their reaction and attention to the child when pain is reported (less secondary again) and to support their child to use their self-regulating skills (Andrasik & Schwartz, 2006).

Nonpharmacologic Interventions

Nonpharmacologic approaches are the cornerstone of treatment of chronic pain and are usually provided on an outpatient basis with frequent visits to the appropriate health care provider's clinic. However, some experts advocate the need for treatment of adolescents with longstanding chronic pain in a specially designed residential interdisciplinary program incorporating CBT and physical therapy with family involvement, demonstrating outcomes of improving social, physical, and psychologic functioning (Eccleston, Malleson, Clinch, Connell, & Sourbut, 2003). Unfortunately, these programs are often difficult to access in local communities and may not be supported by third-party payers.

Cognitive-Behavioral Techniques. CBT can significantly reduce the intensity of pediatric chronic pain. To improve access to CBT treatment when face-to-face sessions between the child and the health care provider are not possible, early work is offered in how to provide these techniques via newer technologies already familiar to children, such as using CD-ROMs or interactive Internet-based techniques (Connelly, Rapoff, Thompson, & Connelly, 2006; Stinson & Bruce, 2009).

Physical Approaches. A return to regular moderate exercise with recommendations from physical therapists if deconditioning has occurred (Anthony & Schanberg, 2007). Because exercise may be counterintuitive for the patients to embrace when increased activity may initially lead to more pain, health care providers need to encourage a commitment to the regimen as gradual improvement in their energy level with the additional benefit of improving sleep, mood, and self-esteem. This will lessen the chronic pain and improve function (McCarthy, Shea, & Sullivan, 2003; Stinson & Bruce, 2009).

Sleep Hygiene. Learning good sleep habits is essential. Pain can interfere with sleep, resulting in daytime fatigue and emotional changes undermining appropriate coping strategies for effective pain relief. Patients are to be taught to avoid napping but to establish a bedtime routine with consistent sleep–wake cycles even during weekends.

Pharmacologic Interventions

Careful consideration needs to be taken when using medications, which are usually used only when nonpharmacologic approaches are insufficient. Information to guide clinical use of these medications is generally extrapolated from adult studies. Acetaminophen, NSAIDs, and coanalgesics administered singly or in combination can be useful. Health care providers are to exercise caution in use of anticonvulsants (Patorno et al., 2010) and antidepressants, especially the selective serotonin reuptake inhibitors, in adolescents because of their association with a risk of suicide (Schechter et al., 2010; Schneeweiss et al., 2010). Serotonin-noradrenaline reuptake inhibitors, such as fluoxetine

(Prozac), may be safer, but health care providers need to consider extensive parental education and close frequent monitoring for side effects (Anthony & Schanberg, 2007).

Opioids. Relatively little research has been done on their long-term use in children with chronic pain (Anderson & Palmer, 2006), and thus, they should be used only for short period.

IMPACT OF CHRONIC PAIN

Unrelieved pain in children may lead to anxiety that becomes more debilitating than the pain itself. In the most severe cases of chronic pain, the child may have signs of catastrophic thinking, including an excessive focus on the sensations of the pain with exaggerated and fearful appraisals leading to more pain, disability, and emotional distress (Miro, Huguet, & Nieto, 2007; Vervoort, Goubert, Eccleston, Bijttebier, & Crombez, 2006). Families may acquire serious economic and social burdens as they use resources while seeking the cause and optimal treatment of pain in their children (Eccleston, Crombez, Scotford, Clinch, & Connell, 2004; Hunfeld et al., 2001; Merlijn et al., 2006).

PAIN RELATED TO NEUROLOGICAL AND COGNITIVE IMPAIRMENT

Although major advances have been made in the assessment and management of pain in children who are otherwise healthy but have an acute illness or injury, pain experienced by children with profound special needs or with intellectual disabilities was not recognized until recently (Hadden & von Baeyer, 2002). Unmanaged pain in children with spina bifida, cerebral palsy, and other significant impairments can have a substantial negative impact on quality of life (Hauer, 2010; Oddson, Clancy, & McGrath, 2006; Parkinson, Gibson, Dickinson, & Colver, 2010). Pain is associated with the many operative procedures or other therapies (i.e., physical therapy) they undergo as part of their medical management to promote flexibility and strength.

Pain has been found to decrease the function of such children across four domains: communication, daily living skills, socialization, and motor skills, resulting in decreased performance even in established skills (Breau, Camfield, McGrath, & Finley, 2007). Over a period of 4 weeks, 78% of children with severe cognitive impairment experienced pain at least once: from accidents (30%), gastrointestinal tract pain (22%), infection (20%), or musculoskeletal pain (19%) (Breau, Camfield, McGrath, & Finley, 2003).

Pain is often underrecognized because of their impaired communication (Breau et al., 2003). Behavioral assessment scales designed for nonimpaired children are difficult to use because of their motor impairments and spasticity (Hadden & von Baeyer, 2002). See Chapter 2 for recommendations on specific pain assessment tools developed for children with neurological impairments.

REFERENCES

American Academy of Pediatrics and North American Society for Pediatric Gastroenterology, Hepatology, and Nutrition, Subcommittee on Chronic Abdominal Pain. (2005). Chronic abdominal pain in children. *Pediatrics, 115*(3), 812–815.

American Pain Society. (2001). *Pediatric chronic pain: A position statement.* Retrieved February 4, 2010, from www.ampainsoc.org/advocacy/pediatric.htm

American Pain Society. (2002). *Guideline for the management of pain in osteoarthritis, rheumatoid arthritis, and juvenile chronic arthritis.* Glenview, IL: Author.

American Pain Society. (2005). *Guideline for the management of fibromyalgia syndrome pain in adults and children.* Glenview, IL: Author.

Anderson, B. J., & Palmer, G. M. (2006). Recent developments in the pharmacological management of pain in children. *Current Opinion in Anaesthesiology, 19*(3), 285–292.

Andrasik, F., & Schwartz, M. S. (2006). Behavioral assessment and treatment of pediatric headache. *Behavior Modification, 30*(1), 93–113.

Anthony, K. K., & Schanberg, L. E. (2007). Assessment and management of pain syndromes and arthritis pain in children and adolescents. *Rheumatic Disease Clinics of North America, 33*(3), 625–660.

Bakola, E., Skapinakis, P., Tzoufi, M., Damigos, D., & Mavreas, V. (2009). Anticonvulsant drugs for pediatric migraine prevention: An evidence-based review. *European Journal of Pain, 13*(9), 893–901.

Breau, L. M., Camfield, C. S., McGrath, P. J., & Finley, G. A. (2003). The incidence of pain in children with severe cognitive impairments. *Archives of Pediatrics & Adolescent Medicine, 157*(12), 1219–1226.

Breau, L. M., Camfield, C. S., McGrath, P. J., & Finley, G. A. (2007). Pain's impact on adaptive functioning. *Journal of Intellectual Disability Research, 51*(Pt. 2), 125–134.

Cepeda, M. S., Carr, D. B., & Lau, J. (2005). Local anesthetic sympathetic blockade for complex regional pain syndrome. *Cochrane Database Systematic Review, 4*, CD004598.

Connelly, M., Anthony, K. K., Sarniak, R., Bromberg, M. H., Gil, K. M., & Schanberg, L. E. (2010). Parent pain responses as predictors of daily activities and mood in children with juvenile idiopathic arthritis: The utility of electronic diaries. *Journal of Pain and Symptom Management, 39*(3), 579–590.

Connelly, M., Rapoff, M. A., Thompson, N., & Connelly, W. (2006). Headstrong: A pilot study of a CD-ROM intervention for recurrent pediatric headache. *Journal of Pediatric Psychology, 31*(7), 737–747.

Connelly, M., & Schanberg, L. (2006). Latest developments in the assessment and management of chronic musculoskeletal pain syndromes in children. *Current Opinion in Rheumatology, 18*(5), 496–502.

Dadure, C., Motais, F., Ricard, C., Raux, O., Troncin, R., & Capdevila, X. (2005). Continuous peripheral nerve blocks at home for treatment of recurrent complex regional pain syndrome I in children. *Anesthesiology, 102*(2), 387–391.

Damen, L., Bruijn, J. K., Verhagen, A. P., Berger, M. Y., Passchier, J., & Koes, B. W. (2005). Symptomatic treatment of migraine in children: A systematic review of medication trials. *Pediatrics, 116*(2), e295–302.

Eccleston, C., Crombez, G., Scotford, A., Clinch, J., & Connell, H. (2004). Adolescent chronic pain: Patterns and predictors of emotional distress in adolescents with chronic pain and their parents. *Pain, 108*(3), 221–229.

Eccleston, C., Jordan, A., McCracken, L. M., Sleed, M., Connell, H., & Clinch, J. (2005). The Bath Adolescent Pain Questionnaire: Development and preliminary psychometric evaluation of an instrument to assess the impact of chronic pain on adolescents. *Pain, 118*, 263–270.

Eccleston, C., Malleson, P. N., Clinch, J., Connell, H., & Sourbut, C. (2003). Chronic pain in adolescents: Evaluation of a programme of interdisciplinary cognitive behaviour therapy. *Archives of Disease in Childhood, 88*(10), 881–885.

Eyckmans, L., Hilderson, D., Westhovens, R., Wouters, C., & Moons, P. (2010). What does it mean to grow up with juvenile idiopathic arthritis? A qualitative study on the perspectives of patients. *Clinical Rheumatology*, [Epub ahead of print].

Gold, J. I., Yetwin, A. K., Mahrer, N. E., Carson, M. C., Griffin, A. T., Palmer, S. N., & Joseph, M. H. (2009). Pediatric chronic pain and health-related quality of life. *Journal of Pediatric in Nursing, 24*(2), 141–150.

Golden, A. S., Haut, S. R., & Moshe, S. L. (2006). Nonepileptic uses of antiepileptic drugs in children and adolescents. *Pediatric Neurology, 34*(6), 421–432.

Grazzi, L. (2004). Headache in children and adolescents: Conventional and unconventional approaches to treatment. *Neurological Sciences, 25*(Suppl. 3), S223–225.

Greco, C., & Berde, C. (2005). Pain management for the hospitalized pediatric patient. *Pediatric Clinics of North America, 52*(4), 995–1027.

Hadden, K. L., & von Baeyer, C. L. (2002). Pain in children with cerebral palsy: Common triggers and expressive behaviors. *Pain, 99*, 281–288.

Hamalainen, M., & Masek, B. J. (2003). Diagnosis, classification, and medical management of headache in children and adolescents. In N. L. Schechter, C. B. Berde, & M. Yaster (Eds.), *Pain in infants, children, and adolescents* (2nd ed., pp. 707–718). Philadelphia, PA: Lippincott Williams & Wilkins.

Hauer, J. (2010). Identifying and managing sources of pain and distress in children with neurological impairment. *Pediatric Annals, 39*(4), 198–205.

Hershey, A. D. (2010). Recent developments in pediatric headache. *Current Opinion in Neurology, 23*(3), 249–253.

Hunfeld, J. A., Perquin, C. W., Duivenvoorden, H. J., Hazebroek-Kampschreur, A. A., Passchier, J., van Suijlekom-Smit, L. W., & van der Wouden, J. C. (2001). Chronic pain and its impact on quality of life in adolescents and their families. *Journal of Pediatric Psychology, 26*(3), 145–153.

Jordan, A., Eccleston, C., McCracken, L. M., Connell, H., & Clinch, J. (2008). The Bath Adolescent Pain–Parental Impact Questionnaire: Development and preliminary psychometric evaluation of an instrument to assess the impact of parenting an adolescent with chronic pain. *Pain, 137*(3), 478–487.

Kashikar-Zuck, S., Swain, N. F., Jones, B. A., & Graham, T. B. (2005). Efficacy of cognitive-behavioral intervention for juvenile primary fibromyalgia syndrome. *Journal of Rheumatology, 32*(8), 1594–1602.

Kondev, L., & Minster, A. (2003). Headache and facial pain in children and adolescents. *Otolaryngologic Clinics of North America, 36*(6), 1153–1170.

Kulas, D. T., & Schanberg, L. E. (2003). Muscloskeletal pain in children. In N. L. Schechter, C. B. Berde, & M. Yaster (Eds.), *Pain in infants, children, and adolescents* (2nd ed., pp. 578–598). Philadelphia, PA: Lippincott Williams & Wilkins.

Larsson, B., Carlsson, J., Fichtel, A., & Melin, L. (2005). Relaxation treatment of adolescent headache sufferers: Results from a school-based replication series. *Headache, 45*(6), 692–704.

Lewis, D., Winner, P., Saper, J., Ness, S., Polverejan, E., Wang, S., et al. (2009). Randomized, double-blind, placebo-controlled study to evaluate the efficacy and safety of topiramate for migraine prevention in pediatric subjects 12 to 17 years of age. *Pediatrics, 123*(3), 924–934.

Lynch, A. M., Kashikar-Zuck, S., Goldschneider, K. R., & Jones, B. A. (2007). Sex and age differences in coping styles among children with chronic pain. *Journal of Pain and Symptom Management, 33*(2), 208–216.

McCarthy, C. F., Shea, A. M., & Sullivan, P. (2003). Physical therapy management of pain in children. In N. L. Schechter, C. B. Berde, & M. Yaster (Eds.), *Pain in infants, children, and adolescents* (2nd ed., pp. 434–448). Philadelphia, PA: Lippincott Williams & Wilkins.

Meier, P. M., Zurakowski, D., Berde, C. B., & Sethna, N. F. (2009). Lumbar sympathetic blockade in children with complex regional pain syndromes: A double blind placebo-controlled crossover trial. *Anesthesiology, 111*(2), 372–380.

Merlijn, V. P., Hunfeld, J. A., van der Wouden, J. C., Hazebroek-Kampschreur, A. A., Passchier, J., & Koes, B. W. (2006). Factors related to the quality of life in adolescents with chronic pain. *Clinical Journal of Pain, 22*(3), 306–315.

Miro, J., Huguet, A., & Nieto, R. (2007). Predictive factors of chronic pediatric pain and disability: A Delphi poll. *Journal of Pain, 8*(10), 774–792.

Oddson, B. E., Clancy, C. A., & McGrath, P. J. (2006). The role of pain in reduced quality of life and depressive symptomology in children with spina bifida. *Clinical Journal of Pain, 22*(9), 784–789.

Olsson, G. L., Meyerson, B. A., & Linderoth, B. (2008). Spinal cord stimulation in adolescents with complex regional pain syndrome type I (CRPS-I). *European Journal of Pain, 12*(1), 53–59.

Parkinson, K. N., Gibson, L., Dickinson, H. O., & Colver, A. F. (2010). Pain in children with cerebral palsy: A cross-sectional multicentre European study. *Acta Paediatrica, 99*(3), 446–451.

Patorno, E., Bohn, R. L., Wahl, P. M., Avorn, J., Patrick, A. R., Liu, J., & Schneeweiss, S. (2010). Anticonvulsant medications and the risk of suicide, attempted suicide, or violent death. *Journal of American Medical Association, 303*(14), 1401–1409.

Perquin, C. W., Hazebroek-Kampschreur, A. A., Hunfeld, J. A., Bohnen, A. M., van Suijlekom-Smit, L. W., Passchier, J., & van der Wouden J. C. (2000). Pain in children and adolescents: A common experience. *Pain, 87*(1), 51–58.

Pintov, S., Lahat, E., Alstein, M., Vogel, Z., & Barg, J. (1997). Acupuncture and the opioid system: Implications in management of migraine. *Pediatric Neurology, 17*(2), 129–133.

Scharff, L., Leichtner, A. M., & Rappaport, L. A. (2003). Recurrent abdominal pain. In N. L. Schechter, C. B. Berde, & M. Yaster (Eds.), *Pain in infants, children, and adolescents* (2nd ed., pp. 719–731). Philadelphia, PA: Lippincott Williams & Wilkins.

Schechter, N. L., Palermo, T. M., Walco, G. A., & Berde, C. (2010). Persistent pain in children. In S. M. Fishman, J. C. Ballantyne, & J. P. Rathmell (Eds.), *Bonica's management of pain* (4th ed., pp. 767–780). Philadelphia, PA: Wolters Kluwer/Lippincott Williams & Wilkins.

Schneeweiss, S., Patrick, A. R., Solomon, D. H., Dormuth, C. R., Miller, M., Mehta, J., . . . Wang, P. S. (2010). Comparative safety of antidepressant agents for children and adolescents regarding suicidal acts. *Pediatrics, 125*(5), 876–888.

Stinson, J., & Bruce, E. (2009). Chronic pain in children. In A. Twycross, S. J. Dowden, & E. Bruce (Eds.), *Managing pain in children: A clinical guide* (pp. 145–170). Oxford, United Kingdom: Wiley-Blackwell.

References **333**

Uziel, Y., Chapnick, G., Jaber, L., Nemet, D., & Hashkes, P. J. (2010). Five-year outcome of children with "growing pains": Correlations with pain threshold. *Journal of Pediatrics, 156*(5), 838–840.

Varni, J. W., Seid, M., & Kurtin, P. S. (2001). PedsQL 4.0: Reliability and validity of the Pediatric Quality of Life Inventory version 4.0 generic core scales in healthy and patient populations. *Medical Care, 39*(8), 800–812.

Vervoort, T., Goubert, L., Eccleston, C., Bijttebier, P., & Crombez, G. (2006). Catastrophic thinking about pain is independently associated with pain severity, disability, and somatic complaints in schoolchildren and children with chronic pain. *Journal of Pediatric Psychology, 31*(7), 674–683.

Wicksell, R. K., Melin, L., & Olsson, G. L. (2007). Exposure and acceptance in the rehabilitation of adolescents with idiopathic chronic pain—a pilot study. *European Journal of Pain, 11*(3), 267–274.

Wilder, R. T. (2003). Regional anesthetic techniques for chronic pain management in children. In N. L. Schechter, C. B. Berde, & M. Yaster (Eds.), *Pain in infants, children, and adolescents* (2nd ed., pp. 396–416). Philadelphia, PA: Lippincott, Williams & Wilkins.

Appendix of Select Websites

PAIN SCALES

Pediatric Pain Scales

- For Faces Pain Scale-Revised (FPS-R): www.usask.ca/childpain/fpsr/
- For FACES Pain Rating Scale: www3.us.elsevierhealth.com/WOW
- For Oucher Scale: www.oucher.org

Infant Pain Scales

- For CRIES Pain Scale: www.scielo.br/img/revistas/rba/v57n5/en_12t3 .gif
- For Neonatal Pain, Agitation, and Sedation Scale (N-PASS): www .n-pass.com/index.html

Pain Assessment for the Physically Impaired

- www.aboutkidshealth.ca/Shared/PDFs/AKH_Breau_everyday.pdf

MANAGEMENT OF PAIN

Management of Acute Pain

- For American Academy of Pediatrics (AAP) position statement: aappolicy.aappublications.org/cgi/reprint/pediatrics;108/3/793.pdf

Management of Chronic Pain

▓ For American Pain Society (APS) statement on pediatric chronic pain: www.ampainsoc.org/advocacy/pediatric.htm

FACTS ABOUT ADOLESCENT PRESCRIPTION AND SUBSTANCE DRUG ABUSE

▓ 2008 National Adolescent Drug Abuse Report: www.monitoring thefuture.org/pubs/monographs/overview2008.pdf
▓ 2008 Partnership Attitude Tracking Report: www.drugfree.org

Facts About Drug Abuse in General

▓ Drug Abuse Warning Network: dawninfo.samhsa.gov
▓ National Institute for Drug Abuse list of commonly abused drugs: www.drugabuse.gov/PDF/CADChart.pdf

SPECIALIZED TRAINING IN CLINICAL HYPNOSIS

▓ For National Pediatric Hypnosis Training Institute: www.nphti.org
▓ For American Society of Clinical Hypnosis: http://www.asch.net/

RESOURCES FOR PATIENTS, PARENTS, AND ADOLESCENTS

▓ The Partnership for a Drug-Free America: www.drugfree.org
▓ Prescription Drug Abuse: Not in My House: www.drugfree.org/notinmyhouse
▓ Home Medication Inventory Card: www.nfp.org/PDFs/HomeMed InventoryCard.pdf
▓ List of high schools in United States with programs for students with a history of substance abuse: http://recoveryschools.org

PATIENT EDUCATION MATERIAL

- St. Jude Children's Research Hospital: www.stjude.org/caregiverresources

PEDIATRIC PALLIATIVE CARE

- Children's International Project on Palliative/Hospice Services (ChIPPS): www.nhpco.org
- The Association for Children's Palliative Care (ACT): www.act.org.uk
- Initiative for Pediatric Palliative Care: www.ippcweb.org

PAIN MANAGEMENT PROFESSIONAL ORGANIZATIONS

- American Society of Pain Management Nursing: www.aspmn.org/
- American Pain Society: www.ampainsoc.org/
- Mayday Pain Project: Pediatric Pain: http://www.painandhealth.org/maydaypediatricpain.html
- IASP Special Interest Group on Pain in Childhood: http://childpain.org/

Index

Note: Page numbers followed by *f* indicate figures, *t* indicate tables, and *e* indicate exhibits.